PRAISE FOR THE FIRST AND SECOND EDITIONS OF WOMEN'S CANCERS

Oncology nurses are often the best people to write such books, combining as they do their scientific knowledge, practical experience, and close inter-actions with patients. I've never advised this before, but I say now that everyone should rush out and buy this book for each woman in their fam-ily. I will. Any woman would do well to have this book on her personal ref-erence shelf. As she gets older (as this book points out), it is probable that she will need it.

— Merle O'Rourke Thompson, Reviewer,
Journal of the National Cancer Institute

This book also promotes primary prevention, including diet, exercise, and smoking cessation, all of which are in the patient's control—again empow-ering the patient to take an active role in the healthcare system. The con-tent is organized in short sections, which makes it easy to pick up and put down; this much material can be overwhelming for the newly diagnosed cancer patient. The book offers definitions of medical terms throughout the text, again, promoting better understanding for the lay reader.

— Katherine M. Zahasky, R.N., Certified Nurse Practitioner, Reviewer,
Journal of Pelvic Surgery

Discussions of exactly what happens during surgery or while getting chemotherapy are excellent . . . and so are explanations of how different can-cers develop. The authors suggest reasonable explanations for why people get cancer—the mix of cancer-causing factors in each woman's life will be unique—thereby downplaying fear-mongering news reports that say the cause of cancer is this chemical or that bad habit.

Women's Cancers will benefit women and their families, and should help some beat their disease.

— *Natural Health*

Of all the concerns by women I see in my medical practice, cancer is at the top of the list. This book will be very helpful to all women, not just those who have diagnosed with cancer. It will also be a resource for women who want to know what they can do to help prevent this all-too-common disease. [The authors] have written a book that will prove very useful to women. I highly recommend this book for all women concerned about their health.

— Customer Review, Amazon.com

They take pains to make the content as easy to understand as possible, including a glossary of technical terms highlighted in the text, illustrating procedures and findings with clear line drawings, and listing questions to ask physicians about each disorder or therapy. Their guide is also significant for its encouragement of women's self-empowerment, advice on pursuing a healthy lifestyle, and advocacy for women's health funding and research.

— *Booklist*

Readers will find all the answers to questions either patients are afraid to ask their doctors or that doctors don't know how to answer themselves.

— *The Richmond Review*

The authors, both oncology nurses, seek to empower and encourage women to be assertive health-care consumers.... *Women's Cancers* is fully comprehensive, helpful to patients and health-care workers alike. Recommended.

— *Library Journal*

Discussions of exactly what happens during surgery or while getting chemotherapy are excellent ... and so are explanations of how different cancers develop. The authors suggest reasonable explanations for why people get cancer—the mix of cancer-causing factors in each woman's life will be unique—thereby downplaying fear-mongering news reports that say the cause of cancer is this chemical or that bad habit.

Women's Cancers will benefit women and their families, and should help some beat their disease.

— *Natural Health*

OTHER BOOKS IN HUNTER HOUSE'S CANCER & HEALTH SERIES:

Breast Implants — Everything You Need to Know (Bruning)
Cancer Doesn't Have to Hurt (Haylock & Curtiss)
Cancer — Increasing Your Odds for Survival (Bognar)
The Cancer Prevention Book (Daniel & Ellis)
Estrogen and Breast Cancer (Rinzler)
The Feisty Woman's Breast Cancer Book (Ratner)
How Women Can Finally Stop Smoking (Klesges & DeBon)
Lymphedema (Burt & White)
No Less A Woman (Kahane)
The Prostate Health Workbook (Malerman)
Recovering from Breast Surgery (Stumm)
Men's Cancers (Haylock)

Project Credits

Original cover design and illustration by Teresa Smith, 3rd edition design by Jil Weil
Book Production: Hunter House & Jil Weil
Copy Editor: Victoria Sant'Ambrogio
Proofreader: John David Marion
Indexer: Nancy D. Peterson
Acquisitions Editor: Jeanne Brondino
Editor: Alexandra Mummery
Publicity Coordinator: Earlita K. Chenault
Sales & Marketing Coordinator: Jo Anne Retzlaff
Customer Service Manager: Christina Sverdrup
Order Fulfillment: Lakdhon Lama
Administrator: Theresa Nelson
Computer Support: Peter Eichelberger
Publisher: Kiran S. Rana

THIS BOOK IS DEDICATED TO THE MANY WOMEN
WHO HAVE TAUGHT US THE MEANING OF COURAGE
AND HOPE.

WOMEN'S CANCERS

How to Prevent Them,
How to Treat Them,
How to Beat Them

Kerry A. McGinn, R.N., M.N., N.P.
&
Pamela J. Haylock, R.N., M.A., E.T.

Hunter House
PUBLISHERS

Hunter House Inc., Publishers
PO Box 2914
Alameda CA 94501-0914

Acknowledgment is made for permission to reprint illustrations on pp. 44, 53, 58, 59, 214, 215, 216, 217, 218 by Ken Miller from Kerry A. McGinn, *The Informed Woman's Guide to Breast Health,* Palo Alto, CA: Bull Publishing, rev. 2001; illustrations on pp. 356, 357, 358 from Judy Sandella, *Oncology Nursing Forum* 14(6): 71–73, Oncology Nursing Press, Inc., 1987; illustrations on pp. 189, 270, 277, 380, 381, 401 courtesy the National Cancer Institute; illustrations on pp. 57, 230, 231, 240, 256, 258, 259 courtesy Susan Schoen; illustration on p. 406 courtesy of the American Cancer Society, Inc.

Library of Congress Cataloging-in-Publication Data

McGinn, Kerry Anne.
    Women's cancers: how to prevent them, how to treat them, how to beat them /
    Kerry A. McGinn and Pamela J. Haylock.— 3rd edition.
    p.cm. — (Cancer & health)
    Includes bibliographical references and index.
        ISBN 978-1-63026-801-5
        1. Cancer in women—Popular works. 2. Breast—Cancer—Popular works.
    3. Generative organs, Female—Cancer—Popular works. I. Haylock, Pamela J.
    II. Title. III. Hunter House cancer & health series.

RC281.W65 M36 2002
616.99'4'0082—dc21   2002075933

Manufactured in Canada by Transcontinental Printing

        9 8 7 6 5 4 3 2 1   Third Edition   03 04 05 06 07

CONTENTS

Acknowledgments xi

Foreword xiii

PART ONE: "YOU HAVE CANCER..." 1

CHAPTER 1 Cancer Basics 4
The Wrong Kind of Cells — Too Many Cells — How Cancer Cells
Behave — How Cancer Comes About — Searching for Cancer
Causes — How Cancer Grows — Cancer Metastasis

CHAPTER 2 Causes and Prevention 15
Physical Activity — Chemoprevention — Tobacco — Diet —
Environment — Infections — Immune System — Medications —
Age — Race and Ethnicity — The Cancer Personality — Hereditary
Factors — Cancer Risk Analysis

CHAPTER 3 Detecting a Change 37
Early Detection — Laboratory Tests — Imaging Techniques

CHAPTER 4 Diagnosis and Beyond 51
Informed Consent — Fine Needle Aspirations, Core Biopsies, and
Guided Needle Biopsies — Biopsies with a Scope — Dilatation and
Curettage (D&C) — Conization (Cone Biopsy) — Open Biopsy —
Needle Localization Biopsy — Feelings about a Biopsy — Timely
Diagnosis — Staging a Cancer — Grading a Cancer — Prognosis

CHAPTER 5 A Woman and Her Doctors 66
Joining the Treatment Team — Cancer Doctors — The Patient–Doctor
Relationship — Second Opinions

CHAPTER 6 The Rest of the Team 77
Family and Friends — Mentors and Support Groups — Information
Sources — The Hospital Experience

CHAPTER 7   Local Treatments for Cancer 86
What Local Therapies Do — Surgery — Radiation

CHAPTER 8   Systemic Treatments for Cancer 99
Chemotherapy — Hormonal Therapy — Biological Therapy — Clinical
Trials — Paying for Cancer Treatment

CHAPTER 9   Complementary and Alternative Therapies
             for Cancer 120
Who Uses These Forms of Treatment? — What Is Unconventional
Cancer Therapy? — Traditional Eastern Healing — Metabolic and
Dietary Therapy — Herbal Therapy — Psychological Approaches —
Physical Approaches — Spiritual Approaches — Pharmacologic Agents:
Drugs and Special Preparations — Programs Using Complementary
Therapies — Separating Hope from Hype

CHAPTER 10   Feelings 171
Numbness and Denial — Regaining Control — Experiencing
Feelings — How We See Ourselves

PART TWO: BREAST CANCER 185

CHAPTER 11   Questions about Breasts 188
Who Gets Breast Cancer? — Preventing Breast Cancer — Making
Sense of Risk Statistics — Breast Changes that Are Not Cancer —
Breast Pain

CHAPTER 12   Detecting and Diagnosing Breast Changes . . 209
Detecting Breast Changes — Performing BSE — Professional Breast
Examination — Diagnosing Breast Changes — If Breast Cancer Is
Diagnosed — Carcinoma in Situ: The In-Between Diagnosis

CHAPTER 13   Treating Invasive Breast Cancer 228
Local Treatments: Mastectomy or Lumpectomy/Radiation — Questions
to Ask Your Physician — Surgery — Radiation Therapy — Systemic
Treatment — Special Situations

CHAPTER 14   Beyond Basic Treatment for Breast Cancer . . 251
Regaining Arm Mobility after Breast Surgery — Body Image after
Mastectomy — The Breast Prosthesis — Breast Reconstruction —
Follow-Up after Breast Cancer — Local Recurrence and Metastasis —
Stem-Cell Transplants

PART THREE: THE GYNECOLOGIC CANCERS   267

Self-Advocacy in Women's Health Care — The Normal Female
Reproductive System — Cancers of the Female Reproductive System

CHAPTER 15   Cancer of the Ovary 272

What Is Cancer of the Ovary? — The Natural History of Ovarian
Cancer — Who Gets Cancer of the Ovary? — Preventive Measures —
Early Detection — Diagnosis — Staging — Treatment — When
Ovarian Cancer Recurs — The Future

CHAPTER 16   Cancer of the Uterus (Endometrial Cancer) . 299

Fibroid Tumors — Endometrial Hyperplasia — Risk Factors for Uterine
Cancer — Prevention — Early Detection — Diagnosis — Types of
Uterine Cancer — Treatment — Questions to Ask Your Physician —
Hormone Replacement Therapy

CHAPTER 17   Cancer of the Cervix and Cervical
                       Dysplasia (CIN) 316

Normal Structure of the Cervix — Dysplasia or Cervical Intraepithelial
Neoplasia (CIN) — Prevention — Diagnosis — Treatment for CIN —
Carcinoma in Situ — Cancer of the Cervix — Treatments for Cervical
Cancer — Advanced and Recurrent Cervical Cancer — Questions to
Ask Your Physician

CHAPTER 18   Cancer of the Vagina 341

Risk Factors — Prevention — Benign Vaginal Disease — Vaginal
Cancer — Questions to Ask Your Physician — DES (Diethylstilbestrol)

CHAPTER 19   Cancer of the Vulva 354

Risk Factors — Prevention — Benign Vulvar Disease — Vulvar
Cancer — Questions to Ask Your Physician

CHAPTER 20   Rare Gynecologic Cancers 365

Cancer of the Fallopian Tube — Gestational Trophoblastic Neoplasia

PART FOUR: LUNG CANCER   371
AND COLORECTAL CANCER

CHAPTER 21   Lung Cancer 373

Who Gets Lung Cancer? — Prevention — Normal Lung Anatomy
and Function — Cancerous Changes in the Lung — Types of Lung
Cancer — Early Detection — Diagnosis — Treatment — Superior Vena
Cava Syndrome — Follow-up and Recurrence — Quality of Life, Lung
Cancer, and Women — The Future

CHAPTER 22   Cancer of the Colon, Rectum, and Anus 400

Precancer Conditions — Prevention — Screening — Signs and
Symptoms — Diagnosis and Workup — Treatment — When Colorectal
Cancer Recurs — The Future

PART FIVE: LIFE AFTER CANCER 421

CHAPTER 23   Long-Term and Late Effects of Cancer
             and Cancer Treatment 422

The Nature of the Problem — Survivorship — Interventions:
Long-Term Wellness Planning for Survivors

CHAPTER 24   Feelings after Treatment Ends 432

General Strategies — After-Treatment Fears — Other Predictable
Difficult Times — Anger and Sadness — How We Feel about
Ourselves — Relationships — Setting Goals

CHAPTER 25   After Treatment Ends: The Other Issues 447

Sexuality — Pregnancy — Lymphedema — Menopause–Without
Hormone Therapy — Employment and Insurance

CHAPTER 26   Cancer Is Still a Political Issue 466

Who Pays? Who Profits? — Technology and Policy — Tobacco —
Cancer Research — Cancer Policy — Managed Care — No Money?
No Mission! — What You Can Do

Afterword 484

Glossary 485

Bibliography 496

Resources 508

Index 516

ACKNOWLEDGMENTS

No book—especially one as extensive as this—happens without plenty of help. Many people helped in pulling it together, and our special thanks go to the following health and social work professionals for the interviews they graciously gave (note: the affiliations listed are those the professionals had when they gave the interviews): Susan Diamond, L.C.S.W., psychotherapist, group therapist, Stanford University; Lyssa Friedman, R.N., O.C.N., oncology nurse, Pacific Hematology-Oncology, San Francisco; Jerold Green, M.D., radiation oncologist, California Pacific Medical Center (CPMC), San Francisco; I. Craig Henderson, M.D., chief, Oncology Center, University of California, San Francisco; Peter Richards, M.D., oncologic surgeon, CPMC; Diane Scott, R.N., Ph.D., nurse-psychotherapist for women with cancer, San Francisco; Helene Smith, Ph.D., researcher/director, Geraldine Brush Cancer Research Institute, San Francisco; Ange Stephens, M.F.C.C., clinical director, Cancer Support Community, San Francisco; and Kelly Van Bokkelen, M.S.W., social worker, radiation oncology, CPMC;

— Theresa Koetters, R.N., M.S.N., oncology specialist, who efficiently and helpfully reviewed the manuscript; and Saskia Thiadens, R.N., founder of the National Lymphedema Network, and Bryant A. Toth, M.D., reconstructive surgeon, CPMC, for reviewing specific sections;

— Artist Susan Schoen, who drew many original illustrations;

— Our publisher Kiran Rana, who believed in the project, and Lisa Lee, our initial editor, who kept pushing gently, and Alex Mummery, editor, and Victoria Sant'Ambrogio, copy editor, who helped make the third edition better.

We also thank each other for mutual support and, last—but definitely not least—we thank our families, who put up with all the tribulations of being around authors on deadline.

IMPORTANT NOTE

The material in this book is intended to provide a review of information regarding the cancers that affect women. Every effort has been made to provide accurate and dependable information, including an overview of what is new and often speculative and a review of unconventional and unproven therapies. The contents of this book have been compiled through professional research and in consultation with medical professionals. However, health-care professionals have differing opinions and advances in medical and scientific research are made very quickly, so some of the information may become outdated.

Therefore, the publisher, authors, editors, and professionals quoted in the book cannot be held responsible for any error, omission, or dated material. The treatments described should be undertaken only under the guidance of a licensed health-care practitioner The authors and publisher assume no responsibility for any outcome of applying the information in this book in a program of self-care or under the care of a licensed practitioner. If you have questions concerning your care or treatment, or about the application of the information described in this book, consult a qualified health-care professional.

FOREWORD

Nearly everyone is touched by cancer in some way. One in four families in the United States is directly affected by this illness. Reports of new information about different cancers, cancer therapy, and research appear almost daily. Changes in our health-care system frequently shift the burden to the consumer to understand treatment options and advocate for effective care. In spite of increasing consumer awareness, the incidence of women's cancers like breast cancer and lung cancer continue to rise. Currently, one in eight women is at risk to develop breast cancer by age eighty. The incidence of lung cancer in women continues to increase despite our knowledge that cigarettes cause cancer. The need for accurate and timely information has never been so great. Women and those who care about us must be informed and empowered to make wise health choices. *Women's Cancers* can help.

Even though the health care available in the United States is among the most sophisticated in the world, most breast lumps are discovered by women themselves or by their partners. The individual with any cancer is often the first to alert doctors that something is wrong. As more attention is focused on women's health issues and we become stronger partners in our health care, women must know about cancer and cancer therapy to make informed decisions, seek care early, and give ourselves the best opportunities for health. No longer can we rely on the familiar family physician who has known us for a lifetime. Our choice of doctors can change rather quickly in our ever-changing health-care system, and insurance coverage for specialists and new innovative therapy is sometimes denied. Personal knowledge, advocacy, and determination are often the keys to obtaining the coverage for care each person considers best. Early detection and early treatment of cancer offer the best chances for long-term survival. Some cancers can be found through regular self-examination and screening, and these account for about half of all new cancers. If all of these cancers were diagnosed at early stages through regular screening, The American Cancer Society (ACS) estimates that the five-year survival rate for these cancers would be close to 95 percent. And, yes, the words "survivor" and "cancer" do go together! The ACS estimates that the five-year survival rate from *all* cancers combined is 62 percent. Early breast cancer has a 96 percent survival rate, and other cancer types, diagnosed early, respond equally well. The diagnosis of cancer is not always a death sentence. Both short-term and long-term survivors need accurate information to advocate for effective therapy and to carry on with life to the fullest while living with cancer. *Women's Cancers* provides a comprehensive, easy-to-use resource to help readers choose healthy lifestyles, ask the right questions about cancer, and advocate for quality cancer care.

Despite amazing advances in detection and treatment, cancer remains one of the most feared diseases in the United States. The diagnosis is a blow that causes confusion, shock, and disbelief and changes lives forever. Important treatment decisions must be made during this stressful time. These decisions are often complicated by the need to choose from seemingly equal options. There is rarely only *one* right choice. Only by approaching cancer and its treatment with accurate information and a clear understanding of your personal lifestyle and life goals can you reduce anxiety and fear and make positive choices. The clear, concise information in *Women's Cancers* helps sort out the options.

Women's Cancers explains what cancer is all about and details common reactions to hearing the news that cancer has entered your life. Authors McGinn and Haylock use their expertise as experienced oncology nurses and patient advocates to give comprehensive information about the cancers that affect women most often. The book gives practical information about risks, prevention, and early detection, and details conventional and complementary therapies used to treat cancer. The authors provide advice for joining the treatment team and finding the care that's best for you. The book also gives tips for success for cancer survivors: coping with a chronic illness, returning to work, facing others, preventing discrimination from insurers and employers, and finding and using self-care strategies that promote optimal wellness after a cancer diagnosis.

This longer, more detailed third edition of *Women's Cancers* addresses important new information. The authors explain the newest advances in the science of cancer as well as the applications of new treatments. A new chapter will help women understand some of the physical, emotional, and social challenges experienced even after treatment ends. This edition also deals with current controversies like hormone replacement therapy and breast cancer, genetic research, risks and testing, and the ongoing issues of health-care reform. Haylock and McGinn include updated information about new medicines, bone-marrow and stem-cell transplant, alternative and complementary therapies, and clinical trials. This book provides a valuable and comprehensive resource for women, for their families and friends, and for doctors, nurses, social workers, and other health-care professionals caring for people with cancer.

This book also speaks to the personal experience of cancer. McGinn and Haylock generously and sensitively share their own experiences with cancer and cancer therapy. They describe the frustration, turmoil, and confusion that an encounter with cancer can cause, and give hints to overcome obstacles in our health-care system. They include practical advice for coping with fear, depression, anxiety, and grief, and share their personal strengths and techniques for success.

Women's Cancers is not just a book for women with cancer. Health professionals and women of all ages and those who care about them can learn from this easy-to-read guide and share the important information with others. In today's health-care system, this book is an important resource to help women make knowledgeable and involved choices that have a lasting impact on their lives.

— Carol P. Curtiss, R.N., M.S.N.
Clinical Nurse Specialist Consultant, Greenfield, Massachusetts
Past President (1992–93), Oncology Nursing Society

PART ONE

"YOU HAVE CANCER..."

"I felt like Alice down the rabbit hole..."

"... as if this had to be a horrible dream, and if I just tried hard enough, maybe I would wake up."

"... as if my emotional circuit breaker was overloaded and had tripped."

It was a reunion potluck of my cancer support group sisters, and we were comparing notes on how we felt when we first heard that we had cancer. As we munched appetizers and caught up on everyone's news, we paused for a moment to look back.

"You have cancer." Such a short statement—but it marks an absolute division between *before* and *after*. We could recall the doctor's words with painful clarity, eerily etched in our memories, like those first words from New York City on 11 September 2001 that told us that the World Trade Center had been attacked.

What the doctor said next we remember less well. There is a blank there, or a recollection of a sense of unreality and doom, of thoughts and feelings tumbling over themselves too fast to be caught.

Take it back. It can't be true. The report must be wrong. You can't be serious! Why me? Why don't we wait a few months and check it again? Am I going to die? What am I going to do? What will happen to me? Even years later, the memory is still painful.

For me, the news was not a complete surprise. The breast lump just felt "different" from the many not serious lumps I'd had over the years. I had one of those gut feelings about it and spent sleepless nights fretting. I persuaded my surgeon to withdraw a few cells through a needle to find out what the lump was—and learned that I had cancer. To this day I have not figured out how I carried on a seemingly intelligent conversation with the surgeon and then drove myself home.

However "prepared" I was for the news, it was not enough. No one among my immediate family and close friends had been diagnosed with breast cancer. I felt I wanted to protect my family and not upset them any more than necessary. But my wayward feelings bewildered me, and so did all the immediate decisions I had to make. I roller-coastered from moment to moment, between being in perfect control and collapsing in fear, anger, and uncertainty. Some mornings I woke up feeling fine—until I remembered. There I was: a registered nurse, who had even written health books (including, ironically, one about breast changes that were not cancer). But what I knew could not save me from feeling very frightened. Cancer was just too overwhelming an experience to go through without help.

There was also a vague but growing inner sense that something good ought to come about as a result of this experience. Cancer is a crisis. Like other crises, it is also an opportunity for us to look at who we are and what we really want. It is a pressure-cooker situation that forces us to change. If I had to change, I wanted it to be for the better.

Plainly, I needed help, and it was my good fortune to find it. My health-care professionals, my family and friends and co-workers, a breast cancer support group, a nurse-psychotherapist, and others all pitched in. Sometimes I felt as if there were an immense network of joined hands buoying me up in deep waters during the times when I was too exhausted to swim. (Of course, there were moments when I wanted them all to just leave me alone!) At other times, I became part of that network, offering a hand to someone else.

Cancer is scary for any human being. Even the word itself, *cancer*—the crab—makes us think of sharp claws, pincers, and pain. And each of us experiences cancer in an individual way, based not only on the specific disease we get but also on who we are, where we have been in life, and what our environment is like. My particular combination of temperament, available support, and past coping techniques, for instance, helps to create my own experience.

But there are common threads. Despite infinite variations among women, most of us tend to bring some "womanness" with us as we face cancer: how we talk about the experience, how we cope, what we value. Being a woman does not necessarily make cancer easier or harder to bear, just different. On occasion, we may complain about some aspect of being a woman, but we are women. Having a "women's cancer" seems to strike at the heart of this womanness, to threaten a crucial part of what makes us who we are.

Next week, my cancer support group plans to gather again for another reunion dinner. We will laugh and cheer each other on and enjoy each other's company, as we have done together for years now. We will also mourn our losses, because that is part of the picture. We will remember yesterday—which makes today all the sweeter—and we will look toward tomorrow.

We cannot change the fact that we have had cancer. But, as I look around the room at my support group "sisters," I know that I will be awed and amazed yet again by how we have risen to that challenge.

— *Kerry McGinn*

CHAPTER 1

CANCER BASICS

What is cancer, anyway?

It is an abnormal growth of cells in the body that do not obey the rules. To be considered "cancer," the cells must

+ look different from normal cells

+ divide rapidly enough to upset the body's status quo

+ have the potential both to invade adjoining cells and tissue and to spread to other parts of the body

Cancer is not one disease but more than one hundred different diseases. Each has its own personality, from slow-growing, sleepy "lapdogs" of cancers to those that move quickly and aggressively, but that may also be better targets for some of our current anticancer therapies.

THE WRONG KIND OF CELLS

A normal body cell viewed under a microscope looks rather round, oblong, or cubelike and has certain predictable parts. Cells that have similar functions in the body look alike because a particular kind of cell does a specific job best. Thus, normal breast duct cells look like each other, but very different from normal red blood cells.

Sometimes, in all the trillions upon trillions of cells in the body, a glitch occurs in the quality control, producing a cell that looks different, or *atypical* (abnormal), under the microscope. The shape may be irregular, the components (such as the cell membrane and the nucleus) broken or disrupted, and there may be extra or missing parts.

Some of these cells are only slightly atypical, while others are wildly different from normal cells. A group of cells that is slightly abnormal is still considered *benign* (not cancer); the very deviant ones are called *malignant* (cancer) cells.

Even among malignant cells, there is wide variation in just *how* abnormal the cells are. Many cancer cells somewhat resemble the normal cells from the same organ or tissue; at the other extreme are cells that look utterly bizarre. How abnormal these cancer cells appear under a microscope provides clues to how they are likely to behave.

Cancer cells are not "super" cells. In fact, they are poor-quality cells: weaker, less resilient, and less functional than normal cells. They are not invincible and they can be killed.

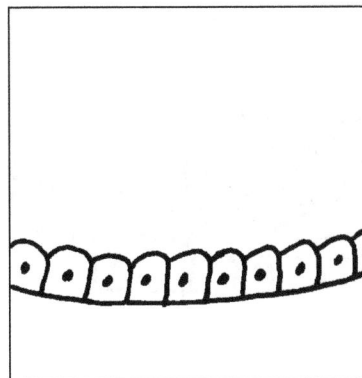

Normal cells

TOO MANY CELLS

The life cycle of every normal cell in the body follows a particular timetable. Each breast duct cell, for instance, divides about as often and lasts about as long as every other breast duct cell, but has a totally different pattern from that of a red blood cell. When a normal cell reproduces, on schedule, it divides into two daughter cells just like itself. The daughter cells mature to do whatever they are supposed to do, wherever they are supposed to do it, and then reproduce in turn. Because normal cells also wear out and die on schedule, the adult body maintains a "zero population growth" cell balance.

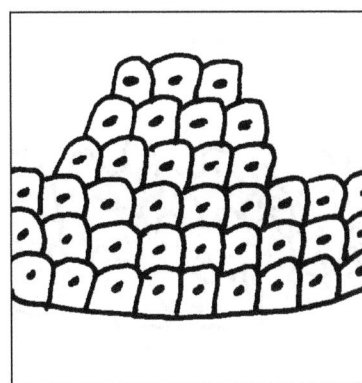

Proliferative change without atypia: too many cells (hyperplasia)

If, for any reason, the status quo is upset and there are too many cells, the resulting overgrowth is called **neoplasia,** or new growth. These cells can clump together as a **tumor,** one kind of neoplasm. Tumors and neoplasms can be benign or malignant.

Benign neoplasms include those in which older (but normal) cells pile up because they are living longer than they should and/or the body is not disposing of dead cells quickly enough. As long as the buildup in cells is not caused by the cells reproducing more often than they should, this is called **nonproliferative change.** If some cells begin dividing more often than normal, but the cells themselves are normal, the result is **proliferative change without atypia;** this condition is also called **hyperplasia,** meaning "too much" growth. A freckle, a wart, an ovarian cyst, and most benign breast tumors are examples of one of these two kinds of benign neoplasms.

If those cells that are dividing too quickly include some that are abnormal—but not too abnormal—the condition is still benign and is called

Cancer Basics

5

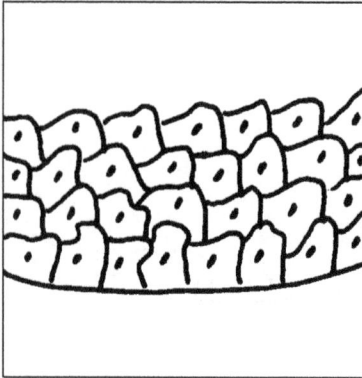

Proliferative change with atypia
(dysplasia)

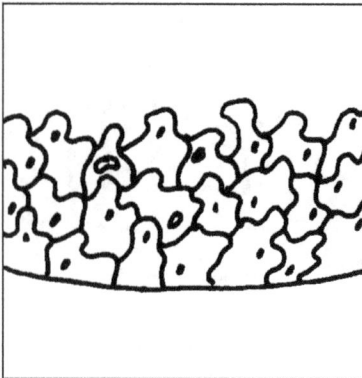

Carcinoma in situ

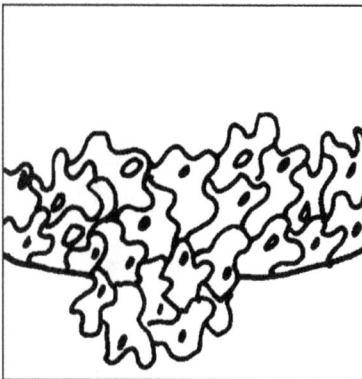

Invasive cancer

proliferative change with atypia or dysplasia (for "bad" or abnormal growth). This kind of change may reverse itself during the normal turnover of cells, may stay the way it is, or may grow worse. A change like this is not in any way cancer, but it is a warning that a quality control problem exists that can be temporary and minor, or more serious. It can somewhat increase the chance that a cancer will develop in that organ later.

If the cells look quite atypical, but are confined to one limited site such as the duct of the breast or the top layer of the cervix, the changes are called **carcinoma in situ** or **noninvasive carcinoma,** among other names. The labels—*"carcinoma"* means cancer—are a holdover from earlier years when doctors considered this the very earliest stage of cancer. While some doctors still believe this, others believe that the cells have not shown that they are abnormal enough to behave like cancer cells (that is, invade neighboring tissues); they may never become that atypical. In any case, while the area needs to be removed or destroyed, carcinoma in situ is not in itself life-threatening. However, carcinoma in situ does significantly increase the risk of an invasive cancer developing in that organ later.

An **invasive** (or **infiltrating**) **cancer** means that the cells that are dividing too often are sufficiently abnormal to behave in ways that can threaten the body. The doctor can see under the microscope that the cells have invaded adjoining tissues. A cell that can do this has the potential to spread elsewhere in the body.

HOW CANCER CELLS BEHAVE

At best, the cancer cell is a parasite, taking up space, devouring nourishment, and crowding out the normal cells. Because it is abnormal, the cancer cell lacks the capacity to function as a full team member. Depending on how abnormal it is, the cancer cell may continue to do some of the things that normal cells are supposed to do, but it usually contributes little or nothing to the body community. It works less efficiently than a normal cell and thus needs larger amounts of cell nutrients to keep going. The cancer cell exists primarily to eat and reproduce.

What is more dangerous is that the cancer cell pays little heed to the body's territorial rules. Normal cells with intact cell parts keep to themselves and stay at a distance from other kinds of cells. Even when benign cells overgrow and jostle or push against neighboring tissue, which is what is happening when benign tumors cause discomfort, they still respect the boundaries of other cells.

Not so the cancer cell when it gets pushed into adjoining body tissue. Lacking a normal "wall" and needing to survive in this new terrain, it penetrates and takes over the cells there for its own use. This is invasive cancer.

These maverick cancer cells can break away, hitch a ride through the circulatory system, and wander elsewhere (**metastasize**) in the body. Extremely abnormal cells are able to plant themselves and grow elsewhere in the body, away from the organ where they originated. This spread is called **metastatic cancer**.

HOW CANCER COMES ABOUT

We do not know yet what causes cancer, but we are learning more about how it happens. For cancer to develop, there must be an abnormal cell, a mechanism through which it can divide rapidly and establish a colony, and a body immune system that does not destroy it.

Inside the nucleus, or command chamber, of each body cell are twenty-three pairs of chromosomes along the double helix ("twisted ladder") molecule of DNA. DNA contains the general information for any living cell. The pairs of chromosomes contain millions of genes; each gene carries the code for a specific characteristic, rather like a bar code that identifies a piece of merchandise for a scanner at a supermarket. This genetic code, which is passed from each cell to its offspring, tells the daughter cell which parts of the DNA message it should read and follow: what kind of cell it is, what it is supposed to do, when to divide, and how to repair itself.

When the cell divides, the DNA "ladder," along with its chromosomes, splits down the middle through the rungs. Each half of the ladder is made whole again using material brought to it by the cell's supply source (RNA), whereby it becomes the DNA for one of the two daughter cells.

A mistake in one of the millions of genetic messages in a cell produces a change, or **mutation**. The change may be for the better and make the cell function more effectively, or it may be so catastrophic that the cell dies immediately. It may also be a flawed message that can get passed down from generation to generation of daughter cells without noticeable effect. But a cell with a flawed genetic message—the atypical cell—is more vulnerable than the normal cell to additional mutations and may eventually become a cancer cell. The more atypical the individual cell is, and the more atypical cells there are, the greater the chance for a cancer to develop.

Most cancer researchers now believe that cancer occurs not because of a single major event that turns a normal cell cancerous, but as a result of *multiple* hits to the genes. Thus, damage accumulates until it reaches a kind of critical mass, at which point the cancer "switch" turns on. The result of a combination of hits may be far greater than the sum of the individual effects. So, whether or not cancer occurs seems to depend not only on how many hits there are, but also on what kinds they are, how often they come, how strong they are, and how much chance the body has to recover between them.

Some hits are called **initiators** because they can cause direct damage to the genes. Substances that produce these hits are called **carcinogens** or mutagens because they can produce cancer or cell mutations. Tobacco is a known initiator for lung cancer, for example, as is the hormone DES for one kind of vaginal cancer. Other hits, like alcohol, are **promoters**—they encourage atypical cells to grow. Then there are miscellaneous hits such as a family history of a certain cancer, for instance.

The likelihood of developing most cancers increases with age. The longer a person lives and the more genetic messages that get passed on, the more opportunities there are for a message to get scrambled.

The total number of cells in the body is normally controlled by a balance of growth genes that urge a cell to divide and suppressor genes that tell it to wait. Current thinking about genes and cancer focuses on three types of genes, all related to how often cells divide.

The first type is the **proto-oncogene**. "*Onco*" means tumor, but proto-oncogenes are the ordinary healthy genes that control how often a cell divides. Cells in the body normally reproduce very rapidly while a person is growing (from a fertilized egg to a baby in nine months is impressive!), is repairing a broken bone, or is pregnant or breastfeeding. Except at these times, cells divide on a strict schedule: They replace only those that die and thus maintain the body's status quo.

The second type of gene is the **anti-oncogene** (tumor suppressor or growth suppressor gene), the normal gene that keeps the brakes on the proto-oncogenes so that cells divide on just the right timetable. For instance, anti-oncogenes seem to "switch off" or suppress the "rapid growth" genes that program cells to divide so frequently during the first nine months of life. Healthy anti-oncogenes also detect abnormal cells and do not give them "permission" to divide. The problem arises when one or more anti-oncogenes mutate so that they can no longer keep the brakes on—and cells begin dividing too often. With this speedup, cell quality control suffers.

A proto-oncogene may mutate to become the third type of gene: the **oncogene** (or carcinogenic oncogene), an abnormal gene that gives its cell the message to make more growth factors so it matures faster and divides sooner. When the cell divides, it passes this genetic message to the two daughter cells. These cells, both flawed and dividing too often, are at high risk for becoming more abnormal through more mutations. Meanwhile, the mutated anti-oncogene no longer withholds permission for the flawed cell to divide and no longer keeps the rate in check. The result is often cancer.

But how and why do proto-oncogenes "switch on" to become carcinogenic oncogenes? What causes anti-oncogenes to mutate? Are there ways to prevent or even reverse these mutations? These are key puzzles in basic cancer research.

For example, researchers have focused on a particular gene, p53, one of the genes that normally acts as an anti-oncogene, or tumor suppressor. If the DNA in p53 is damaged (perhaps by tobacco smoke or some other carcinogen), it mutates and may no longer be able to hold the proto-oncogenes in check, beginning a quality control breakdown.

Scientists looking for a common mechanism in the development of various cancers have found that p53 appears to be damaged in about 90 percent of all human cancers. The mutation may occur decades before cancer appears and is only one of several genetic changes that move the cell along the path toward cancer—but it appears to be a necessary step. If this step could be prevented or reversed,...

Scientists researching p53 are looking for the "fingerprints" of factors that may have led to the original mutation. During the last several years, publicity has linked mutated copies of several genes (BRCA1, BRCA2, and others) to family clusters of breast cancer and ovarian cancer. These genes, mostly anti-oncogenes or tumor suppressor genes, may mutate at any time during a woman's life, but the greatest concern is that a mutated copy of one of these genes may be passed down in some families. The baby who receives one of these mutated genes has already, before birth, taken a major step toward cancer.

Only 5 to 10 percent of all breast cancers seem to fall into this category, with the disease striking many people from several overlapping generations in a family, all at an early age. This is not usually the problem if a woman has a family history of one or two people diagnosed with the same cancer after age fifty-five or so. A woman who receives the gene may also never develop cancer, because this is only one mutation in a series required for the disease. (For more information, see "Who Gets Breast Cancer?" in Chapter 11.)

A big factor in whether a person develops cancer is the body's immune system. Our bodies defend us against atypical cells all the time. The cell itself may repair some small mutations. Some abnormal cells may lose the ability to reproduce. Normal cell turnover disposes of abnormal cells as well as normal ones.

Throughout our lives, the body's immune system recognizes atypical cells (including cancer cells) as "enemy" and destroys them. Unfortunately, some cancer cells seem able to slip through the body's surveillance: They pass for normal cells or disguise themselves. Others may divide so rapidly or are so aggressive that they overwhelm even the strongest body defenses.

Or, the immune system may be exhausted or operating at partial power. People with AIDS or people on certain medications that suppress the body's immune system (to keep it from rejecting a transplanted organ, for instance) are especially vulnerable to cancer. When the immune system is stressed severely and continuously by anything, such as poor diet, personal losses, or relationship difficulties, it may become less effective, less able to search out rogue cancer cells and destroy them.

SEARCHING FOR CANCER CAUSES

With our current level of knowledge we cannot say, "Such-and-so caused this cancer." If we were to try to indicate the causes of an individual cancer on a pie-shaped chart, we would have to draw a piece for the person's inherited vulnerability, a piece for age, a piece for possible initiators (many of which we do not know yet), a piece for a weakened immune system, and so on. Each person's chart would be different and, knowing what we do now, we could only guess at how big each section of the pie would be.

But more information about possible causes of cancer comes in all the time, much of it from researchers working at the molecule and gene level. Statisticians and epidemiologists (scientists who study patterns of disease in large populations of people) continue searching for common factors among women diagnosed with a particular women's cancer. The challenge for all these researchers lies in clarifying which factors actually contribute to the disease, which are effects of the disease, and which are innocent bystanders.

Every day medical stories report this or that astonishing research finding, often contradicting what was believed yesterday. Research is the way scientists verify their proposed answers to questions; but not every research study is equally valuable. The woman trying to make sense of all the conflicting medical research needs to ask these questions:

+ Was the research conducted on animals or on humans? (Humans often react quite differently from animals.)

+ How many individuals were studied? (The results of larger studies are influenced less by chance or coincidence.)

+ How large or significant was the effect? (Did women with a particular factor develop cancer slightly more often, for instance, or five times as often?)

+ How common is the condition being studied? (It is generally not worth worrying about a factor that significantly increases the risk for a specific cancer that almost no one gets.)

+ Was the study a reasonable way of exploring the question? (Did it study the right population and change one factor—and only one—that might be expected to make a difference?)

+ Are there other possible explanations for the findings?

+ Has the study been repeated to confirm the findings?

HOW CANCER GROWS

If enough changes happen to the genes of a cell that it becomes a cancer cell (**malignant transformation**), and that cell then divides, the result is two cancer cells, a doubling. If those two daughter cells survive, they in turn divide so that there are four cells. Eventually, unless something happens to stop the process, there will be a trillion cells doubling at the same inexorable rate. The time it takes for the number of cells in a tumor to double is called the **doubling time**.

Each cancer has its own doubling time, coded in its genetic message. The doubling time for one cancer may be one week; for another, six months. Barring another change in the genetic message, this doubling time will remain constant. For instance, a cancer with a doubling time of four months will take four months to double from two cells to four, but also four months to double from two billion cells to four billion.

It takes ten doublings to reach about one thousand cells, twenty doublings to reach about one million cells. It takes about a billion cancer cells to form a lump that can be felt. That represents about thirty doublings, which means that a long silent period—often several years—may have passed since the first cancer cell began dividing.

Every cancer has the potential to invade adjoining tissues and metastasize to other organs, but each follows its own timetable. Some tend to stay in their own local area where they can grow quite large, while others begin metastasizing very early.

When cancer penetrates adjoining tissues within the organ where it started, it is called **local invasion**. The logical way to treat a local problem is with local therapies: removing the cancer cells surgically or destroying them in that area with controlled high-energy nuclear beams of **radiation therapy**.

If the cancer cells continue to invade neighboring tissues, they may reach a new organ (ovarian cancer cells may begin invading the nearby bladder, for instance). This is called **regional extension**, and it can sometimes be treated at the same time and/or with the same therapies as a local invasion.

CANCER METASTASIS

Distant metastasis is a serious problem that occurs when cancer cells break off from the parent tumor, transplant themselves to another organ, and continue doubling there. This continues to be the same kind of cancer, though. For example, if breast cancer spreads to the lung, it still looks, behaves like, and is breast cancer; it does not behave like a cancer that started in the lung.

How do cancer cells travel to distant organs? Even if they do reach a distant organ, where the cells will generally be very different from those in the original site, only a tiny percentage of cancer cells are abnormal enough to settle there and grow successfully. About a century ago, a scientist developed the "seed and soil" theory of distant metastasis, and it still seems true: For cancer cells to grow in a distant organ, a particular kind of cancer cell (seed) has to reach a particular kind of tissue (soil) where it might have a chance to grow; anywhere else, it will die.

The cancer cell can begin the metastatic journey through either of the body's two parallel circulatory systems, the **artery–vein system** or the **lymphatic system**. These eventually join into one system, so the later steps in the journey are the same.

What might happen when a rogue cancer cell leaves the original tumor? To feed their voracious appetites, cancer tumors develop their own connections with the body's artery-vein blood supply and often even develop new blood vessels of their own, a process called **angiogenesis**. With the help of some genes in the cell that turn on to produce enzymes, the cancer cell may invade the blood vessel wall, break loose, and travel along with the rapid flow of the bloodstream. Since the bloodstream exists to transport materials through the body, it forms beds of tiny blood vessels (capillaries) near body organs where blood flow can slow down for efficient delivery and pick up before speeding on again. If the cancer cell slows down enough in a capillary, it may lodge against the wall of the vessel and use enzymes to penetrate the wall into the organ, which may be a place where it can settle.

At every point along the journey, the cancer cell faces death. Most die a natural cell death, are hunted down and killed by specific kinds of defender blood cells, or never find an appropriate place to settle.

Currently, unless doctors know that there is a distant metastasis, they cannot be certain whether cells from an invasive cancer have made their way into the bloodstream. When they look at slides of the tumor under a microscope, however, they may be able to make a knowledgeable guess based on the blood supply near the cancer.

In the lymphatic system, a fluid called **lymph** flows through a network of small vessels, scavenging and draining substances that the body recognizes as used up, foreign, or dangerous. A series of lymph nodes, way stations along the lymph system, filter the lymph. They trap and often destroy escaping cancer cells. Circulating white blood cells in the lymphatic system also kill cancer cells. The lymph eventually empties into a large vein near the heart and thus joins the artery–vein system.

The lymph nodes are a fallback defense system for the body. When a lymph node is positive for cancer (has cancer cells in it as seen under a microscope), that may mean either that all the cancer cells straying from the original organ have been trapped and have died in the lymph node, or that some of the cells have been trapped there while others have traveled beyond the node.

Unless there is clear evidence of distant metastasis, it is impossible to know whether any cancer cells have evaded this filter system. The more positive lymph nodes there are, however, and the more cancer cells there are in each one, the greater the chance that some cancer cells have escaped, although it may be years before a metastasis shows itself.

If **medical oncologists** (cancer doctors) either know that there is distant metastasis or suspect that there might be cancer cells in transit that could eventually establish a distant colony, they may prescribe systemic treatment, which treats the whole body and backs up the body's own defenses. **Chemotherapy** uses powerful medicines to kill rapidly dividing cells (such as cancer cells) anywhere in the body. **Hormone therapy** changes the hormone balance in the body to create a hostile environment for cancer cells. **Biological therapy** bolsters the body's own defenses so they are better able to destroy cancer.

Obviously, the best strategy for beating cancer is to prevent it. Until we learn how to prevent it, however, we must try to detect and treat it early, before any cancer cells have a chance to metastasize. If some cancer cells escape from the organ where they originate, we try to destroy them before they can settle and grow in a vital organ, an organ necessary for life. (Breast and gynecological cancers do not arise in vital organs. Lung cancer, on the other hand, arises in a vital organ and does not need to metastasize to be deadly.) Cure is possible up until this point. Even in the case of distant metastasis, treatment can often buy a woman time, comfort, and a good quality of life. And sometimes more.

Some of our weapons against cancer have been around for centuries. Some are as new as today. Having them all available and being open to whatever new ones tomorrow brings give a woman a real chance of surviving cancer.

"Died in her sleep . . . natural causes . . . age 102?"
Why not?

— Kerry McGinn

CHAPTER 2

CAUSES AND PREVENTION

In each section of this book, we describe risk factors that are linked to each of the women's cancers. There are many other cancers, in addition to the cancers specific to women, to which women are susceptible or that will affect them in some way. Women are also likely to be affected by the cancers of loved ones—friends, husbands, children, sisters, and relatives. So, in this chapter, we have included a general overview of known risk factors related to the development of cancer and information on what you can do to help prevent cancer.

The entry of managed care organizations (also called health management organizations or HMOs) into our lives may or may not alter access to preventive care and early detection services, but this is an all-important issue. For prevention to be a valued activity, insurance companies and managed care organizations must see prevention as a long-view issue. The investment in preventive care that a company (or individual) makes today will not deliver a benefit until twenty to thirty years down the road. In some managed care organizations, the greatest rewards go to doctors and other providers who offer minimal care, do not encourage cancer screenings, and avoid giving time-consuming counseling.

When considering a new insurance policy or signing on with a new HMO, be aware that good policies and health plans will include prevention and screening services. Such services address smoking cessation, alcohol cessation, nutritional counseling, weight loss, fitness, and cancer risk assessment and counseling. Other preventive and early detection services in a quality health plan include access to and coverage for chemoprevention trials, mammography, Pap smears, digital rectal exams, sigmoidoscopy and colonoscopy, skin assessment, and education about how to prevent or at least reduce environmental exposures. Employers, insurance companies, and managed care organizations must know the facts: It is estimated that between $60,000 and $120,000 *per case* can be saved when cancer is found and treated early rather than at a later, less manageable stage. These estimates are based on direct costs of medical care, disability associated with illness and treatment, use of temporary help to replace a sick employee, and other ongoing employee benefits. It is well worth employers' efforts to include good prevention and early detection services in their company's health plan benefits.

Sometimes it seems like everything causes cancer. Cigarette smoke almost certainly causes cancer, despite the tobacco industry's denials. This is pretty frightening for those of us who have inhaled secondhand smoke for many years. We know that toxic chemicals cause cancer and that there are several carcinogenic pollutants in rivers, lakes, drinking water, and the air we breathe. Too late to do anything about it, I discovered I had been exposed to asbestos dust throughout my childhood. It is entirely possible that the fresh country air in Iowa where I grew up was loaded with toxins from farm supplies—fertilizers, pesticides, and weed killers. Just when I thought I had found an acceptable diet soda, I learned that saccharin may cause cancer. More recently, and more critical to my current tastes, I read that wine might be related to the development of breast cancer. Alcohol intake at moderate to high levels is risky. (The good news is that red wine might prevent some forms of heart disease.)

Is there anything any of us can do to decrease our risk of getting cancer? Sure there is. But remember that cancer results from a combination of factors: heredity, exposure to toxic chemicals and environmental hazards, and personal and social habits, such as cigarette smoking, alcohol consumption, and a high-fat diet. Just as there is no one cause of cancer, there is not likely to be one method of prevention.

Knowledge and awareness are key to people having some control of their own health. **Primary prevention** can help us to avoid exposure to cancer-causing agents, or **carcinogens,** and to make healthful behaviors a routine part of our lives. Of course, the best way to prevent cancer is to avoid exposure to carcinogens altogether. For most of us, this is unrealistic. It is useful to be aware of the risks we take and the substances we are exposed to and, when possible, to make informed decisions about the risks. We can also adopt personal habits (like decreasing dietary fat and increasing physical exercise) that promote wellness.

Secondary prevention involves identifying people with more risk factors and following them closely to assess for precancerous conditions and early cancers. **Risk factors,** traits that are linked to increased numbers of certain cancers, can be divided into two classes—those a person can control (such as diet, smoking, and exercise) and those not under a person's control (genetics, age, menstrual history, and some environmental exposures). In the early 1990s, **chemoprevention**—prescribing specific preventive medicines to people thought to be at high risk for cancer—entered the picture.

Many studies suggest that 80 to 90 percent of all cancers are somehow related to lifestyle and occupational exposures. Most people agree on the need to regulate exposure to environmental carcinogens, but disagree on who should impose the regulations and how and what to regulate. A person's lifestyle exposures are determined by choice or circumstance or both. Decisions about what risks are acceptable are personal and are best made with good, solid facts and clear information. Each of us needs to consider the relative risks that accompany certain choices, certain exposures.

For example, the decision to smoke cigarettes must be considered in light of the risks associated with smoking: the chance of nicotine addiction, the certainty of permanent lung damage, the possibility of heart disease, and the increased risk of developing cancers of the lung, cervix, bladder, lip, mouth, nose, and throat. In other words, the "relative risk" associated with cigarette smoking is pretty high. On the other hand, the relative risk that goes with using the artificial sweetener saccharin is probably quite low. Rat studies used to define the cancer-causing potential of saccharin involved massive doses over a short time span—much more than a human would consume in a lifetime.

The occurrence of different types of cancer varies in different countries. Different ethnic and cultural groups have their own social, dietary, and environmental risk factors. Migrant populations develop types of cancer that are characteristic of where they live, rather than those of their ethnic group. For example, native Japanese have a higher incidence of stomach cancer but lower rates of colon cancer compared to Americans. After one or two generations in America, Japanese Americans have the same lower incidence of stomach cancer and higher incidence of colon cancer that affect other American populations.

PHYSICAL ACTIVITY

While the cause and effect is unclear, it is known that active women are less likely to develop cancer than are women who are inactive "couch potatoes." Obesity and some dietary factors are known risk factors for breast, endometrial, and colon cancers. And clearly, obesity and low levels of exercise are closely related.

The risk of breast and endometrial cancers in women who are markedly overweight is thought to be related to the estrogens that come from andro-estrogens and estrones found in fat (or adipose) tissues. There are actually more estrogens in the blood of obese women, and many cancers affecting women are linked to this hormone's activities over a lifetime.

Colon cancer has been closely linked to high-fat diets as well as diets with limited fiber content. Colon cancer is also associated with the time it takes food to digest and travel through the bowel. We know that exercise stimulates bowel activity, and this may well be a factor in the prevention of colon cancer, although this theory has not yet been proven. But, with the physical and mental benefits of exercise so obvious, incorporating regular, enjoyable physical activities into our daily routines makes sense.

CHEMOPREVENTION

Chemoprevention is the use of natural or synthetic chemicals or medications to prevent precancerous conditions from becoming full-blown cancer. Chemoprevention is based on the theory that cancer develops only after a series of events or steps occur—generally believed to be events that cause a cell's genes to mutate, producing the original cancer cell—and that this change can be reversed, at least in the early stages. Nearly forty research studies and clinical trials are in progress worldwide that test nutritional elements and chemical agents for their benefits in preventing cancer. One study is designed to assess the value of dietary fiber in preventing colon polyps. Another will evaluate whether dietary fat content relates to the chance of breast cancer **recurring,** or returning, after initial treatment.

The Women's Health Initiative (WHI), launched in 1991, is a government-sponsored, nationwide research effort conducted by the National Institutes of Health. Its goal is to determine whether hormone replacements, low-fat diets, and vitamin supplements (calcium and vitamin D) play roles in the prevention of cancer, heart and vascular diseases, and osteoporosis. Over 161,000 postmenopausal women fifty to seventy-nine years of age are participating in the WHI. Sixty-eight thousand post-menopausal women are enrolled in a clinical trial with three components: hormone replacement therapy, dietary modification, and calcium/vitamin D. Women who are not part of the clinical trial are involved in the observational study which is designed to examine the relationships between lifestyle, health and risk factors, and health outcomes. Recruitment was completed in 1998, and participants will be followed for eight to twelve years, after which time data will be analyzed and finally reported.

The most publicized of the chemoprevention studies is probably the Breast Cancer Prevention Trial, organized by the National Surgical Adjuvant Breast and Bowel Project (NSABP)—a program funded by the National Cancer Institute. Tamoxifen, used to treat women with breast cancer, was studied for its potential use in preventing breast cancer in healthy women who are at high risk. The Breast Cancer Prevention Trial in the United States and Canada enlisted sixteen thousand women; half were given tamoxifen and half received a placebo. The study was expected to contine well into 2002, but it was apparent quite early that tamoxifen reduced the risk of invasive breast cancer by almost 50 percent. The study was concluded early and led the NSABP to launch the STAR trial (Study of Tamoxifen and Raloxifene), designed to compare the effects of these drugs, especially in their abilities to reduce the occurrence of breast cancer, bone fractures, heart attacks, and changes in cognitive abilities. The STAR trial, which began in 1999, will recruit a total of 22,000 postmenopausal women or women at least thirty-five years old who are at increased risk of breast cancer. Another chemoprevention trial involves the drug finasteride, used to treat noncancerous enlargement of the prostate gland in men, to determine whether the drug can prevent prostate cancer. An "accidental" finding is that this drug increases hair growth for some men; thus it is now being touted as a drug to prevent baldness!

TOBACCO

Tobacco is the major carcinogen in industrialized nations. *Smoking tobacco causes at least 85 percent of lung cancer deaths and 30 percent of all cancer deaths.* The risk of lung cancer is ten times greater by middle age for smokers than for lifelong nonsmokers. Cigarette smoking is also linked to cancers of the mouth, larynx (voicebox), pharynx, esophagus, breast, bladder, pancreas, kidney, stomach, and liver. Smokeless tobacco (chewing tobacco and snuff) is also related to cancers of the mouth. Making a decision *not* to use tobacco products—smokeless tobacco, cigarettes, and cigars—is the major action any woman can take to decrease her chances of developing cancer.

In recent years, it has become fashionable for young men *and* women to smoke cigars. Columnist Ann Landers called cigars a "trendy way for tobacco to kill." Just like cigarette smokers, cigar smokers risk permanent lung damage and emphysema, and also put themselves at risk for cancers of the mouth, larynx, and esophagus. Cigar smokers should be aware that cancer death rates for cigar smokers are 34 percent higher than for nonsmokers. In addition, the carbon monoxide fumes from one cigar are thirty times those from one cigarette, and secondhand cigar smoke is even more deadly than secondhand cigarette smoke.

At least 85 percent of deaths from lung cancer could have been prevented, which means of the 170,000 people in the United States diagnosed with lung cancer every year, at least 145,000 could have prevented it. Currently, about 79,000 women are diagnosed with lung cancer, and over 65,000 women die from it—meaning over 55,000 women died who might otherwise have led normal, healthy lives. There is some encouraging news: The number of lung cancer cases among women peaked in 1998 and is now just slightly declining.

Some molecular biology studies suggest that women are more susceptible to the carcinogens in tobacco smoke than men—making smoking even more dangerous for women. Tobacco and alcohol used in combination create a higher risk for cancer than when either substance is used alone. In other words, a woman who smokes and drinks alcohol is more likely to develop a cancer than a woman who drinks alcohol but does not smoke.

So what about those people we all know who smoke and never get cancer? Everyone has a story about a relative or friend who smoked a couple of packs a day, lived to a ripe old age, and died of "natural causes." We also know of people who have never smoked who get lung cancer. These individuals do throw a wrench into the theory, but they seem to be the exceptions to the rule.

Ironically, thousands of women are up in arms about claims that the government has not funded enough studies on breast cancer and other diseases that affect women—yet almost 30 percent of American women continue to smoke (probably even a greater percentage in European countries, and there is an alarming increase in smoking among girls and women in China and other Asian countries) and continue to be exploited by the tobacco industry. Although more than 203,000 women in the United States are diagnosed with breast cancer yearly, most can be treated. On the other hand, lung cancer is especially deadly for women. Lung cancers are not usually found early and most cannot be effectively treated. Most lung cancers and at least 30 percent of other cancers could be prevented by women changing only one behavior: smoking.

People who quit smoking, regardless of age, live longer than people who continue to smoke. Smokers who quit before they are fifty have half the risk of dying in the next fifteen years as those who continue to smoke. Quitting smoking decreases risks of cancers of the lung, larynx, mouth, pancreas, bladder, and cervix. Keep in mind, too, that stopping smoking can also help prevent other serious diseases: heart disease and strokes, emphysema and bronchitis, and peripheral vascular disease (poor circulation in the legs).

DIET

Both undernutrition and overnutrition have been linked to various types of cancer. Low-fiber diets have been blamed for cancers, but how fiber actually prevents cancer has not been defined. Researchers think that fiber decreases the time it takes food products to move through the colon, which in turn limits the time the interior of the colon is in contact with carcinogens contained in foods or that develop during digestive processes.

High-fat diets are also linked to cancer. As fats are digested, some chemicals are produced that are thought to be carcinogenic. Additives used in food processing in the United States and other industrialized countries may also be related to the development of cancer.

It is estimated that in the United States about one-third of all cancers can be linked to dietary factors. The National Research Council recommends that our fat intake not exceed 25 percent of total daily calories (the average American diet is composed of more than 40 percent fat) and that we increase the amount of fruits, vegetables, and wholegrain cereals in our diet. In 2001, The American Cancer Society (ACS) updated its guidelines for nutrition and physical activity. Important changes emphasize the related roles of physical activity and diet in reducing cancer risks. Complete information can be obtained through the American Cancer Society (www.cancer.org), but basic recommendations include the following:

1. Eat a variety of healthful foods, emphasizing plant sources: Eat five or more servings of vegetables and fruit daily; eat more whole grains and less processed grains and sugar; limit your consumption of red meats; and maintain a healthful weight.

2. Adopt a physically active lifestyle, defined as at least thirty minutes of exercise on five or more days each week. Recommended activity levels are higher for children and adolescents.

3. Maintain a healthful weight throughout life: Balance calories with physical activity.

4. Limit consumption of alcohol to no more than two drinks per day for men and one drink per day for women.

ENVIRONMENT

Our environment includes where we live and work, and most cancers in the United States seem to be linked in some way to our physical surroundings. Certain occupations have known cancer risks: Chemicals and other substances used in some industries are known to cause cancer. For example, arsenic compounds are linked to lung and skin cancer. Aromatic amines, which are man-made chemicals used in dye and drug manufacturing, increase the risk of bladder cancer. Asbestos is a factor in several cancers, including lung cancer—especially mesothelioma. The additive effects of asbestos and tobacco smoke are especially deadly. Dioxin from chemical plant emissions or inadequate chemical waste disposal and pesticide residues in food products are environmental exposures that may or may not contribute to the overall human cancer problem. These exposures are man-made and therefore should be controllable through regulatory safeguards.

Radiation

Radiation exposure increases the risk of leukemia and cancers of the breast and lung. Sources of radiation occur in the natural environment in such minerals as radon, uranium, and radium. As these sources decay naturally, some radiation is released into the air and water. We can be exposed to radiation through foods or water contaminated by a radioactive substance. Other types of radiation can be inhaled—as people in Nevada discovered after early nuclear bomb testing.

Radon, a gas that occurs in nature as a decay product of radium and uranium, has been recognized as a possible cause of lung cancer. It is present in nearly all soil and rock and may be linked to lung cancer in people who mine uranium and other underground minerals. Radon seeps into the indoor air from the soil below and around a building. Many houses built on certain geologic formations, such as the Reading Prong in Pennsylvania, have been found to have high radon levels. In seven states surveyed by the Environmental Protection Agency, nearly one of three houses had high radon levels. Advisory warnings first issued in 1988 from the U.S. Public Health Service urge that all housing be tested for radon. You can contact the EPA for the pamphlet, "A Citizen's Guide to Radon," which provides guidelines for monitoring and sets a national standard for the annual average radon concentration in the living space of homes. Copies of the pamphlet are available directly from EPA offices. Radon detection services can be located through county building departments and through listings in local telephone directories and yellow pages.

Cancers related to radiation exposure include those of the breast, thyroid, and blood-forming tissues. Certain leukemias have been related to radiation, most of them occurring two to four years after exposure. The occurrence of certain tumors and blood-system cancers among Japanese citizens increased after the use of the atomic bomb in Japan near the end of World War II. A similar increase in the rate of radiation-related cancers is already being observed as a result of the 1986 nuclear accident in Chernobyl in the former Soviet Union.

Minor exposure to radiation occurs through diagnostic X rays and the use of radioactive substances in treatment, but the risk of developing cancer from a diagnostic test is estimated to be one out of a million tests per year. Even though the risk is low, there is concern about the risk of radiation exposure. Medical centers take care to select people who truly need diagnostic X rays and limit routine procedures where the risks outweigh the benefits.

Therapeutic radiation, such as the radiation used to treat various forms of cancer, can be a risk factor for the development of new cancers and is just one of the reasons that follow-up after cancer treatment is so important. Although modern technology limits the amount of normal tissues exposed to the radioactive beam, there is as yet no way to completely protect normal tissues from the DNA damage that radiation causes. Radiation-associated leukemia is a concern after a large area of bone marrow has been exposed to radiation. Lymphomas and solid tumors (tumors involving the breast, thyroid, salivary glands, skin, gastrointestinal tract, bone, or brain) are associated with direct radiation to these tissues. The actual risk is higher with larger doses of radiation, but it has also been linked to a person's age at the time of radiation exposure. For example, among women who received radiation to the breast and/or chest at a relatively young age (34–42 years of age), there is an increased risk of developing breast cancer. Ultraviolet radiation sources include the sun and industrial equipment like welding arcs and germicidal lights. It is thought that this radiation causes damage to DNA and eventually leads to skin cancer.

Radiofrequency radiation, the radiation emitted from cellular telephones, has been implicated as a cause of cancer since a report in 1993. Television, radio, and cell phone transmission facilities are other sources of radiofrequency radiation emissions. At this time, there is neither epidemiologic nor laboratory evidence of an association between radiofrequency radiation and cancer.

Exposure to the Sun

Most of the one million cases of skin cancer diagnosed each year can be traced to exposure to the sun. There is some suggestion that the diminishing ozone layer is increasing skin cancer rates. Most of these cancers (the majority of which are basal-cell or squamous-cell cancers) are both preventable and curable. Malignant melanoma is the exception. **Melanoma** is a deadly form of skin cancer that is not as responsive to treatment as other skin cancers are. The number of melanoma cases in the United States has risen steadily—increasing at a rate of 3 percent each year—and the death rate is growing.

While it is true that melanoma is more common in older people, it is now being found more often among people as young as twenty years of age. People who develop melanoma are most often white with fair skin that sunburns easily (the rate is ten times higher for whites than it is for blacks). In fact, a history of blistering sunburns early in life is common among people who develop melanoma. Hereditary factors seem to play a role here as well: At least one gene is linked to a form of melanoma.

Preventing skin cancer starts with limiting exposure to the sun's ultraviolet rays. The sun's rays are strongest from 10:00 A.M. to 4:00 P.M., so you should avoid exposure at these times, use sunscreens with a solar protection factor (SPF) of 15 or higher, and reapply them frequently. It is especially important to protect children from sunburn, not forgetting that they need sunglasses to protect their eyes, too.

Skin cancer presents an interesting cultural dilemma. It has become very fashionable—particularly among Caucasians—to have what is marketed as a "deep, dark tan." Teenage women seem particularly susceptible to this idea. One study surveyed people thirty and younger about their use of sunscreens and knowledge of sun protection factors and sun exposure risks. The study revealed that knowing the risks did not improve their use of sunscreens.

Electromagnetic Fields

The notion that exposure to electromagnetic fields might cause cancer has been under study for over twenty years. Studies cover two basic areas: (1) monitors of cancers of children and adults in various home and work conditions and (2) experiments that attempt to re-create the cancer-causing effects of electromagnetic exposure in cells, tissues, and laboratory animals. To date, there is no scientific evidence that electromagnetic exposure causes cancer. Still, there is a great deal of interest in this idea because electric power is everywhere—from the electric power lines that bring electricity into our homes to the radios and televisions in our living rooms and bedrooms and the microwave ovens in our kitchens. Given the ongoing public interest and speculation, many scientists continue to explore questions about the effects of electric frequencies on our health in general and its potential to cause cancer in particular.

An electromagnetic field (EMF) is created by the flow of alternating electric current (AC). When current flows, electric and magnetic fields are created. The electric frequencies people are exposed to range from extremely low frequencies, including a wide range of radio, television, radar, and microwave frequencies, to the high end of the range, including ultraviolet rays and X rays. Electric fields are easily shielded by all kinds of materials, including buildings and even the human body. Magnetic fields, however, pass through most of these substances. Because they can move through tissues, magnetic fields are the major focus in studies attempting to link electromagnetic fields to cancer. But, even though EMFs move through or penetrate tissue, evidence shows they are *not* able to disrupt or damage structures in the cells that cause gene mutations.

The first scientific study of a link between an EMF and cancer was published in 1979. Since that report, thirteen more studies have been published describing EMF exposure in home settings (primarily assessing home electric wiring) and the risk of cancer. Eight others look at cancer risks relating to EMFs from such household appliances as electric blankets, hair dryers, heated water beds, electric razors, and massage units. Several others have explored EMF exposure in work settings. One theory gaining the attention of scientists is that EMF exposure alters the body's normal rhythms—also called the circadian rhythms—and decreases the body's production of the hormone melatonin, a decrease that, in turn, promotes the development of cancer, especially breast cancer. Some laboratory animal studies just hint at a link, but this idea has not been confirmed.

Studies done in the United States, France, Canada, Great Britain, and the Scandinavian countries have focused most of their attention on leukemia, brain cancer, and lymphoma. All of the studies put together tell us only that exposure to EMFs may or may not cause cancer. The findings are not strong in any of the studies, and many of the findings are contradictory. In some studies, the people who developed cancer following EMF exposure had several other risk factors that complicate the picture. The frequency of each exposure has not been (or cannot be) controlled, and the naturally occurring EMFs cannot be eliminated or controlled. It is not known whether there is a cumulative effect to exposure over time. At this point, it is impossible to prove whether a risk exists or not.

INFECTIONS

Infections with viruses, parasites, and bacteria are linked to various kinds of cancers. The ability of viruses to cause cancer is evident through the relationship of the hepatitis B virus to liver cancer; the Epstein-Barr virus (EBV) to Burkitt's lymphoma and nasopharyngeal cancer; the human T-cell lymphotrophic virus to adult T-cell leukemia and lymphoma; the human papillomavirus (HPV), or "venereal warts," to cervical cancer (see Chapter 17); and the human immunodeficiency virus (HIV) to lymphoma and Kaposi's sarcoma. Current theory is that the virus becomes part of the DNA or RNA of the cells, which results in cell mutation.

Liver flukes are parasites that have been linked to liver cancer, and blood flukes are implicated in bladder and colon cancers. In 1991, it was found that infection of the stomach with the bacteria *Helicobacter pylori* is linked to stomach cancer. The fungus *Aspergillus* produces toxic substances called aflatoxins that are thought to be a risk factor for liver cancer.

Overall, few infections thought to actually *cause* cancer have been identified. As with other carcinogens, the actual agent or event that leads to cancer is difficult or impossible to pinpoint.

IMMUNE SYSTEM

The immune system protects the body from things it recognizes as "foreign," such as bacteria, viruses, and cancer cells. People who have deficient or damaged immune systems are more likely to develop cancer. Nearly 70 percent of people with AIDS develop certain cancers, such as Kaposi's sarcoma, lymphoma, and cancers of the central nervous system. Children younger than two years and adults older than sixty have immune systems that function at a less than optimal level, and often have above-average cancer rates. People who take immunosuppressive drugs to reduce the chance of organ rejection also have a higher chance of developing cancer.

MEDICATIONS

At least a few of the medicines we use to treat illnesses or conditions are themselves carcinogens. The most common are drugs that fall into the category of sex hormones. The hormone women use in the hormone replacement therapy often prescribed during and after menopause—estrogen—is associated with uterine and breast cancer. For over a decade, it was believed that the addition of progestin would offset the risks of estrogen alone. But in mid-2002, an analysis of data from the Women's Health Initiative revealed a slight increase in breast cancer for women using this combination of hormone replacement therapy. In addition, heart attacks, strokes, and blood clots occurred more often among the WHI participants using the estrogen and progestin combination. Fewer women using these hormones were found to develop colorectal cancer or suffer hip fractures, and the risk of endometrial cancer was found to be about equal to that of women not using these hormones. This component of the WHI study was discontinued immediately, and participants were told to stop taking the estrogen plus progestin study pills. Study participants taking estrogen alone were asked to continue taking their study pills, while the importance of yearly mammograms and clinic examinations was reinforced. The number of questions to be addressed with regard to hormone replacement therapy seems to be increasing, and these questions include whether hormone replacement is needed at all, the recommended length of time a woman who decides to use HRT should continue therapy, which therapy should be used, and what benefits and risks are inherent in hormone use.

Tamoxifen, a synthetic "anti-estrogen" hormone, has been weakly linked to liver tumors and uterine cancers. Another hormone, diethylstilbestrol (DES), was given in previous decades to women to prevent miscarriage. In 1971, it was reported that DES was linked to cancer of the vagina in the female children of women who had used DES, and the drug is no longer used for this purpose.

Medicines made from arsenic, more common in the past than today, are linked to skin cancers. Some of the cancer chemotherapy drugs commonly used today are known to cause the development of new or second cancers (specifically, leukemia and lymphoma, which occur after treatment for a solid tumor). Coal-tar ointments (sometimes used in the treatment of psoriasis) might be connected to skin cancer, amphetamines to lymphoma, and phenacetin (used to reduce fever and relieve headaches) to kidney cancer.

AGE

Many women believe that their risks for the "female cancers" decline after the childbearing years. This could not be farther from the truth. Age is the single most important risk factor for cancer. Over half of all cancer occurs in people over sixty-five. Studies indicate that cancer in this older population, as in most other population subgroups, is related to exposure to carcinogens and other known risk factors.

The knowledge that increasing age is related to cancer risk cannot help us prevent cancer, but it can help us be more watchful for signs. Spotting cancer early is the second-best defense against it—which is why early detection is referred to as "secondary prevention."

Fewer women over sixty-five have Pap smears and, as a result, older women with cervical cancers are diagnosed at a much later stage of disease than younger women. When women over sixty-five are screened, they tend to have more abnormal Pap smears—primarily because they have not been screened often or have never been screened at all. The "law of averages" catches up with them. In other age groups, things like chronic infections would be found and treated earlier, before they convert to dysplasia.

After a woman passes the childbearing years, she may not get screened for cervical cancer as regularly. Women who have had a hysterectomy often neglect Pap smear screening—and doctors often fail to suggest them after hysterectomy. This can be a grave error in thinking: Remnants of cervical tissues left after hysterectomy can and do develop cancers that must be detected and treated. Nongynecological doctors may think of cervical cancer screening as the territory of the gynecologist. Some general practitioners may not have good skills or any interest in gynecologic care. More than a few older women cannot do the gymnastics required during the gynecologic exam (bending at the waist, flexing at the ankles and knees, and flexing and rotating the hips). Doctors may need to use special examination techniques and skills because of these normal changes in aging women.

This issue has increasing importance, as many managed care plans limit women's access to specialists such as gynecologists—leaving important screening decisions to general practitioners. This is especially true for women who have found it necessary to change doctors (or health-care providers such as the nurse practitioner) to comply with a new managed care plan. For these reasons, a woman needs to know what screening tests are appropriate for her age and unique medical history.

Breast cancer is the most common kind of cancer found in women over sixty-five, lung and colon cancers the second and third. The American Cancer Society recommends that women over sixty-five be examined yearly. The exam should cover general health counseling and a cancer checkup that includes examination of the thyroid, ovaries, lymph nodes, mouth, and skin; breast exam and mammogram; Pap test and pelvic exam; digital rectal exam; and a test for blood in the stool.

RACE AND ETHNICITY

Cancer rates and the ways cancer affects people vary among races and ethnic groups. For example, African Americans generally have lower survival rates than other racial or ethnic groups. Many people believe the differences can be explained by delays in detection and differences in access to various forms of treatment, but new data tells us that these differences are not totally explained by poverty or wealth, insurance coverage, stage or severity of disease, or availability of health services. African Americans and Hispanics are more likely to be diagnosed at later, more advanced stages of cancer. This is particularly true with regard to prostate cancer among African-American men: 35.4 percent of African-American men diagnosed with prostate cancer have metastases at diagnosis as opposed to 22.2 percent among whites. Fewer African-American women develop breast cancer than Caucasian women, but African-American women are more likely to die from breast cancer after it is diagnosed. Cancers of the stomach and liver are diagnosed more often among Asian-American populations, indigenous people from the Pacific Northwest have higher rates of colon and rectal cancers, and Hispanic and Vietnamese-American women develop cervical cancer more frequently than Caucasians. Even though the major cancer sites are the same among all races, the ranked order is slightly different. Of new cancers found among African Americans in the United States, lung cancer was the most common, followed by breast cancer in women, prostate cancer, and cancers of the colon and rectum. Cancer rates for Hispanics and other ethnic minorities are lower than for the Caucasian and African-American populations. This could be attributed to cultural, socio-economic, and other life expectancy factors.

When we think about the risks for developing cancer, we cannot consider race and genetics in isolation. Behaviors of a culture or ethnic group, diet, and economic and social factors all have to be taken into account. Cancer rates and survival are also very often related to economic factors, like access to health-care services.

It is impossible to separate geographic and racial factors from other factors that define a person or a group of people. People in our modern world are very mobile—moving from one town or from one continent to another. For example, the Chinese population in San Francisco, California, has a high incidence of nasopharyngeal cancer. The incidence drops in later generations of Chinese Americans. It is unclear whether the high rate of this cancer is related to social or environmental factors (the nitrite content of prepared foods is suspect) or to the Epstein-Barr virus, which is also often found in people with nasopharyngeal cancer.

THE CANCER PERSONALITY

Speculation about personality traits, emotional reactions, and development of disease is not new. Some people believe that cancer develops, at least partly, as a result of several serious life changes, continued demands for readjustment, and the potential for wear and tear on the body's protective systems. As early as 1956, Hans Selye showed that body structure and function could change in response to stress. Work by several researchers demonstrated that negative events or negative stressors are related to the onset of some illnesses. Some have even demonstrated a relationship between loss experiences and onset of cancer. Onset of illness in these studies usually follows experiences of greater than normal life change within a year.

In *Heal Your Body,* Louise Hay calls illness "dis-ease," which reflects her belief that illness is caused by an inability to be at ease with one's self. She reveals in the introduction that she had vaginal cancer, and she describes her background of being raped and battered as a five-year-old child. She says, "It was no wonder I had manifested cancer in the vaginal area." Hay

Causes and Prevention

believes that "cancer comes from a pattern of deep resentment that is held for a long time, until it literally eats away at the body." She advocates the power of self-healing. She is a metaphysical counselor, known for her workshops and books using affirmations, visualizations, meditation, and forgiveness.

Dr. Bernie Siegel, author of *Love, Medicine, and Miracles,* has said that the most powerful stimulant for the immune system is love, and that love heals. Many methods of natural healing derive from ideas about self-care, self-love, getting rid of old resentments and hurts, and achieving a state of balance in the body. The question that follows is, what wears the immune system down and makes us sick—ourselves? All of these ideas imply the existence of a cancer personality.

On the other hand, it can be pretty hard for someone to think she is responsible for causing her own cancer. Some interpret Louise Hay's teachings to mean that a person with cancer should forego traditional medicine and instead invest her time in working out deep resentments and go through body detoxification. I am a proponent of maintaining a balance between traditional and complementary medicine. Complementary treatment has a role, but I would hate to see anyone give up her medical options while exploring methods of natural healing and metaphysical renewal.

HEREDITARY FACTORS

Some cancers occur with greater frequency among relatives. Breast cancer occurs at rates higher than expected in daughters and sisters of women who have been diagnosed with breast cancer before menopause. We now know that there are at least three genes that are passed from mothers and fathers to sons and daughters that increase the likelihood of developing some forms of breast and ovarian cancers. Similarly, genes have been found to be a factor in some forms of colon cancer, accounting to some extent for the fact that colon cancer is more likely to be found in relatives of people who have had colon cancer. Some families are known to have higher rates of different types of cancer than would normally be expected. The role of environment, diet, and other factors in the development of cancer in these families is difficult to determine. At this point in time, less than 10 percent of all cancers are thought to be strictly linked to hereditary factors alone.

A few cancers occur because a flawed gene is inherited from one parent. A cancer might develop at a later time, when that gene is exposed to a carcinogen. Such cancers include retinoblastoma, a tumor starting in cells of the retina of the eye, and Wilms' tumor, a tumor in the kidney that affects mostly children.

Other conditions caused by genetic flaws are linked to the development of cancer. For example, children with Down's syndrome have a higher than normal risk of developing leukemia. Nearly all people (95 percent) who develop myelocytic leukemia have an inherited chromosomal change called the Philadelphia chromosome. Other chromosome alterations have been noted in people with other forms of leukemia, lymphoma, and solid tumors. Familial polyposis, an inherited condition in which polyps develop in the colon and rectum, is strongly linked to colon cancer.

There are clues as to whether or not a cancer can actually be considered hereditary. The most important of these clues are as follows:

1. The cancer has occurred in two or more first-degree (mother, daughter, sister) or second-degree (cousin, aunt) relatives.

2. The cancer occurred at an earlier age than would be expected for that kind of cancer.

3. Several cancers (primary cancers) have occurred in the same person.

4. The cancer occurred in a person who is not normally thought to be at risk (for example, a male with breast cancer).

5. The cancer is usually associated with an environmental risk, but the person with the cancer has not been exposed to that factor (for example, lung cancer in a person who has never smoked or been unduly exposed to secondhand smoke).

6. The cancer occurred in a person who also has other unusual traits (for example, a person with birth defects or mental retardation).

These clues are just a few pieces in the cancer risk puzzle.

CANCER RISK ANALYSIS

Cancer risk is an estimate of a person's chances of developing cancer. Access to cancer risk analysis is increasing, but for the most part, sophisticated cancer risk analysis is available only at major cancer centers and teaching hospitals. A cancer risk analysis complete with genetic testing is expensive, costing as much as $6,000. Genetic testing and cancer risk analysis are not covered in most insurance plans, so women at high risk who *don't* get risk analysis and genetic testing are likely to be those who cannot afford it or who don't know about it.

Cancer risk analysis can be performed by medical doctors, medical geneticists, and nurses. Regardless of their background, the people providing the service must have advanced training in molecular genetics, family history taking, risk assessment and analysis, and the ethical, legal, psychological, and social issues related to having access to genetic knowledge. Cancer genetics is rapidly evolving into a subspecialty area that requires special training and education in genetics and counseling. The Oncology Nursing Society recommends that nurses in this field have a master's degree in nursing with a specialty in genetics.

At the present time, there are no federal rules or standards that guide the practice of cancer risk analysis and genetic testing. Some states and a few individual facilities have established clinical practice guidelines for genetic testing for single genes. For example, the Roswell Park Cancer Institute and Kaiser Permanente have developed clinical practice guidelines for testing of specific genes. In these institutions, each time a new gene is identified, new testing guidelines are developed. The American Board of Genetic Counselors is a certification body that identifies "board-certified genetic counselors." A similar entity, the Association of Genetic Nurses and Counselors (AGNC), exists in the United Kingdom. Generally, individuals wishing to obtain certification by either of these two organizations must have a graduate degree in genetic counseling, substantial clinical experience including verification by a supervisor, and must have completed general and specialty certification examinations. Some states (New Jersey was the first) are rushing to enact legislation to regulate the profession of genetic counseling—qualifications, how competence in the field is verified, and who can legally call themselves "genetic counselors." (Similar state regulations govern who can call themselves "registered nurses" or "licensed medical doctors.") Presently, however, certification is something qualified individuals obtain by choice since there is no legal mandate to do so.

Cancer risk analysis is controversial: Many doctors do not believe it is worthwhile, and some think it causes people to worry more. There may well be a burden associated with knowing. One writer calls this sort of information "toxic knowledge." For some people, such knowledge could be depressing and could severely affect the quality of their lives. Others believe that knowledge of cancer risk can relieve unnecessary fear by providing useful information that can serve as a base for a solid wellness program uniquely tailored to an individual's needs and background.

There are questions about who should have genetic testing. At present , the costs and the social and emotional implications of genetic testing preclude its use as a general screening tool. The American Society of Clinical Oncology currently recommends genetic testing for people who have a strong family history of cancer or have had a very early onset of cancer or when the results of such testing might affect cancer treatment decisions.

Other concerns surround the use of the information gathered during cancer risk analysis and genetic testing. While genetic information can help a woman make decisions about prevention and early detection, it might also increase the risk of discrimination against her and her children by insurers. Though genetic testing is becoming widely available, important social protection is not currently in place. Legislation being considered in the U.S. Congress just begins to address the social issues that arise as a result of access to genetic information. If passed, these new laws would restrict employers' ability to obtain or disclose genetic information gathered during the genetic testing of an employee, prohibit health insurers from denying coverage or varying the cost of premiums based on genetic information, and define the situations in which genetic information could be disclosed. Despite the importance of these issues, this legislation is progressing at a snail's pace. As of the fall of 2002, the legislation entitled the "Genetic Nondiscrimination in Health Insurance and Employment Act" has received no attention beyond the preliminary hearings that took place in 2001 and 2002.

Risk involves both the probability of an event happening and the seriousness of the event's effects. There is no such thing as zero risk—we cannot avoid some gambles, and we must sometimes make trade-offs between quality of life and quantity of life. The major risk factors thought to be responsible for nearly 80 percent of all cancers in Western industrial societies can be placed in the following categories:

A. Environmental
  1. Nonoccupational
    a. Habits
      — smoking
      — alcohol consumption
      — sunbathing
      — diet
    b. Customs
    c. Air and water pollution
  2. Occupational
    a. Chemical (for example, asbestos)
    b. Physical (for example, radiation)

B. Sex differences (hormonal, anatomical)

C. Virus

D. Race

E. Habitat: rural versus urban

F. Genetics

G. Marital status

H. Psychological
    1. Personality profile theory
    2. Stressful life events

I. Socioeconomic class

J. Medical therapy–related cancers

(Cohen & Frank-Stromberg, 1990)

Genetic testing is a new piece in the puzzle of risk analysis. The 1994 discovery of the BRCA1 gene that is linked to breast and ovarian cancers is a milestone in the understanding of cancer biology. The identification of BRCA1, BRCA2, p53, hMLH1, and other genes confirms for many scientists what they had assumed: Every cancer is genetic, but *not* every cancer is inherited. Cancer is a disease that arises from a flaw in a gene. Just having a flaw in a gene does not automatically cause cancer, but if the flawed gene is affected by a carcinogen, it can trigger the development of cancer.

It is estimated that 10 to 25 percent of all cancers develop as a result of the combined effects of genes and environment. Only 5 to 10 percent of all cancers are thought to be related to hereditary factors alone (i.e., susceptibility or increased risk by a single inherited flawed gene).

For now, the knowledge of having an inherited flawed gene allows a woman a better chance of finding cancer in early, more curable stages. Using information about inherited risk, some women may be able to take steps to prevent these cancers from developing. Some research suggests that the prognosis, or therapeutic outcome, is better for women with BRCA1-associated ovarian cancer and women with hMLH1-associated colon cancer than for women with other types of ovarian and colon cancers. Eventually, the identification of these and additional genes should lead to new therapies.

A good cancer risk analysis takes time and the full cooperation of a woman and her family. The features of a comprehensive cancer risk analysis are as follows:

1. Detailed personal and family history for cancer risk assessment that includes information about at least three generations of family members, the perception of risk, and other emotional and social factors. From this history, a pedigree is developed that includes

— personal risk factors
— medical risk factors
— environmental risk factors
— family risk factors

2. Physical examination and assessment

3. Multidisciplinary evaluation to develop a plan for risk management and control

4. Assessment of the educational needs of the woman and her family

5. Development of a program of care with respect to the identified risk factors

6. Genetic counseling that gives the woman the support and information she needs to make health-care decisions

7. Access to clinical trials

8. Possible genetic testing, including evaluation of the woman's emotional and physical responses to the testing, diagnosis, and treatment, and ongoing communication and coordination of services relating to the identified risks

A cancer risk analysis might suggest that a woman with a history of infection with the human papillomavirus (HPV) have Pap smears at least yearly, with testing done by a doctor or nurse who is aware of her risk for cervical cancer. Or it might suggest that a woman who is at high risk for breast cancer look for ways to increase her knowledge and practice of breast self-examination skills. She would also likely want more frequent mammograms, or at least clinical breast examinations by a nurse or doctor who specializes in breast care and is familiar with her unique history and risks. Some women at extremely high risk for breast cancer opt for **prophylactic mastectomy**—having the breasts removed even before a cancer appears. A woman at high risk for ovarian cancer might develop a screening program that includes not only a pelvic examination every six months, but also regular use of a special tumor-marker blood test for ovarian cancer, ultrasound (soundwave) studies of the pelvic region, and perhaps experimental tests of blood flow in the area of the ovaries. Similarly, women at high risk for ovarian cancer sometimes consider having their ovaries removed—**prophylactic oophorectomy**—before ovarian cancer occurs. Prophylactic mastectomy and oophorectomy procedures are very controversial; neither guarantees that cancer will not develop in tiny bits of breast or ovarian tissue left behind.

Knowing cancer risk factors can help a woman develop a personal cancer risk profile. She can alter some risk factors to decrease the chance of developing cancer. When risk factors cannot be altered, she can create a plan for actions that will help find cancers early, in the most curable stages. Cancer risk analysis may also identify options to help a woman make realistic decisions about her own health care. A total health plan can be tailored to a woman's risk and ability to live with that risk. It is also important that a woman know that the risk of developing cancer is not the same as the risk of dying from that cancer.

We are exposed to cancer risks all the time—in our food, environment, and lifestyle. The key to cancer prevention and early detection lies in making informed decisions. By balancing acceptable risks in our lifestyle choices, we can have some control over the risk factors around us.

— *Pamela Haylock*

CHAPTER 3

DETECTING A CHANGE

For me, it was finding a tiny lump in my breast. Something was different. What did it mean?

Finding the answer to that question is what the diagnostic process is all about. It has three phases:

1. **Detection,** in which a woman or her health-care professional finds a change from normal. The doctor gathers enough information about it to decide whether it is necessary to proceed further.

2. **Diagnosis,** in which cells or tissues from the "different" area are removed and examined under a microscope to see what the change means.

3. If the diagnosis is cancer, doctors determine as much about it as they can, including how extensive it is (**staging**) and how it looks and behaves (**grading**), so that they can treat it most effectively.

This chapter is about detection. The next chapter is about diagnosis, staging, and grading.

As it grows, cancer eventually becomes large enough to show itself in some way: It can be felt as a lump, causes pain as it presses on nearby tissues, leads to bleeding as it grows into blood vessels, or in some other way changes how the body works. On the other hand, many things that have no connection at all with cancer can cause identical signs or symptoms. (To a health professional, a sign is something that can be detected by someone besides the woman, such as a lump or bleeding, while a symptom is something only the woman can feel, such as pain.)

Regardless of how a change is detected, the physician (or nurse practitioner, osteopath, or other health professional) assesses it by taking a "history"—listening to the woman and asking her questions—and performing a physical examination. Additional information can come from imaging procedures, such as mammograms or other X rays that picture the area, and from laboratory tests such as blood counts.

Since we do not know how to prevent many cancers, we try to detect them as early as possible. If a cancer is discovered during its silent period, we will be dealing with a smaller tumor that has had less time to cause damage.

Does early detection really make a difference? "*Early*" is a relative term since most cancers have been growing in the body for quite some time before we can detect them. Cancer is a whole range of diseases, from those that grow very slowly and spread late to those that grow very aggressively—and early detection probably has little effect on the outcome at these two extremes. There is plenty of time to find a slow-growing cancer that does not metastasize for twenty years while, until our ways to treat it improve, no detection that we have now can be early enough for some rapidly spreading cancers. But many cancers fall between these extremes, and those are the targets for early detection.

How early a cancer is diagnosed and treated is not the only factor in cancer **prognosis** (the statistically likely outcome), but it is an important one. Sometimes "early detection" simply finds a cancer a little earlier, which then progresses the way it would have in any case. That is, if a test detects a cancer two years earlier than it would have been found otherwise but, despite full treatment, the woman dies of cancer the same day she would have died if it had not been found "early," it will make a difference in the *statistics*—because she lives longer after diagnosis—but does it make a genuine difference in the length of her life? In statistics, this "extra time" is called **lead-time bias,** and it is always something to consider when looking at early detection measures. To be truly effective, early detection must make a real difference in how long a woman lives.

Early detection includes screening measures that check for cancer in the woman who is asymptomatic (without signs or symptoms of disease). A sensible screening program balances the woman's risk of developing a particular disease with the ability of current tests to detect the disease at a stage where it makes a consistent difference in survival and ease of treatment—as well as with the safety, cost, convenience, and availability of tests.

Thus, a woman considered at high risk for ovarian cancer because of family history might undergo various sophisticated and expensive screening tests every year. Although these may be appropriate for her, they have not yet met the cost-benefit criteria for mass screening. On the other hand, it makes sense for a woman at average risk for ovarian cancer to be screened with regular pelvic examinations.

Terms that health professionals use when they evaluate a screening test for cancer are how **sensitive** it is (how well it detects everyone who has the cancer, or how many **true positives** it gives) and how **specific** it is (how rarely it looks at someone healthy and incorrectly indicates that the person has cancer, or **false positives**). Thus, a test that is not very sensitive would miss many people who really have cancer, indicating they are healthy when they are not (**false negatives**). A test that is not very specific would force many perfectly healthy people to unnecessarily undergo further testing, with its anxiety, cost, inconvenience, and so on (**false positives**). No screening test we have now is 100 percent sensitive and 100 percent specific, but the goal is to balance sensitivity and specificity so that, as much as possible, those with a real abnormality—and only those—go on for further testing and treatment.

Pap Smears and Similar Tests

The **Pap smear** is an appropriate screening test for large groups of women with no symptoms. This simple test of the cervix (the necklike opening of the uterus or womb) has saved countless lives. It was named after Dr. Papanicolaou, who first came up with the idea that some cancers can slough off cells into surrounding fluid. For the Pap smear, a few cells from the cervix are examined under the microscope for any sign of abnormal cells. This is one of several uses of **cytology,** the study of cells under the microscope for signs of disease. The Pap smear does not diagnose a specific cancer; it simply shows when something is abnormal somewhere on or near the cervix. This alerts the health professional to the need to look further.

The best time for a Pap smear is at the midpoint of a woman's menstrual cycle, when the cervical canal is most open, so that better samples can be taken. For example, if a woman menstruates every twenty-eight days, the best time for a Pap smear is at or around fourteen days after the first day of her last period. Women are instructed not to douche or use a contraceptive jelly before having a Pap smear because these could make it harder to collect a good specimen.

To do a Pap smear, a health professional often uses a small, plastic brush (cytobrush) and a flat, wooden spatula to obtain a sample of the fluid from the cervical canal and to gently scrape the surface of the cervix. The cells are then "fixed" with a chemical on a microscope slide or added to a vial containing a chemical solution that preserves them until they can be examined under a microscope. Pap tests should not cause pain, but women often feel some pressure during the procedure, which is usually done during a full pelvic examination.

The **cytotechnologist** (a person with special training in examining cells under the microscope) looks at the Pap smear first and reports whether it is obviously normal. If there is *any* question about its normality, a

pathologist, a medical doctor who is an expert on cells and tissues in disease, examines the slide next.

Results of a Pap smear classify cells within several categories ranging from clearly normal to, at the other extreme, two categories for carcinoma in situ and invasive cancer. The problem is how to classify the cells that fall in the middle ranges—abnormal, but not that abnormal. One very common naming system subdivides these "somewhat abnormal" cells into three grades of cervical intraepithelial neoplasia (CIN): I, II, and III, for mild, moderate, and severe dysplasia. "*Intraepithelial*" means that the abnormality affects only cells within the surface layers of the cervix. The initials and numbers depend on the classification system that the laboratory uses, with some differences in how the systems categorize cells that appear somewhat abnormal.

Many women develop these CIN cervical changes that may progress to cancer if they are not treated. Finding and treating these changes early makes a major difference in the survival rate as well as the ease of treatment. The vast majority of women with dysplasia, carcinoma in situ, or cancer that has not spread beyond the cervix survive, often with minimal therapy. But only a very small percentage of those diagnosed with advanced cervical cancer survive for five years or more. The Pap smear finds these changes reliably and conveniently, with minimal cost and risk.

The Pap smear is very specific; if a smear shows invasive cancer, that information is almost always correct. But its sensitivity is not as good, with many false negatives. These usually occur because either the smear is obtained incorrectly or the technologist reading the slide lacks training or adequate time to examine the smear carefully. A woman can help ensure the most accurate Pap smear by using a provider who performs the test often (such as a gynecologist, family doctor, or women's health nurse practitioner) and by asking how satisfied her provider is with the lab processing the smears. A woman also protects herself by making sure that she is notified about the results of any Pap smear—"We'll call you if there is a problem" is not enough. She receives the test at recommended intervals so that even if suspicious changes are missed once, they will be found on the next Pap before they have progressed to invasive cancer.

Researchers are exploring new ways to improve both the collection and the interpretation of Pap smears. A special light bar, inserted into the vagina to visualize the cervix at the time of the Pap test, may increase the detection of precancerous changes. The laboratory may use a computer program to evaluate the cells, or may compare the DNA content or the spectrum of light rays of the specimen with that of normal cells.

For many years, scientists have been studying ways to examine cells from a drop of breast fluid suctioned from the nipple to screen large groups of women for breast cancer. **Nipple discharge cytology** is essential for women with a spontaneous nipple discharge on bra or night clothes, but does not work yet as a screening test for actual disease. (On the hopeful side, at least one large recent study suggests that testing suctioned nipple fluid for the presence of certain kinds of cells might show whether women are at average or greater risk for developing breast cancer later. If more studies show the same findings, this could become a screening test for increased risk.)

Researchers would also love to find a cytology screening test for people at high risk for lung cancer that would make a real difference in survival. So far, however, although pathologists examine cells from sputum (coughed-up mucus from the lungs) to diagnose lung cancer in some patients with symptoms, this procedure has not met the criteria for a good screening test.

LABORATORY TESTS

Standard blood tests can show nonspecific suspicious changes. Along with a regular physical examination, health professionals sometimes routinely order a complete blood count to show the numbers of red cells, white cells, and platelets in the blood, and perhaps a blood chemistry panel, which measures several components of blood against a normal range of values. With changes in the health-care system, however, ordering routine laboratory tests is becoming less common, partly because they have not proven to be of much benefit for most people.

If test results are too high or low, the doctor focuses on certain body systems to see what is wrong. A high "alkaline phosphatase" value on a standard blood chemistry panel, for instance, is a clue to possible bone or liver disease. Bone or liver metastasis from a cancer could cause this change —as could many other conditions that have nothing to do with cancer.

Other blood tests are more cancer-specific because they measure levels of certain chemicals called **serum (blood) tumor markers**. These are proteins found in the blood after they are produced (or produced in greater than normal amounts) by particular cancers. Ovarian cancer may give off a protein called CA 125, for instance; the blood of the woman with breast cancer may show higher than normal amounts of CA 27-29, CA 15-3, and/or one of the more recently discovered serum tumor markers. Colon or rectal cancer may cause a rise in carcinoembryonic antigen (CEA) in the blood.

Unfortunately, the blood tests we have now cannot trace these proteins early enough and reliably enough for them to be appropriate screening techniques for large groups of women. If the blood level becomes elevated at all, it may not do so until the cancer is beyond the early detection stage.

However, the serum tumor marker counts still have very important uses. They can provide additional information when a doctor suspects cancer. Often, repeated tumor marker assays can "follow" a cancer during treatment to evaluate how effective the therapy is. For example, a CA 27-29 that is high when a breast cancer is diagnosed and then drops to normal after chemotherapy indicates that the treatment is working. In addition, some doctors use tumor marker assays every few months or every year after the end of therapy in the hope of getting an early warning if cancer recurs so that it can be treated as soon as possible.

IMAGING TECHNIQUES

Imaging studies provide a picture of the inside of the body. The doctor can visualize body organs without having to cut through the skin. Imaging studies, however, detect changes rather than diagnosing cancers. No matter how abnormal an imaging study may look, cells or tissues from the suspect area are still necessary for firm diagnosis.

Imaging studies can be used to screen asymptomatic women, to give more information when cancer is suspected or has been diagnosed, to help check the effectiveness of treatment (is a tumor gone, or is it smaller?), and to follow up over the years after a cancer diagnosis to check for any changes.

Used wisely, imaging studies can save a woman's life, protect her from unnecessary surgery, or define the scope of her treatment. They can also be overused. Before any imaging study, a woman can ask, "Will the results of this examination influence what treatment I receive?" and "If I do need an imaging study, is this the most appropriate one for my situation?"

Standard X Rays

The most common imaging studies are **X rays,** which show bones and certain tissues well. Chest X rays, for instance, can show changes that might be lung cancer; unfortunately, they do not show these changes early enough or reliably enough to be a good screening test for people without symptoms. With the addition of a **contrast medium** (which is injected into a vein, swallowed, or given as an enema), X rays can outline some additional organs. A barium enema, in which a white liquid is given as an enema to outline the lower digestive tract in X rays, might detect a cancer in the colon or rectum of a woman complaining of digestive problems. While they do not image the organs in the pelvis well, X rays can indicate whether a cancer has spread to other organs that do show up well on film, such as the lungs.

Before major abdominal/pelvic cancer surgery, X rays using a contrast medium can provide the surgeon with a road map of where organs in the abdomen and pelvis are located. Thus, a woman might have an intravenous pyelogram (IVP), which uses dye injected through an arm vein to outline the urinary tract. Or she might be asked to swallow barium before upper gastrointestinal X rays (UGI series).

Mammograms

Mammograms are special X rays of the breasts. They can image lumps or thickened areas in the breast tissue as well as places where the normal "architecture" of lacy fibers in the breast may be distorted by a tumor. The particular magic of mammograms, however, is their ability to show the tiny white specks of calcified tissue called **calcifications** or **microcalcifications**. These accompany many completely innocent breast changes, but clusters of microcalcifications with certain shapes may be the only sign of carcinoma in situ or may signal the presence of an early invasive cancer before there is a lump to feel.

The mammograms done today usually look like large black-and-white film negatives. To obtain mammograms, the technologist uses a plastic "paddle" to compress each breast in turn against the platform of the machine. Breast and machine are repositioned to provide pictures of each breast from the side and from top to bottom. A **radiologist,** a doctor who specializes in "reading" imaging, views the mammograms after they are taken, compares them to any earlier ones, and checks for abnormalities.

The radiologist who needs more information about a specific area asks for **cone views**, which use a cone-shaped compressor to focus on the suspicious area and show it in more detail, or for **magnification views**, additional mammograms that show the suspicious area enlarged. These views often let the radiologist see whether the edges of a suspicious area are smooth (much more likely with a benign change, which tends to evenly and gently push away surrounding tissue) or ragged (more likely when cancer cells at the borders invade surrounding tissues).

Mammography can be briefly uncomfortable because the breast must be firmly compressed. This compression thins and spreads the breast tissue, making it easier to see the structures inside. Compression also decreases the scatter of radiation so that the dose can be smaller and safer, one reason that mammography can use minimal amounts of X-ray energy and be considered quite safe. Finally, compression keeps the breast from moving so that the pictures are not blurred.

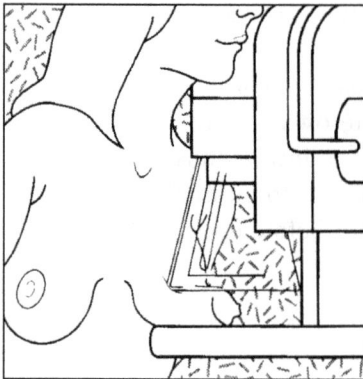

Mammography
(courtesy of The Informed Woman's
Guide to Breast Health)

Women who are still menstruating can make mammography more comfortable by scheduling the X rays during the first half of their menstrual cycle, when their breasts are softer and less hormonally active. Some women say cutting out coffee, tea, and other caffeine for a week or two before their mammograms makes the procedure more comfortable.

It makes sense for a woman to tell the technologist before the test if she is worried about pain, which is often the result of a previous bad experience, so that they can work out a plan together. The technologist may be able to compress the breast just until the woman signals that it is uncomfortable, and then immediately release the compression slightly. Some places are even experimenting with teaching the woman to control the compression herself.

Technically, mammograms do not diagnose cancer because they do not obtain actual cells to examine under the microscope. Still, radiologists often call mammograms performed to obtain more information about a specific breast change **diagnostic mammography**. This is different from **screening mammography**, routine mammograms of women without symptoms. Diagnostic mammograms take more technologist and radiologist time and usually cost more; they are also the right mammograms for women with breast implants or those who have had previous breast cancer surgery.

How useful is mammography as a screening test? The jury remains out. If a woman finds herself bewildered by conflicting reports, she has plenty of company.

The controversy heated up in October 2001 with an article by Danish researchers Ole Olsen and Peter Gotzsche in the *Lancet*, a British medical journal. They were puzzled by a 1999 Swedish study that seemed to show no decrease in breast cancer deaths over many years as mammography use increased. This conclusion contradicted not only the published results of earlier studies but also the general expectation that finding cancer early with mammograms would save lives. Was the Swedish study flawed—or was the problem with the earlier studies?

Curious, Olsen and Gotzsche went back to take a second look at eight large earlier studies from different countries. In most of the studies, they found flaws in *randomization*: The women who had mammograms differed in other ways (such as age and other breast cancer risk factors) from the women who did not have mammograms, which made the two groups hard to compare. Combining the studies they considered well randomized, the researchers failed to find believable evidence that mammograms reduced breast cancer deaths. Too, they voiced concern about possible disadvantages of mammography, such as false positives and cost.

Just about everyone leaped into the fray, with thousands of impassioned articles and editorials and television mentions. A 3 February 2002 letter to the editor in *The New York Times* was signed by nineteen large U.S. cancer organizations who urged a careful consideration of all the evidence before changing current mammography guidelines. Within the same month, the Physician Data Query (PDQ) screening and prevention editorial board, which writes information for the National Cancer Institute's website, admitted it did not know whether the benefits of screening mammography outweighed the disadvantages for groups of women without symptoms. Meanwhile, the U.S. Preventive Services Task Force not only affirmed its confidence in mammography, but also recommended increased mammography screening in women between forty and fifty. Both the U.S. Congress and the major players in the breast cancer community scheduled huge hearings.

The blunt facts: The studies we have now are open to different interpretations, depending on who is interpreting them. For several reasons, it is unlikely that we will *ever* have a perfect study to prove that mammography does or does not save lives of groups of women. (In fact, the big issue in this controversy is that the studies did not provide sufficient evidence, one way or the other.)

We do know that mammography can save many individual lives by finding suspicious changes well before there is anything to see or to feel with the fingers. Mammography remains the best way we have now to detect breast carcinoma in situ, a condition that is almost 100 percent curable but which can progress to invasive breast cancer. With a carcinoma in situ that is destined to become invasive breast cancer eventually (not all of them are), finding and treating it early might well save the woman's life.

Detecting invasive breast cancer earlier with mammography than it would be discovered otherwise may make no difference, some difference, or a decisive difference in a woman's longtime survival. How much of a difference mammography makes depends on the individual cancer and the individual woman. For the very slow-growing cancer or the very agressive cancer, the benefit may be minimal. For the in-between cancer, finding it relatively early can spell long-term survival. In some cases, earlier detection can decrease the amount of treatment needed.

Those are the pluses of mammography, important ones indeed.

But even in the best of hands, mammography still misses about 10 percent of breast cancers. These false negatives are probably lower than 10 percent in older women—and considerably higher than that in younger, premenopausal women. Mammograms "see" best through fatty breast tissue, which makes them ideal for viewing the breasts of older women. Younger women, on the other hand, normally have large amounts of glandular tissue in their breasts. In some women this may image clearly, but in others this normal breast tissue is so dense that the mammograms look as if they were filmed through a heavy cloud cover. A cancer or a cluster of calcifications might show up, or it might not.

Plainly, relying too much on an imperfect technique can be disastrous—and might even cost lives. The doctor or woman who ignores a suspicious breast lump, skin change, or spontaneous nipple discharge because "the mammogram didn't show it so it must be okay" is asking for trouble. Any suspicious and persistent breast change needs thorough evaluation, whether or not mammography shows it.

Almost as troubling for the mammography researchers are the large numbers of false positives, the changes detected by mammography that prove to be completely benign, but only after the anxiety, hassle, expense, and discomfort of a diagnostic procedure. Some experts worry too about possible overtreatment of breast changes that might never become cancer, such as some carcinomas in situ. Others point to the price tag for mammograms, associated diagnostic tests, and treatment and ask whether the money and time might be spent better elsewhere.

The positive side of the controversy is that good questions are being asked. As uncomfortable as it is to tolerate uncertainty, it helps to remind everyone that mammography is a very useful tool (currently the "gold standard" of breast imaging techniques), but not a perfect one; that screening techniques carry a hefty price tag; and that "early" detection may help, but is no substitute for research into prevention.

Meanwhile, what is a sensible course of action for a woman and her health-care providers? As of early 2002, the National Cancer Institute, the American Cancer Society, and the U.S. Preventive Services agree on the prudence of a screening mammography every one to two years for women from forty to seventy, but these organizations have slightly different schools of thought about the ages at which annual mammograms are recommended. After seventy, there is no standard recommendation.

These guidelines could stay the same—or change at any time as new evidence accumulates. It makes sense for a woman to discuss her personal situation and feelings with her health-care provider so that they can decide together what is best for her. The website www.breastcancer.org presents clear, helpful, and very up-to-date information on the whole mammography question.

Just about everyone agrees that most women over thirty-five with a breast symptom or a strong family history of breast cancer should undergo mammograms, and some doctors recommend them for even younger women in these situations.

Women who are pregnant or breastfeeding should not have screening mammograms, and it is wise to wait three months or more afterward for the breasts to return to their prepregnancy state. However, if there is a lump to evaluate, mammography can be used safely as long as the uterus is well shielded. Women whose breasts have been augmented with implants can get clear mammograms from a technologist who takes extra views and uses a special technique to bring the breast tissue forward, in front of the implant.

As a rule, the greater the number of mammograms done at an institution, the better: Getting the best films and reading them correctly takes constant experience as well as state-of-the-art equipment. Because quality varied so much among mammography facilities, in 1994 the Food and Drug Administration (FDA) began certification and annual inspection for all mammography facilities in the United States (except those in veterans' health facilities, which must follow their own similar set of standards). In 1999, the final comprehensive regulations of this **Mammography Quality Standards Act** (MQSA) went into effect, calling for facilities to meet specific standards for training personnel, equipment, quality control, records, notification of patients, and follow-up of abnormal mammograms in order to continue being accredited. Accreditation must be renewed every three years.

Mammograms can detect some breast cancers long before they can be felt. But, because the technique is not fail-proof, the wise woman combines mammography with monthly breast self-examination (see Chapter 12) and regular, thorough breast examinations by a health professional.

Other Imaging Techniques

Normal tissue differs from cancerous tissue. All imaging techniques work by capitalizing on one or more of these differences. Mammograms work because X rays move differently through normal tissue than through cancer. Other techniques explore how sound, electricity, and other forms of energy move through tissue. The 1990s and early 2000s brought a new surge in imaging techniques, largely because of the growing technological ability to translate body information into digital images on monitors.

A relative newcomer in breast imaging is **digital mammography,** which captures its images with an electronic X-ray detector that converts the image into a digital picture that can be read by a computer. Like other digital technology, digital mammography distinguishes only two values, such as off and on, or 0 and 1, or no dot and dot. Long strings of these digits are "read" as a picture.

The pluses of digital mammography: The radiologist can increase the contrast in the picture with a simple computer manipulation; computers can be programmed to spot abnormal areas as a backup for the radiologist; digital images can be transmitted easily to radiologists at a different location for second opinions; and computer images take much less storage space than film X rays do. But there are minuses as well, including expensive equipment and training. It also appears that digital mammography doesn't image microcalcifications quite as well as standard mammograms do, although the increased contrast helps make up for this. This technology is slowly spreading from clinical trials into communities.

Ultrasound, or **sonography,** projects high-frequency sound waves into the body. These sound waves bounce off different kinds of tissue in characteristic ways. A computer reads the pattern of echoes and generates a picture from them. Ultrasound images the ovaries and uterus well, is useful for telling whether a breast lump is solid or fluid-filled and for revealing the area close to the chest wall, and can often show whether a breast implant has ruptured. It is considered safe to use during pregnancy and for women under thirty if a suspicious lump is found on breast exam. However, sonography does not show microcalcifications or changes in breast architecture and it requires a suspicious area as a clear destination, so it is not useful for most screening.

For conventional ultrasound tests, a technologist or radiologist applies a slippery gel or cream to the skin over the organ to be imaged and then glides a handheld instrument over the skin to produce the sound waves and pick up the echoes. The process takes about fifteen minutes. Transvaginal sonography involves inserting an ultrasound probe into the vagina. This can give a more precise image of the ovaries than conventional ultrasound. As with mammography, researchers are experimenting with ways to digitize ultrasound, producing images in computer "numbers."

Doppler studies use sound waves to image blood flow to an area. These may be able to detect increases in blood vessels around a "hungry" cancer, and researchers are trying this special ultrasound technique to detect ovarian cancer.

Computerized tomography (CT, CAT, computed tomography) and **magnetic resonance imaging** (MRI) have revolutionized cancer detection and treatment because they show clear cross-sectional images of body parts that do not show up sharply in standard X rays and that could not be seen well before without surgery. Neither test shows moving parts of the body well (such as the intestine), but they can provide distinct pictures of "quieter" organs.

The woman undergoing CT lies still on a narrow table while a CT scanner (inside what looks rather like a giant, flat doughnut) rotates rapidly around the table and takes X-ray images of narrow "slices" of the body (**tomograms**) from different angles. A computer then assembles these images into pictures. Sometimes a contrast material is swallowed or injected into an arm vein before the test. CT is relatively expensive and uses higher doses of radiation than do regular X rays, which makes it a poor screening tool.

Instead of X rays, magnetic resonance imaging uses a magnetic field to align radio waves and provide its pictures. For a standard MRI, the woman, lying on a stretcher, is wheeled head first into a narrow tube. She lies without moving for periods of several minutes and hears loud clicking noises while the computer collects its data. Again, she may receive a contrast material, either swallowed or injected into a vein, to increase the contrast between normal and abnormal tissues. Anyone who is somewhat claustrophobic can ask for a sedative before the test or can ask about the availability of "open" MRI equipment, built so the person can see out and feels less enclosed. Do take into consideration, though, that this method may be less effective for some tests.

For breast MRI examinations, the woman usually lies on her stomach with her breast hanging freely into a cushioned pocket with a signal receiver (breast coil), and she receives an injection of gadolinium through the vein. There is no long, narrow tube. Expensive as breast MRI is, it can be especially useful for examining the dense breasts of younger women after a cancer diagnosis or when cancer is strongly suspected or to see the extent of disease in older women in certain situations or sometimes to measure the response to treatment. It can also help evaluate the breast when an implant rupture is suspected, although mammography or ultrasound may be all that is needed. One problem with breast MRI is that it shows contrasts so well that healthy tissue might look cancerous, which can lead to biopsies of normal tissue. Doctors may order **nuclear scans** after diagnosis of a woman's cancer to see whether the disease has spread to a particular organ. They are sometimes used for routine follow-up (occasional bone scans after breast-cancer treatment, perhaps), although this is becoming less common. For a bone, liver, or brain scan, a tiny amount of radioactive substance is injected into a vein, travels through the body, and is absorbed by the target organ. A scanner then moves back and forth, looking for "hot spots" in the target organ, where cancerous areas have absorbed more radioactivity. A computer assembles the information into a black-and-white film negative.

The injection is given well before the scan. Depending on the organ being scanned and how long it takes the radioactive substance to reach it, the woman may leave the nuclear medicine department for a time. She

Detecting
a Change

49

needs to drink lots of water or other fluids and urinate frequently during this period (about three hours for a bone scan) to dilute the radioactive substance and move it safely through the body and out through the urinary tract. The dose of radioactivity is minuscule, and it is safe to be near other people during this time. The woman then returns to the nuclear medicine department and lies as directed on a table while the scanner moves back and forth over her (or under the table) for about an hour.

Although researchers continue to search for the perfect imaging technique, none of the other imaging techniques developed so far fits the bill as a good screening test for women without breast symptoms, since the tests tend to be relatively expensive and do not show microcalcifications. However, they may prove quite useful when mammography cannot be used or does not give enough information. For instance, **T-scan imaging** (electrical impedance imaging or EIS/T-scan) measures the passage of tiny amounts of low-level electrical current—about the amount in a penlight battery—through the breasts while a computer reconstructs the information and displays it on a monitor. For **scintimammography** (sestamibi nuclear medicine breast imaging), the nuclear medicine doctor or technician injects into the woman's vein a tiny amount of a radioactive substance called technetium sestamibi along with another agent that makes the sestamibi collect in the breasts. A scanner then passes over the breasts and "reads" the information, displaying an image of the breast on a computer.

Thermography and other heat-sensing techniques try to identify "hot spots" in the breast where a "hungry" cancer has developed an increased blood supply to nourish itself. Early efforts that used some kind of heat-sensitive material placed against the breast were never considered very accurate. **Computerized thermal imaging** (CTI), a newer technology being tested in clinical trials, uses a highly sensitive, high-speed infrared camera, with the findings analyzed by computer and a colorful digital image produced on a monitor. A useful website for all these imaging techniques is www.pinnacleimaging.com/procedures.

Breasts are not the only body organs for which imaging technologies continue to emerge. There are lung spiral CT scans for smokers and other people at risk for lung cancer. Virtual colonoscopy and even a swallowable pill-size camera to image the digestive tract are being tested for possible value against colon cancer. (More about these in Chapters 21 and 22 on lung and colon cancers.)

The goals, as always: Find a real problem when it exists, do not find a problem when none exists—and do it all inexpensively, simply, and safely. Not an easy task, and the work is ongoing.

— Kerry McGinn

DIAGNOSIS AND BEYOND

After a change has been detected, diagnosis requires obtaining a specimen of cells or tissue from the suspect area and examining it under a microscope to see if cancer is present. The surgeon, gynecologist, or other doctor collects the cells or tissues, but it is the pathologist, the physician who specializes in examining cells and tissues under the microscope, who looks at the specimen and makes the diagnosis. Even if a doctor is 99.99 percent sure that a cancer exists because of the history, physical examination, imaging, and laboratory studies, there can be no firm diagnosis without a pathologist's analysis of a specimen of cells or tissue.

The challenge with any diagnostic procedure is to obtain the right tissue or cells. If cancer cells in a suspicious area are clustered in one small spot, a diagnostic procedure that samples the wrong spot will miss the cancer entirely. Plainly, any diagnostic procedure must be performed as carefully and completely as possible.

How is the specimen obtained? Sometimes the doctor can see an obviously suspicious area and reach it easily to get a specimen. During a routine pelvic examination, for example, the gynecologist may notice an abnormal-appearing spot outside the vagina or, after spreading the vaginal walls with a speculum, may see something worrisome inside. The doctor then takes a biopsy, snipping or scraping out a small piece of tissue for the pathologist to look at under the microscope.

Depending on the organ and the situation, if the area is not obvious and accessible, the doctor may

- ✦ use a needle through the skin to withdraw cells or tissue (the needle size determines whether this is a fine needle aspiration or a core biopsy)

- ✦ take a biopsy with the aid of some kind of scope (**colposcope, sigmoidoscope,** or **laparoscope,** for instance) to see better than or beyond what could ordinarily be seen

- scrape out the surface layer lining the uterus and remove it through the cervix (dilatation and curettage) so that the pathologist can examine it

- cut out a cone-shaped piece of the cervix through the vagina (conization, also called cone biopsy)

- perform an "open" biopsy of some kind, surgically cutting through skin to reach and remove the suspicious area

Sometimes there is no separate biopsy at all. For instance, the surgeon may perform a hysterectomy when a large tumor in the uterus must be removed in any case because it is causing symptoms. Afterward, the pathologist examines the removed uterus to see whether the tumor is benign or cancerous.

INFORMED CONSENT

Before surgery or any other "invasive" procedure and before a patient participates in any experimental study, doctors must explain what they are doing, what they expect to achieve, and what the risks and options are. Thus informed, the patient agrees in writing to the procedure; this is called **informed consent**. Some states have other requirements, such as California's law that all women diagnosed with breast cancer must receive certain information about treatment options.

No doctor can predict how a particular procedure or therapy will affect an individual woman. There are no guarantees. What the doctor is responsible for is telling her the statistically common outcomes and risks.

FINE NEEDLE ASPIRATIONS, CORE BIOPSIES, AND GUIDED NEEDLE BIOPSIES

With some breast lumps, the doctor or other specially trained health professional can simply **aspirate** (withdraw) some cells through a thin needle to obtain a specimen. This **fine needle aspiration** (FNA) is especially appropriate for on-the-spot diagnosis of a lump that feels as if it might be a cyst, a benign fluid-filled lump that is common in the breast. The doctor scrubs the skin with an antiseptic, stabilizes the lump with the fingers of one hand, inserts the needle of a regular hypodermic syringe through the skin into the lump, and then tries to withdraw whatever is inside. The syringe may have a special holder that makes it easier for the doctor to perform the procedure. The aspiration may smart a bit and may leave a temporary bruise; sometimes a little local anesthetic is injected under the skin before the doctor begins the procedure.

If the lump is a cyst, it will collapse as the fluid is sucked out, giving both instant diagnosis and treatment. As long as this fluid clearly looks like cyst fluid, it does not need to be examined under the microscope. If the lump is solid, the doctor inserts the needle through the skin and then moves the needle up and down in various locations within the area to sample cells or bits of tissue from several places for the pathologist.

Quite often today, with a lump that feels solid, the doctor will perform a **core biopsy,** an in-between procedure that does not require a skin incision but uses a wider-bore "cutting" needle. This needle allows the doctor to obtain one or more small cylinders (cores) of tissue so that the pathologist can see not only individual cells but also how they fit together. This core needle may be attached to a special "biopsy gun" that "fires," instantly inserting and then withdrawing the needle, now filled with its core sample, through the skin. Another system, Mammotome, uses ultrasound to locate the suspicious area before the doctor makes a tiny (quarter-inch) cut in the skin and inserts a probe with a high-speed rotating cutter attached to a small vacuum pump. This system allows the doctor to withdraw a substantial specimen without leaving a big scar.

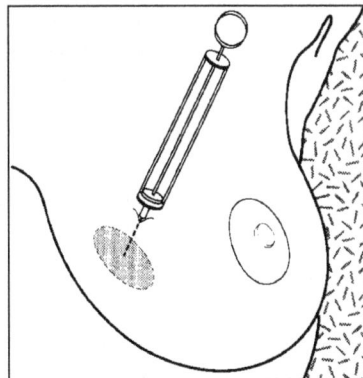
Needle aspiration into cyst

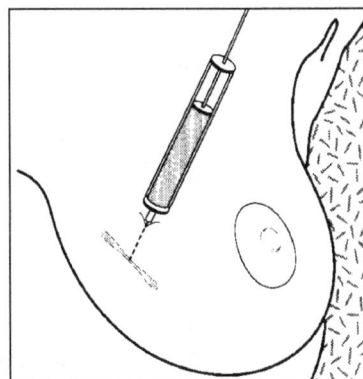
Needle aspiration with fluid
(*courtesy of* The Informed Woman's Guide to Breast Health)

Most women prefer a local anesthetic for a core or a Mammotome biopsy, and often a surgeon or pathologist performs it in the doctor's office. The final report from the pathologist may take twenty-four hours or longer.

Newer technology often makes it possible to perform a fine needle aspiration (or a core biopsy with a larger needle) for breast abnormalities, such as clusters of microcalcifications that can only be seen on a mammogram, so there is nothing that the surgeon can feel.

With a **stereotactic guided needle biopsy,** a computer system uses mammogram views to aim the biopsy gun needle toward the suspicious area. The radiologist, who commonly performs the procedure, views this area like an imaginary clock face and withdraws samples from the center and from other areas evenly spaced around it (such as at three, six, nine,

Diagnosis and Beyond

53

and twelve o'clock). With one kind of equipment, the woman lies face down on a special table with her breast(s) hanging through an opening on the table. A variation on the stereotactic biopsy uses breast MRI rather than mammography to localize the suspicious area; for the woman, the procedure feels about the same. A local anesthetic is often injected, but some women notice discomfort and bruising afterward.

Other procedures combine another imaging technique with an FNA or core biopsy. For instance, a doctor might locate a cyst deep in the breast with a portable ultrasound and then watch the screen while inserting the needle to be sure it reaches the right place and causes the cyst to collapse. Often a radiologist uses a CT scan to guide a core biopsy of a suspicious area in the lung.

Women tend to prefer FNAs and core biopsies to open biopsies for several reasons. Standard FNAs and core biopsies can often be performed on the spur of the moment, although the more complex procedures like stereotactic guided needle biopsies usually take time to schedule. Also, FNAs are much cheaper, and stereotactic biopsies are considerably cheaper than surgical biopsies and leave little or no scarring. The big questions for the doctor and the woman to ask are whether they will believe a benign report—or will still want a surgical "open" biopsy to remove all the suspicious tissue. The woman needs to ask how often the doctor performs the specific procedure. In most cases, with a doctor experienced in the technique, the woman can trust the results. If any question remains, or if atypical or cancerous cells are found, she will probably need either an open biopsy or other surgery.

BIOPSIES WITH A SCOPE

Abnormal Pap smears of the cervix are graded by how abnormal the cells look. If they appear quite abnormal, the gynecologist knows that a source somewhere in the cervix, vagina, or uterus is sloughing off "different" cells, and this area needs to be located and perhaps treated. But if, even after washing the vaginal canal with a stain to show abnormalities better, the gynecologist still cannot find anything obviously strange, what then?

To see the area better, the gynecologist may spread the vaginal wall with a speculum and use a **colposcope,** an instrument that looks like a glorified pair of binoculars mounted on a stand with wheels. The colposcope provides a powerful light and a set of magnifying lenses that can enlarge the area up to twenty times. It can be wheeled into place and raised and lowered to give the best view.

Looking through the colposcope, the gynecologist can perform a **punch biopsy,** taking pinhead-size specimens of tissue for biopsy using an instrument somewhat like a paper punch. This can be done without anesthesia in the doctor's procedure room. If the woman is prompted to cough at the moment of the biopsy, she often avoids the brief, sharp pain of the procedure. The whole process takes only a few minutes. The woman may have slight bleeding afterward or some cramping "periodlike" pain.

Another kind of scope is the **endoscope,** an instrument inserted through a body opening to see an internal area. Different types of endoscopes, each named after the Greek word for the part of the body viewed, allow a doctor to see and reach into the body without having to cut through the skin.

To look into the uterus, for example, the gynecologist may be able to insert a **hysteroscope,** a narrow, lighted magnifying probe, through the cervix to see into the uterus. This can be done in the doctor's office, and a specimen of abnormal-appearing endometrium, the tissue lining the uterus, can be scraped out in an endometrial biopsy.

A doctor who wants to check the bowel wall for signs of cancer can look at it directly through a **sigmoidoscope** (or **proctosigmoidoscope**), a long, flexible, lighted tube that is threaded up through the anus into the sigmoid colon. A **colonoscope** is a longer tube through which the doctor can see the whole large intestine. Both sigmoidoscopy and colonoscopy usually require laxatives and/or enemas beforehand to clean out the lower intestines so that the walls can be seen clearly.

To see into the bladder, the doctor can insert a **cystoscope** through the urethra, the opening of the bladder. A **bronchoscope** threaded through the mouth and throat into the broad tubes, or bronchi, of the lung lets the doctor see the lungs. Through these and other scopes, the doctor can snip out a piece of tissue for biopsy.

Still another kind of scope, the **laparoscope,** requires a tiny slit in the skin around the navel (this is sometimes called "Band-Aid" surgery). Through this slit the doctor can examine and remove tiny specimens from the pelvis or abdomen. A **culdoscope** is similar to a laparoscope except that it is inserted through a small slit in the vagina rather than through the skin so that the doctor can see the area in the cul-de-sac between the uterus and the rectum.

Many scopic exams can be performed in the doctor's office or a special procedures room. Depending on the exam, the woman might not need medication or might receive a sedative or anesthetic. For a laparoscopy, she might be hospitalized briefly and given a general anesthetic.

DILATATION AND CURETTAGE (D&C)

When the doctor needs a pathology specimen from the uterus or inside the cervix, a dilatation and curettage (D&C) can provide it without any incision into the skin. In this procedure, the gynecologist dilates (widens) the cervical canal and then inserts a **curette,** an instrument with a sharp, spoon-shaped tip, to scrape off the surface layer of the uterus. This whole layer is then sent to the pathologist to be checked for cancer cells (or other changes, since D&Cs are used to diagnose and sometimes treat a wide array of non-cancer-related gynecologic problems).

A D&C is often performed in a special procedures room in the gynecologist's office. The woman has the D&C and can return home in a few hours. She lies on an operating table with her feet in stirrups in the standard pelvic exam position while the vaginal area is thoroughly cleansed with a solution to kill any germs. She is usually put to sleep with a short-acting general anesthetic injected through an arm vein for the fifteen minutes or so that the procedure takes; sometimes, a local anesthetic is used instead to numb the cervical area, perhaps along with a sedative.

When the woman is asleep and her muscles are completely relaxed, the doctor performs a careful bimanual (two-handed) examination of the pelvic organs, using the fingers of one hand in the vagina and the other hand on the outside of the pelvis. Then the doctor inserts a speculum, grasps the cervix with a special clamp to hold it steady and, if using a local anesthetic, injects this into the cervix and the area around it.

A "dipstick" rod is threaded through the cervix to measure the depth and position of the uterus. The doctor then inserts a tapered rod into the cervix and begins to stretch the opening, using progressively larger rods until the opening is dilated to about half an inch. Finally, the curette is inserted and the endometrium and possibly part of the lining of the cervical canal is gently scraped out. After the curette and other instruments are removed, the woman rests in a recovery room until she is fully awake. The final pathology report is usually available within a week.

The cervix may take a week or two to close to normal. In the meantime, many women experience some bleeding and cramping. Most doctors recommend that a woman not use tampons or douches during the period the cervix is still open. While some doctors allow sexual intercourse with a condom if the woman is not actively bleeding, many others ask their patients to abstain for ten days or so to prevent infection. The woman who still menstruates may have heavy or irregular periods for a few months after a D&C.

CONIZATION (CONE BIOPSY)

In a cone biopsy, the gynecologist surgically removes a cone of tissue from the center of the cervix—rather like one would core an apple. This used to be standard procedure after an abnormal Pap smear. With the advent of colposcopes that can pinpoint small abnormal areas for punch biopsies, it has become much less common. It still has value, however, especially when the doctors cannot tell whether an area is carcinoma in situ or an early invasive cancer, conditions that require different types of treatment.

Conization is done in an operating room at the hospital under local, spinal, or general anesthesia. The woman lies in the pelvic exam position, a speculum is placed in the vagina, the cervical area is washed thoroughly, and anesthesia is given.

The gynecologist steadies the cervix by putting stitches on each side, cuts a shallow circle around the opening that includes all the affected area, and then continues to cut deeper and toward the center of the cervix until a cone of tissue has been loosened. The doctor removes the cone and sends it to the pathologist and then stitches the cut edges of the cervix with sutures that the body will absorb after a few days.

Conization
(courtesy of Susan Schoen)

Heavy bleeding is common, either right after surgery or about ten days later when the sutures are absorbed. Occasionally, a woman finds it more difficult to become or stay pregnant after conization because of scar tissue buildup.

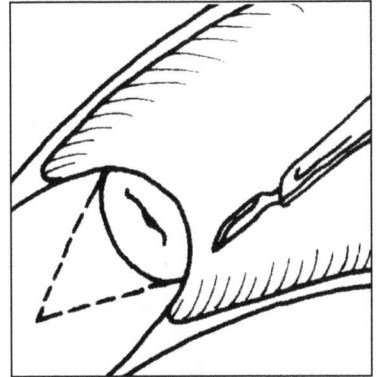

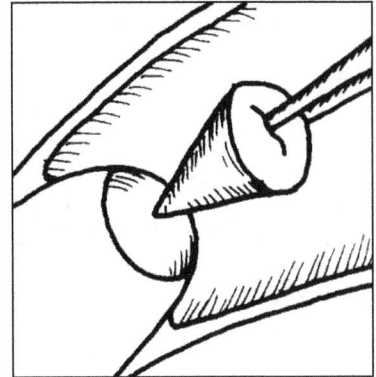

OPEN BIOPSY

In an open biopsy to sample an area of the body that cannot be reached any other way, the doctor cuts through the skin over the suspect area and removes some tissue so that it can be examined by the pathologist. An incisional biopsy cuts into a tumor and takes out a piece, perhaps a wedge from a large tumor. An excisional biopsy cuts out or excises all of the suspect area, along with a margin of nonsuspicious tissue from all around the area.

All open biopsies are performed in an operating room. This could be an area set aside for minor surgery in a doctor's office or clinic, or the woman is admitted to the hospital as a "same-day surgery" patient.

*Diagnosis
and Beyond*

57

In the operating room, the skin is swabbed repeatedly with germ-killing solutions and then draped so that only the area to be cut shows. The surgeon may mark the area where the incision will be.

Depending on the circumstances and her preference, the woman may receive either a general or a local anesthetic. If the woman needs general anesthesia, a short-acting anesthetic is given through the vein. If the surgery will be longer than a few minutes, a tube is passed through the woman's mouth into her windpipe after she is asleep, and a mixture of anesthetic gases and oxygen is administered. The tube is removed before she wakes up, but it may leave her with a temporarily irritated throat and the feeling that she is coming down with a cold.

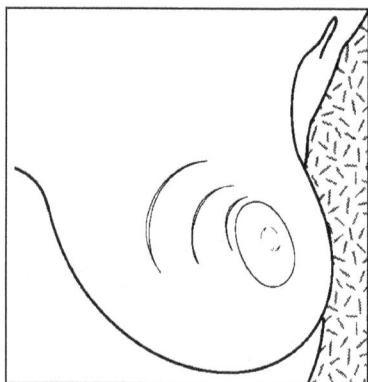

Typical biopsy incisions

(these illustrations—above and on page 59—courtesy of The Informed Woman's Guide to Breast Health)

For a biopsy done under a "local," the surgeon will inject an anesthetic similar to Novocain under the skin; this can sting briefly. The woman lying awake on the operating table during a biopsy probably will not be able to watch, even if she is so inclined, because a screen is placed between her face and the surgical area. As long as the area is sufficiently numbed, she will not feel pain but may feel sensations of pressure and tugging; if there is any pain, it is time to ask for more local anesthetic. She will hear unfamiliar noises, like the faint hiss of the electric cauterizing wand that stops bleeding from tiny blood vessels. Some surgeons explain what is happening during the procedure.

The surgeon cuts through the skin and other layers of tissue to find the suspicious area, removes all or part of it, and sends it to the pathologist. One option, still valuable in some situations but less common now than it used to be, is an immediate **frozen section**, in which the pathologist quick-freezes a piece of the specimen, slices it thinly, stains it, and then examines it under the microscope. This report can tell the surgeon immediately if more tissue needs to be removed, such as a "clear margin" of tissue around a cancer. The disadvantages are that there are many false negatives and that waiting for a report that may add little new information is an inefficient use of the operating room and staff. For a **permanent section**, the pathologist painstakingly prepares the specimen, a process that takes about twenty-four hours. The final report may take two or more days.

The surgeon may stitch the underlying tissues together with sutures that do not need to be removed and then closes the skin with special tape strips or stitches. The tape strips fall off in about two weeks; skin sutures are removed by the surgeon after a week or so. The surgeon bandages the area with a protective, bulky gauze dressing. If the biopsy was performed under general anesthetic, the woman usually wakes up in the postanesthesia recovery room.

The amount of postbiopsy pain, bruising, and scarring depends on the individual surgery and the woman who undergoes it. Pain from a simple biopsy usually subsides within a day or so and can be relieved with pain pills. Complications from a biopsy are rare, but include the possibility of infection, a collection of fluid at the site (**seroma**), or bleeding into the surrounding area (**hematoma**).

NEEDLE LOCALIZATION BIOPSY

What if the biopsy is for a breast abnormality, such as a cluster of microcalcification, that appears only on a mammogram or MRI? Since there is nothing to see or feel, the surgeon must turn to the radiologist for help in localizing the spot. This can be done either with a stereotactic guided needle biopsy (described on pages 53–54) or with a special procedure called a **needle** (or wire) **localization biopsy**.

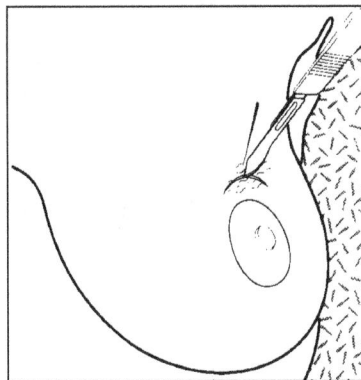

Needle localization biopsy

For a needle localization, depending on the kind of imaging study that showed the abnormality, the woman first goes to either the X-ray department or the breast MRI room. There the radiologist uses mammograms or MRI to decide on the proper spot for inserting one or more wires or needles; these may have tiny hooks to keep them from moving. After their placement is determined, a little dye may be inserted to mark the spot; the dye often stings at first.

Wires and dye in place, the woman is taken to the operating room, where the surgeon follows the track of the wire with a scalpel and removes the marked area as in a regular biopsy. Since the abnormality can be seen only on a mammogram, the biopsy specimen is X-rayed (**specimen radiographed**) so that the pathologist can see if the abnormal area—and all of it—has been removed.

FEELINGS ABOUT A BIOPSY

It is scary to have a biopsy or other diagnostic procedure. Whatever the outcome, most of us feel upset, frightened, and helpless at the prospect. No matter how well we understand intellectually that this is simply a necessary step to find out what is happening, and that most biopsies reveal only benign changes, our feelings may not match our thoughts.

Many women admit to being surprised and horrified by their emotional reactions. One minute they are convinced that all will be well; the next minute they are rehearsing deathbed scenarios. There is anxiety about what the biopsy may show, of course, and every day of waiting makes it worse. To face a biopsy is to confront the possibility of serious illness and our own mortality—but it is also to inhabit an unreal, in-between time of *not knowing*. And we may feel apprehensive about the procedure itself: Will it hurt? What about scars?

It is common to become angry at health professionals, family members, and friends because they may seem insensitive or blasé about what is, for us, a very difficult experience. Professionals sometimes forget that what is everyday for them is not so for us, or they may protect themselves emotionally by pulling away from patients. Family and friends are often so scared that they retreat into themselves or behave in unpredictable ways. Our own strong feelings may also distort what we perceive.

Sometimes, though, our anger is a smokescreen for feelings that are even more painful to accept in ourselves. Thus, "I can't believe what a jerk that doctor is!" or "Why do I have to be cut open to find out that I'm perfectly healthy?" masks "Do I have cancer? Will I die?"

These feelings are strong stuff, but they are normal. It is human to feel scared, sad, and angry before a biopsy. Our emotions may make us uncomfortable, sometimes acutely so, but if we can look at them clearly and talk about them freely, we can also draw on all that energy to help us recover quickly. It is the emotions we do not acknowledge that corrode our souls.

It helps to know that we are normal. It also helps to get information about what the procedure will be like so we know what to expect. If we admit we need someone to talk to, a doctor, nurse, spouse, or friend may be able to help. Biopsies and other diagnostic procedures are not fun. They are physically and emotionally uncomfortable. But the news is often good and, even if the diagnosis is cancer, a biopsy lets us know where we stand so that we can begin to take action.

TIMELY DIAGNOSIS

Nobody wants an unnecessary diagnostic procedure. On the other hand, failing to detect a curable cancer at an early stage because either the doctor or the patient refuses a biopsy is tragic.

One all-too-common scenario is a woman with a "dominant" breast lump and a doctor who says, "You're too young to have breast cancer, so this must be benign. I'll see you in a year." No matter how young the woman, no matter whether or not the lump is painful, if there is a persistent dominant breast lump—or a symptom of any other kind of cancer—it *must* be diagnosed.

Waiting a month to see if the lump goes away with the next menstrual cycle is reasonable and may well save a biopsy. Performing a fine needle aspiration in the doctor's office is also reasonable. Waiting a year to check it again is not.

If a woman has a suspicious symptom, she has a right to timely diagnosis or to referral to another doctor who can diagnose the condition. If she is not content with what is being done, she has both the right and the responsibility to herself to ask for an explanation; if the explanation is not satisfactory, she can ask for a second opinion or change doctors.

STAGING A CANCER

A cancer can behave like a lapdog or like a school of piranhas. If the diagnosis after the biopsy is cancer, the doctors still want to learn much more about it in order to treat it most effectively. This involves learning how extensive it is (its **stage**) and how aggressive it is likely to be (its **grade**).

Cancer is named by the type of body tissue involved. Breast and colon and many gynecologic cancers tend to be **carcinomas,** cancers that develop in the tissues that line internal organs or passageways; more specifically, many are **adenocarcinomas**, from *adeno*, the Greek word for gland. A few women's cancers are **sarcomas,** cancers that grow in the supporting or connective tissues of the body: muscles, bones, tendons, blood vessels, or nerves. Lung cancers are diverse, with some carcinomas or sarcomas, but many are named after the kinds of cells (like small cells or squamous cells) that make up the tumor. The type of tumor makes a difference in how to treat it.

Staging a tumor is based on three aspects: how large the **tumor** itself is (T); how much, if any, the tumor has spread to the lymph **nodes** (N); and whether there is any known **metastasis** or spread to distant organs (M).

A number after each letter answers the question "how much," so a T1 cancer of an organ is smaller than a T3 of the same organ. On the other hand, what falls into each "how much" group varies with each organ. Thus a breast cancer classified as T2 N1 M0, for instance, would be between about 1 and 2 inches (2–5 cm) in diameter, would have one or more lymph nodes from the armpit that show some cancer but not so much that they cannot move freely, and would have no known distant metastasis. A cancer of the same size that appeared in the ovary, however, might have a very different T number.

How do doctors discover a cancer's node and metastasis status? They may be able to feel some enlarged lymph nodes even before surgery, but many nodes are not close enough to the skin to be palpated. Removing the nodes close to the cancer and having them examined by a pathologist is currently the common way to find nodes in which there are tiny islands of cancer cells (**microscopic nodal invasion**).

Because common places for women's cancers to metastasize are the bones, lungs, liver, and brain, these areas are checked especially. Does the woman report any bone pain, shortness of breath, or other complaint that could possibly mean a metastasis? Is there anything the doctor can see or feel, such as a swollen liver? Usually, the woman undergoes a staging work up, including laboratory tests and imaging studies. The doctor also searches for any sign of regional spread, such as bladder changes with ovarian cancer, or spread to the opposite breast with breast cancer. The doctor may request a biopsy if there are suspicious signs or symptoms.

Cancer stages range from 0 or I to IV, with subgroups, and the stages define where the cancer diagnosed fits in the TNM framework. Stage 0 means an in situ carcinoma, a tumor that has not invaded neighboring tissues and thus cannot have spread to lymph nodes or distant sites. Not all cancers have an in situ stage, but breast, colon, cervical, vaginal, and vulvar cancers do. The TNM status for this would be T0 N0 M0; the 0 after the T simply means there is no invasive cancer. Stage I is a relatively small invasive cancer without node involvement or known metastasis. Depending on the organ, Stage I may be subdivided into A and B or more subgroups. Stages II, III, and IV are progressively more extensive cancers, but may represent different TNM combinations. A Stage II breast cancer, for example, has no evidence of distant metastasis, but could be quite small with some spread to nearby lymph nodes, or considerably larger with no known node involvement.

The TNM classification gives doctors a common language. However, there are other classification systems, and gynecologic cancers are frequently classified using the FIGO (International Federation of Gynecology and Obstetrics) system.

While non-small cell lung cancers go by a TNM system, small cell lung cancers are staged simply as "limited" or "extensive," with some controversy about what goes into each classification. TNM can be used for colon cancer, but many doctors use the traditional Dukes' classifications, named after Duke University where the categories were developed.

A pathologist looking at slides of cancer cells under the microscope can tell several things about how this particular cancer might behave. And every year new tests appear that offer more information.

The pathologist sees how different the individual cells are from a normal cell in that organ. The cancer cells that still look quite a bit like a normal cell—typical in the **well-differentiated** cancers—tend to behave more like normal cells and to be less aggressive. The **poorly differentiated** cancers are at the other extreme, and **moderately differentiated** cancers fall somewhere in the middle.

How fast is the cancer growing? The pathologist counts how many cells in the slides are in the process of dividing (mitosis) for an estimate of the cancer's growth pattern. Cancers with a shorter doubling time grow more quickly and have more cells dividing at any one time; for instance, it is likely that the pathologist will catch more cells in the process of dividing in a cancer whose cells are programmed to divide every two weeks than in one with a doubling time of four months.

The pathologist looks at the particular types of cells, the presence of any necrotic (dead) areas, how the cells fit together, what the nucleus and other cell parts look like, how many tiny blood vessels are in the area of the tumor, and so on, and compares the findings with how other cancers with this profile have behaved.

Tumor material can be subjected to assorted tests, some of which are very new. These can provide valuable clues about treatment options. For example, breast cancer cells are tested with hormone receptor assays to see if and how much they respond to the female hormones estrogen or progesterone, because cancers that thrive in the presence of estrogen may be treated by depriving them of that hormone, thereby creating an additional therapy option.

When cancer cells are preparing to divide—during the S-phase of the cell cycle—they make copies of their DNA so it will be available for the daughter cells. Thus a tumor with large amounts of DNA for its size has a lot of cells dividing, which means it is a faster-growing, more aggressive cancer. **S-phase fraction** (SPF) and **Ki-67** are two tests that can be done on a small piece of the tumor specimen to tell quite accurately what percentage of cells are dividing.

DNA Ploidy status looks at the chromosomes in cancer cells. Tumors with a normal number of chromosomes in the cell DNA (**diploid**) tend to be slower growing than those with too many or too few chromosomes (**aneuploid**). **Flow cytometry** is the name of the process which checks both ploidy and S-phase fraction.

Depending on the type of cancer, other tests for specific tumor proteins, oncogenes, or increased amounts of growth factors may be appropriate. Breast cancer tumors, for example, especially those in younger women, are usually tested now for **HER-2/neu receptors**. Breast cancers with too many of these receptors tend to grow very fast and respond better to certain treatments, including a specific drug that works only with this kind of tumor.

The idea behind all these tests is to find out what kind of treatment is most likely to help a woman live longer and better after a diagnosis of cancer. The most aggressive cancers, those with a high **nuclear grade**, require an "elephant gun" approach, while a lazier cancer may be destroyed with a gentler treatment.

If, no matter how aggressive the cancer is or is not, there is only one possible treatment, then it is a waste of time, effort, and money to find out how aggressive it is. On the other hand, for a cancer with multiple variations and many treatment options—such as breast cancer—it makes sense to learn everything we reasonably can before deciding on therapy.

PROGNOSIS

"What are my chances?"

After receiving a cancer diagnosis, many women ask (or wonder silently) about **prognosis**, the statistical odds of what will happen to a woman with this condition. The prognosis depends on the kind of cancer, how extensive and aggressive the individual case is, how successful the current treatments for it are, and whether there are other personal or medical factors that are likely to make a difference.

Postmenopausal women with very early stage breast cancer, for instance, are likely to have an excellent prognosis, a very good chance of being cured. The woman with widespread ovarian cancer faces a poorer prognosis. But prognosis says nothing about what will happen to this individual woman. She may face poorer odds with a certain prognosis, but that is all. Years later, many a woman with a terrible prognosis is still around, enjoying life, thumbing her nose at the prognosticators.

In addition, all it takes is one effective new therapy to turn a bad prognosis into an excellent one. Many years ago, my sister-in-law was diagnosed in her twenties with Hodgkin's disease, a cancer of the lymph system that was then considered almost invariably fatal. Horrified, we searched for information and learned that a doctor at Stanford University Medical Center was getting exciting results treating Hodgkin's with a new program of radiation therapy.

So Chris and her family moved in with us for four months so that she could commute to Stanford. With four adults and six young children in a three-bedroom, one-bath San Francisco flat, it was close quarters, but worth it. Chris just celebrated her fifty-fifth birthday, still vibrantly healthy and a pioneer in one of the treatments that have turned Hodgkin's from a virtual death sentence to a cancer that most people survive.

— *Kerry McGinn*

CHAPTER 5

A Woman and Her Doctors

For most of us, cancer is too big a battle to fight alone. It takes a team effort.

On my team, I wanted

+ myself at the center of the team—after all, it was my body, and I insisted on having a voice and making choices about what happened to it

+ the best doctors I could find: smart, knowledgeable, and the kind of people I could work with

+ lots of other very important people: health-care workers other than doctors (including practitioners of any complementary therapies, such as acupuncture, that I chose to use); people who had "been there" as mentors and perhaps a support group; my family, friends, and coworkers; information resources, and so on

I felt shell-shocked after my diagnosis—vulnerable and overwhelmed by the choices that needed to be made promptly. As I gathered my "get well team," however, I regathered my own strength and sense of control as well. We were not perfect, any of us. We all made mistakes sometimes, failed to communicate, had bad days, or stepped on each other's toes. But at the same time, each person contributed something valuable—the will to get through this, specific chemotherapy drugs, or a care package of paperback mysteries sent with love. Woven together, these strands became far stronger than each alone. A rope? A safety net? A tapestry?

A team.

Some women want to hear as little as possible about their cancer and prefer to leave all the control and decision making in their doctors' hands. (Many women see nurse practitioners, osteopaths, or physician assistants rather than physicians as their primary health providers—or as women's health or oncology specialists—but *doctors* is used for brevity's sake.) They have always trusted their doctors to make the right medical choices for them and see no reason to change that pattern now. This is a legitimate way of coping, and this woman might tell her doctor something like, "I will follow whatever treatment you advise. I really do not want to hear any more about this than I have to."

However, "Yes, doctor," "No, doctor" is simply not enough for a growing number of women. They expect to be functioning members of their own treatment teams, and they do not wish to leave all the decisions to their doctors. As much as they might trust their physicians, these women are profoundly aware that their doctors are not the ones who will have to live day after day with the choices that have been made.

These women expect their physicians to present treatment *options*—including no treatment. The doctors may argue strongly for a particular option, but they must explain the pros and cons of each choice so that the women can understand them. The women, in turn, ask questions, read, tell the doctors what they observe and how they feel—and they seek second opinions when appropriate.

To participate in her own treatment, a woman does not have to become a medical expert, but she does need to trust her intelligence and good sense. She is capable of learning about cancer and its treatment and of making rational decisions. And she can contribute what no doctor can. Since she lives in her body every day, she is in the best position to notice and monitor subtle changes. She knows her own needs and desires better—and cares more about her health—than any doctor can.

Thinking of herself and her doctors as *partners* in a team effort does not mean she has to make all the decisions or always be in control. Part of being on a team is contributing what she can; the other part is welcoming the strengths of her teammates. Before getting cancer, I had grand notions about my role as a member of my health-care team. I envisioned myself briskly making intelligent decisions and participating fully as its center. It worked like that sometimes during my cancer diagnosis and treatment, and I made some good decisions and some crucial observations. In truth, however, there were other times when I was barely slogging along, or was being carried by my teammates. That is what the team approach is all about.

*A Woman
and Her
Doctors*

CANCER DOCTORS

A surgeon, gynecologist, or other health-care provider obtains the biopsy tissue. A pathologist then examines the biopsy specimen under the microscope to tell whether cancer is present. If cancer is diagnosed, some kind of treatment is often necessary, and many doctors might become involved in recommending cancer therapy and carrying out treatment.

A surgeon or gynecologist may perform more surgery (or other local treatment such as freezing or laser therapy) to remove a larger area after the biopsy. This doctor may be a general surgeon or gynecologist, or perhaps a doctor who specializes in cancer treatment: a **surgical** or **gynecologic oncologist**. This is all the treatment some women need. If there is a reasonable possibility that stray cancer cells remain in the vicinity and have not been removed by surgery, a **radiation oncologist** (or **radiation therapist**) may join the treatment team. This specialist has received years of training in how to destroy local areas of cancer with high-beam X-ray energy. (Although the titles sound similar, a radiation oncologist has a very different job from a radiologist, who reads X rays and other imaging studies and thus helps detect cancer, but does not treat the disease.)

But cancer is frequently both a local and a systemic (whole-body) problem—and no single therapy currently available treats both parts of the problem adequately. Doctors often either know or suspect that some cancer cells have escaped from the local area and prefer to play it safe. This means that a woman with cancer may have to deal with a combination of therapies: one or more local treatments (surgery, freezing or burning, and radiation), and one or more systemic treatments (chemotherapy, hormone therapy, and biological therapy).

Many women choose a **medical oncologist** to help fit the pieces together. This doctor not only coordinates care but also specializes in the systemic therapies for cancer. After completing training to become a doctor of internal medicine (internist), the medical oncologist has pursued advanced training in cancer therapy. When people refer to "my oncologist," they usually mean a medical oncologist.

Depending on the situation, any of these specialists, or the woman's primary care provider (such as her internist or family doctor), may assume the role of cancer therapy "chief." This individual prescribes and delivers therapy and/or coordinates treatment and sees the woman frequently during treatment and often at regular intervals afterward for the rest of her life. If she has more than one cancer doctor, a woman often continues to check in with each of them regularly after her treatment is completed, perhaps alternating the appointments so that she sees each doctor at least once a year.

Finding a Doctor

The gynecologist, internist, or family doctor may suggest a particular doctor to treat the cancer. Many women today receive their health insurance through a health maintenance organization (HMO) or some other form of "managed care" in which the internist or other primary care provider acts as a "gatekeeper," deciding when specialist care is needed and which specialists should provide it. If the woman wants her insurance to pay all or most of the hefty costs of her cancer care, she may be limited to doctors in her health plan, although this often includes a choice of physicians; it makes sense to check her health plan *before* beginning the decision process. She might also get recommendations from a nearby medical school, the local medical society or American Cancer Society unit, a nurse on the oncology ward at the hospital, or friends.

These sources may provide further information: Is the doctor aggressive in treatment or more conservative? What about communication skills and bedside manner? Is she or he involved in clinical research? A call to the Cancer Information Service of the National Cancer Institute at (800) 4-CANCER will provide a list of cancer specialists. For Internet users, www.asco.org, the website for the American Society for Clinical Oncology, has a very helpful "Find an Oncologist" section.

Choosing the best doctor from among several candidates may be the problem for the woman with adequate health insurance living in or near a city, but many women do not have easy access to any doctor with expertise in cancer therapy. If there is only one doctor within one hundred miles, for instance, and if this doctor rarely treats cancer patients, the woman with cancer may need to travel or have her records sent to a cancer center for assessment, development of a treatment plan, and perhaps therapy.

Choosing the Right Doctor

If all doctors made the best possible use of the cancer therapies available today, more women would survive cancer. This is too serious a disease and the long-term relationship with the primary cancer doctor is too crucial to settle for the wrong doctor. But how does a woman find the right one?

No doctor is perfect, and no doctor can be expected to combine all the qualities a woman wants all the time. Most women have to choose a cancer doctor under less-than-optimal conditions: Their anxiety levels are sky-high and they are under pressure to start treatment soon. Most women also do not have the time and money to interview several doctors, although they may be able to talk to more than one (by phone if not in person) and can also weigh what they have heard from other people.

With the stakes as high as they are in cancer treatment, however, it makes sense for a woman to think hard about what really matters to her in a doctor: What is essential, what is important but negotiable, and what she would like but could do without in a pinch. In fact, most women seem to find a cancer doctor they both like and trust. As one woman said, "My oncologist is the perfect combination of hope and reality. He does not soft-pedal the bad news, but he can always be counted on to be there and to cheer me on."

Basic credentials are essential. The *Directory of Medical Specialists* and the *American Medical Directory,* available in many libraries, list such factors as a doctor's education and specialty preparation. For instance, is the doctor board certified in the specialty? The doctor or office staff should be willing to supply this information as well. Many women insist that their doctors be members of relevant professional organizations such as the American Society of Clinical Oncology (for medical oncologists).

Before agreeing to help finance treatment, many health plans require that doctors be covered by the woman's insurance plan and that they have admitting privileges at a hospital included in that plan. The woman with Medicare or Medicaid (Medi-Cal in California) coverage needs a doctor who accepts this form of payment.

Competence and experience come next. The doctor must have the basic skills to take care of a patient with this type of cancer. If there is an unusual condition, the woman may need to see a "super-specialist" who has dealt with similar situations before. (If one surgeon is the acknowledged national master of the rare kind of surgery I need, I may bemoan the fact that he or she has the communication skills of a turnip, but I will have that surgeon do my surgery anyway.)

Beyond these essentials, the right doctor for one woman may not fit another woman's needs at all. One woman may place a premium on bed-side manner, while another happily sacrifices empathy for access to clinical trials. If a woman has a choice between two or more well-qualified doctors, she weighs what matters most to her. How clearly and honestly does the doctor communicate the whats, whys, and wherefores of diagnosis and treatment? Are the treatment recommendations backed up with convincing reasons? Is this a doctor who will not gloss over the risks of therapy while being a cheerleader for the benefits? Some doctors rely on their staff (oncology nurses, perhaps) to pass along some of the necessary information, and this can be a satisfactory arrangement.

How carefully does the doctor listen to the woman? Does he or she obviously respect the woman's input and look upon therapy as a shared venture? This is a key consideration for the woman who wants to work *with* her doctor, rather than simply to follow directions. It does not mean that the doctor will always agree with her, however, or say just what she wants to hear.

Is this physician involved in research or clinical trials? Some women prefer a doctor who is on the cutting edge of treatment, while others prefer one with a more conservative approach.

What is the doctor's treatment philosophy? To work well, cancer treatment often must be quite aggressive, but there is still a range of reasonable treatment styles. One oncologist builds a reputation for no-holds-barred treatment, never gives up, and always has another possible therapy to try. Another oncologist ordinarily suggests comfort care when cure is unlikely and is much more ready to say "enough." All oncologists are bound by the individual woman's wishes, but most women will feel more comfortable with a doctor whose treatment philosophy meshes with their own desires.

What about the doctor's bedside manner? Cancer doctors have to present painful news and difficult choices all the time. To protect themselves emotionally—and perhaps save their energies for the long run—some fine doctors distance themselves from patients and may appear somewhat reserved, detached, or clinical. Others fear that a personal relationship will jeopardize their objectivity.

Many oncologists, however, recognize how therapeutic, how vital a part of effective treatment, their manner can be. While a cancer doctor is not a mother, a father, or a buddy, basic friendliness and moral support are important. "Detached" may be adequate; "cold machine" is not. It makes sense for a woman to insist on doctors she can both respect and like enough to follow the treatment plan they suggest.

Susan couldn't stand her oncologist. She spent her whole treatment period quietly rebelling by flushing her chemotherapy pills down the toilet and missing appointments. Her early stage cancer spread soon afterward, and she died quickly. Those of us who loved her will always wonder if things might have been different with a better doctor–patient relationship. Of course, because cancer doctors are often the bearers of bad news and unpopular treatments, they may become the innocent targets of a woman's anger. But if it is more than that, and if the anger seriously interferes with the treatment process, it is crucial to either renegotiate the patient–doctor relationship or find another doctor.

Health care is a product and patients are its consumers. While a woman cannot expect perfection, she has a right to competent, considerate care. This includes reasonably helpful office staff, appointments scheduled so that she does not routinely have to wait long, and adequate telephone access in case of a problem.

THE PATIENT–DOCTOR RELATIONSHIP

Like other relationships, the patient–doctor relationship carries with it both rights and responsibilities. What does this mean for a woman?

First, she listens. Ideally, a few days after diagnosis, when she is past the initial shock, she brings a family member or friend with her, along with a small tape recorder (if the doctor agrees) or a pen and notebook with questions written beforehand, and they sit down with her doctor for a comprehensive treatment-planning session. Doctors know that anxiety blocks a person's capacity to listen and they are accustomed to repeating what they have to say more than once; that is just the nature of communication during a period of high stress and does not indicate deficiencies on the woman's part. However, bringing someone along for any serious appointment, as a backup listener, saves missed information and misunderstanding; a tape recorder also lets the woman replay the conversation later for herself and her family.

Many women complain that they do not understand what the doctor and other health professionals say, that the vocabulary is unfamiliar and the explanations too technical. But medical concepts can all be explained in ordinary words; medical terminology cannot be allowed to become a barrier between doctor and patient.

The right to clear explanations in words she understands must be a woman's nonnegotiable demand. It is always appropriate to ask, "Would you please explain that again in simpler terms?" or "Could you rephrase that?" or "This is what I think you said—is that right?" Many nurses have become proficient at explaining medical concepts; medical book illustrations, drawings by the health professional, and books and booklets can all be helpful. It also makes sense for a woman to ask where she can get more information if she is interested.

The woman needs to think about what she wants and communicate it as clearly as possible. No matter how sensitive they may be, doctors cannot read minds. Unless the woman answers questions honestly and raises issues that concern her, the doctor cannot read her mind. (I have been guilty of that myself, thinking, "He must know that—and if he doesn't, he should.") Cancer treatment is no place for guessing games. In particular, the woman accepts responsibility for either following the treatment plan she and her doctor have devised or communicating any problems she encounters with it so that they can be resolved.

Sometimes, a woman may be too embarrassed to tell her doctor about some sensitive area in her life. Most doctors are virtually unshockable, however, and find their jobs much easier if they can deal with a candid patient.

If appropriate, the woman can request that certain items not go into her medical record.

Many times a woman is reluctant to ask "silly" questions. Focusing on what is important to her is the key to asking sensible questions, and she can ask family or friends for input. Cancer books or booklets often include questions to ask doctors. Many women find it helpful to keep a notebook handy at all times so that they can jot down questions when they arise. A woman can review her list before an appointment and bring it with her. And if she does not know something and wants information, no question she asks is silly.

Many women have problems being assertive with doctors. They do not want to cause trouble or take too much of the doctor's time, and they shy away from anything that might lead to a confrontation. But the woman is fighting for her *life;* it is absolutely necessary that she say what she has to say with enough "oomph" to make her point. This does not mean being rude, but it can mean being very definite. She has the right to insist on appropriate concern for her problems and thoughtful answers to her questions, not only because she is the health-care consumer paying for this service but also because she is a person of intrinsic worth. If a problem arises, remembering that this is a partnership—to which the doctor brings medical expertise and the woman brings the equally valuable contributions of her intelligence, personality, ability to observe, and coping skills—makes it easier for some women to ask for the care they deserve. Many women also find it helpful to rehearse with a mentor or in a support group more effective ways to communicate with doctors and other health professionals.

The woman needs to take time to make treatment decisions. While it is important to begin any therapy reasonably soon, it ordinarily does not make any difference to her long-term survival if a woman takes a few extra days—or even two or three weeks—after a cancer diagnosis to gather information and mull over what she wants before making any serious decisions. Often, in fact, it is not the doctor who is pressing for a prompt decision, but the woman's own urgent sense that something needs to be done.

Excellent—and free—help for any woman going through this process is the award-winning audio program *The Cancer Survival Toolbox.* Available as either audio tapes or compact discs, the *Toolbox* includes a basic skills set: communicating, finding information, making decisions, solving problems, negotiating, and standing up for rights. Three additional programs cover topics for seniors, finding ways to pay for care, and caring for the caregiver. Both authors of this book worked on the *Toolbox,* a joint venture of the National Coalition for Cancer Survivorship, the Oncology Nursing Society, and the Association of Oncology Social Work. To obtain her free copy, a woman can call (877) TOOLS-4U (866-5748) or can order it online at www.cansearch.org, under the "programs" listing.

Most women want to be more than just "that breast cancer in Exam Room Four." They want to be real people to their health-care providers, and that means opening up enough so that their personality shows through. Interests, goals, fears, and stresses are important information to share.

If she expects her doctor to treat her courteously, the woman must return that consideration. That includes taking time before her appointment to collect her thoughts and questions, so that the doctor can meet her needs without having to change the whole day's appointment schedule. It also means such basics as keeping appointments or informing the office if she cannot, using advice phone calls reasonably, and not taking out her anger at the cancer itself on the medical staff.

Both the woman and her doctor are human, and only human. Accepting each other as human beings, sharing their strengths, and acknowledging their mutual fallibility are all part of forging a strong but flexible bond between them.

SECOND OPINIONS

Cancer therapy changes all the time. What was state of the art just last year may be outdated now. In many cases, doctors do not yet know the best way to treat particular cancers. That means that good doctors may legitimately disagree about what therapy to recommend. It often makes sense for a woman to find out what different doctors think about the therapy options for her cancer.

For instance, she might see a medical and/or a radiation oncologist after a biopsy but before any further surgery. If there are several possible acceptable ways to treat a particular cancer (as with breast cancer), the surgeon or gynecologist is more likely to look at surgical solutions, the radiation oncologist to recommend radiation, and the medical oncologist to propose systemic therapy.

This process tells a woman she has choices and helps her clarify what each might mean to her. In the long run, it may save her from having to repent at leisure a decision hastily made. In the short run, however, hearing all these different points of view may be confusing and distressing. If we *have* choices, it means we have to *make* choices. (There were times when I longed for someone to take that responsibility out of my hands. However, after floundering for days weighing imperfect options, I woke with a start at about 3:00 A.M. one morning knowing clearly what my choice had to be—

and I have never regretted it. Had I followed my initial instincts, I doubt that I would have been happy with them six months later.)

A woman can seek a second opinion from another doctor in the same specialty who is not connected with the original doctor, such as another surgeon who practices at a different hospital. This does not mean that she does not trust her original doctor. Most doctors consider second opinions routine and welcome; they are a safety mechanism that protects both patient and doctor. Of course, it is possible to go overboard getting second opinions. Visiting two surgeons makes sense; visiting six is usually too much.

Second opinions are common before surgery or other cancer treatments. Many women never think about getting a review of the biopsy microscope slides from a second pathologist with special expertise in her type of cancer, but slides and other medical records can be safely and quickly mailed for a prompt second look.

A woman can get several second opinions at one time if her case is reviewed by a **tumor board,** a group of health professionals from different cancer specialties who meet periodically at a regional hospital. They listen to a presentation of the case and view any visual evidence, such as imaging films or biopsy slides, and then pool their expertise to recommend a course of treatment. Often the doctor asks for the tumor board review, although some boards invite the patient to request the service; patients are also free to bring up the subject with their doctors, who can then request a review. There may be a fee, sometimes a hefty one.

In the United States, a woman may want to travel to one of the hospitals designated by the government's National Cancer Institute as a "Cancer Center," where new methods of cancer diagnosis and treatment are investigated. The NCI Cancer Centers Program recognizes over twenty-five **Comprehensive Cancer Centers** that meet its criteria for large-scale, balanced programs of cancer research, patient care, and community outreach. Several other NCI-designated Cancer Centers fall into categories with a narrower research focus, but still offer potential resources for certain women. Some other countries have similar programs. Information on NCI Cancer Centers is available from NCI's Cancer Information Service (see Resources) or from its website at www3.cancer.gov/cancercenters/centers-list.html.

Traveling to a cancer center or having her case reviewed there before treatment begins makes special sense for the woman who has limited access to specialized cancer care in her community, has an uncommon cancer, or has a cancer with either no standard treatment protocols or many therapy options. Some women may be candidates for, and choose to participate in, a **clinical trial** (a study to evaluate a new therapy). These are administered by Cancer Centers, or sometimes by oncologists in the community. The experimental portion of the therapy (such as new drugs) may be given at reduced or no cost, although the woman and/or her insurance usually must pay for any standard treatment included; financial arrangements in clinical trials vary widely (see "Clinical Trials" in Chapter 8).

A woman's local doctor benefits from any second opinion information. Also, her doctor can access computer programs such as the online database **Physician Data Query** of NCI for up-to-date research and treatment protocols. The better informed *everyone* is, the better care a woman will get.

— *Kerry McGinn*

CHAPTER 6

The Rest of the Team

And then there are all the other members of the team. Whether they are professionals, like other health-care workers, or contribute in other ways, they can become an indispensable part of a woman's cancer journey.

Depending on the treatments she receives, a woman with cancer can come into contact with a bewildering array of health-care workers in addition to her cancer doctors.

Nurses, whether in the hospital or at the doctor's office, include general nurses, specialist nurses such as oncology certified nurses (OCNs), and clinical nurse specialists (with a master's degree in a specialty). Nurses frequently administer chemotherapy drugs in the oncologist's office or the hospital. Because of their education and focus, nurses may be especially interested in teaching patients and in quality of life issues.

The woman may need the services of several kinds of technicians and technologists, including personnel who draw blood samples, perform imaging tests such as mammograms and bone scans, or administer radiation treatments. A physical therapist can help the woman regain her strength and a full range of movement if she has undergone treatment that has affected these. In the hospital or as an outpatient, depending on her needs and wants, the woman may see a dietitian, respiratory therapist, social worker, volunteers, admissions clerk, office staff, and the hospital chaplain, among others.

Many women value the time spent with a psychotherapist or other mental health professional. Seeking help in coping emotionally with a cancer diagnosis does not mean a woman is maladjusted or crazy; it simply means she is making good use of resources to make her life better in a very difficult situation. (In fact, because they have found it so valuable for all their patients, some cancer centers and breast care centers routinely include in their services an appointment with a psychotherapist experienced in working with women with a new diagnosis of cancer.) Counseling can also come from a social worker or other licensed counselor.

The woman who includes complementary therapies in her treatment package may see such helpers as a relaxation-training teacher, an acupuncturist, an herbal medicine specialist, and so on. Sometimes it seems like a blur of different people, with no time to get to know any of them. Many of them may be unsung members of her team—but they are an essential part of it.

FAMILY AND FRIENDS

Health professionals call them "significant others": spouses, family members, lovers, best friends. However strange the term is, it does reflect the fact that a special person makes a difference. Often, not-quite-so-significant others—friends, acquaintances, coworkers—can play major roles in a woman's cancer journey as well. A diagnosis of cancer is difficult and distressing not only for the woman but for everyone around her. Serious illness changes roles and rules in relationships. Family members may have to face new responsibilities, often with little help or instruction; family and friends may have to cope with their own feelings of fear, sadness, anger, and perhaps guilt.

Some people respond to cancer in someone close to them by being consistently loving, supportive, and helpful. They are there for her, accept her low days, show her that she is still loved and accepted, and bring her news and encouragement from the outside world.

However, cancer treatments often take a long time and it is common for family and friends to react differently at different times. People may be supportive part of the time and run out of steam at other times. No matter how much they love a woman, family members and friends are not immune to fatigue, other responsibilities, and strong and difficult feelings of their own.

I have been both a cancer patient and a close family member of a cancer patient, and I contend that being the patient is sometimes easier. As a patient, no matter how miserable I was, I knew my limits and trusted my strengths; as a family member, often all I could do was look on helplessly.

While it is not her job to make everyone around her feel comfortable, a woman with cancer can encourage a helpful response from others by being frank about what is happening and about what she wants and needs. By talking freely about the cancer, she cues other people that they do not need to tiptoe around the subject. At the same time, if she talks about other subjects as well and avoids concentrating exclusively on her illness, she reminds them—and herself—that she is a person who just happens to have cancer, rather than a cancer that just happens to have a person attached. Of course there are some times, such as right after diagnosis, when the ability to think or talk about anything but cancer may be too much to expect.

The woman may justifiably feel sad or angry, but she will scare off family and friends if she continually makes them the targets of her anger or if she mopes for months and expects them to bear the weight of her depression. A mentor, a support group, or, better yet, a psychotherapist or counselor may help her move out of this emotional tunnel.

Some people just cannot handle being around a person with a cancer diagnosis. This is their problem and is in no way the fault or responsibility of the woman with cancer. Even if they do not believe cancer is contagious (a myth that some people still believe), they may feel scared and vulnerable. They avoid facing the possibility that they might be in the same situation someday by avoiding the woman. Or they may be so afraid that they will not know what to say or will start crying that they just stay away.

On the other hand, a woman may wish that some people *would* stay away, and she may have to communicate this forcefully, if necessary. Some friends become so gloomy, pessimistic, or overly concerned that they make the situation worse. Others hover endlessly or overstay their welcome. My least favorites are the armchair psychologists who try to convince the woman that she "needed" the cancer, that her feelings have caused the cancer, and that she needs to "deal with her feelings" so that she can heal herself.

The woman may not have the stamina during this time to deal with exhausting emotional issues with others, including family members. These can wait until she feels better. And many women find themselves caught between opposing groups—close friends and family, perhaps, who have different ideas of what she should do. She may need to say, "You people resolve this between yourselves. I don't want any part of it." A helpful booklet, *Taking Time: Support for People with Cancer and the People Who Care About Them,* is available free from NCI's Cancer Information Service. It discusses many relationship issues, including coping within the family, sharing the diagnosis and the feelings involved, and maintaining and building relationships.

What about children? I remember driving home from the doctor's office and blurting out the news of my diagnosis to my husband. Together we planned for several days how best to break the news to our grown children and other family. It is crucial that children still at home be told very clearly (and repeatedly, if necessary) that they will be taken care of—and that they are *in no way to blame* for the cancer. Most children are sensitive to undercurrents of emotion. They react better to a simple, reasonably hopeful explanation than to a wall of silence that leaves them imagining the worst. Of course, the explanation needs to be tailored to the situation and the age of the child. A mother beginning chemotherapy who has a young child, for instance, might say something like, "I got sick. I have to take medicine for a while so I will get well. The medicine makes me feel very tired so I can't take you to the park today—but I still love you as much as always."

A useful booklet for older children, *When Someone in Your Family Has Cancer*, is available free from the Cancer Information Service. An informative pamphlet for parents can be found online at www.bacup.org/info/child/child-1.htm.

MENTORS AND SUPPORT GROUPS

Even with the best medical care in the world, many women long to compare notes with someone who has been there: "Did you feel like this?" "What did you do about that?"

A woman may find someone who has been through the experience to act as a mentor for her. The woman who has undergone breast cancer surgery, for instance, can visit with an American Cancer Society "Reach to Recovery" volunteer who has recovered from a similar surgery. Instead of medical advice, the volunteer offers moral support, practical information, a simple temporary prosthesis (breast form) if the woman has had a breast removed—and the living, breathing proof that a woman can live well after breast cancer. This is ordinarily a short-term relationship: a visit and a phone call or two. Some doctors or hospitals automatically refer their breast cancer patients to "Reach to Recovery." Otherwise, a woman can call the local ACS unit and refer herself for this free service.

Some women find a mentor by asking their doctors to recommend a woman who is doing well after treatment for a similar cancer. Referrals from friends can provide mentors, too: "I know this woman who was diagnosed with cervical cancer years ago. I bet she'd be happy to talk with you."

Before cancer, I never thought of myself as the support group type and sometimes even looked down on people who "needed" the help of a group to get through life's troubles. Cancer changed that.

My cancer support group sisters understood what I was feeling without my having to spell out each detail. The group provided information (especially practical tips on dealing with treatment side effects), a safe and accepting place for fears and tears, laughter and celebration, and a strong sense of a shared effort in getting well. Separately, we were all reasonably strong and interesting women; together, we were that—and more. And where else could we go on at length about treatments for vaginal dryness after some kinds of chemotherapy or fantasize about redecorating the oncologist's gloomy waiting room?

Being in a group gave me a sense of perspective and progress. At first, others who were further along in treatment were cheering me on; later, I could lend a hand to those just beginning and could appreciate how far I had come. I saw firsthand the positive changes other women were making in their lives after a cancer diagnosis. I was also forewarned of common emotional potholes so I could avoid some completely and get through others more easily.

By spending a couple of hours each week concentrating intensely on the experience, we began integrating it into our lives, but also we were able to put it out of mind some of the rest of the time. Our group was a place where we could discover how common and normal our feelings were, talk about them without burdening family and friends endlessly, and discover coping strategies that worked for others. The group gave us a chance to rehearse more effective ways of communicating with health professionals, family, and friends. And it provided a chance to help others, to know that we were still contributors to life rather than just takers.

When psychiatrist David Spiegel of Stanford began investigating support groups for women with cancer, he fully expected that the groups would make women feel better but would not affect their survival. To his astonishment, he found that in his research sample of women with advanced metastatic breast cancer, the average survival rate after diagnosis was almost *double* for women who were in a support group as compared to those who were not.

If groups do in fact make a difference in survival, why might this happen? Theories include increased access to information about cancer therapies, support and practical tips so that women persist in difficult treatments, and actual changes in the immune system from the psychosocial benefits of group work.

Follow-up studies have produced mixed results about longer survival but have shown at least a better quality of life in women with metastatic cancer who are in a good support group. Other studies are underway both in the United States and elsewhere. Until we have conclusive evidence one way or the other, Spiegel comments in the New England Journal of Medicine, "...group therapy for patients with cancer can be prescribed for its psychological benefit, if not necessarily for any prolongation of survival. Curing cancer may not be a question of mind over matter, but mind does matter."

Groups may be short-term (six to eight weeks, for instance, or a weekend retreat) or much longer; homogeneous (women currently undergoing treatment for breast cancer, perhaps) or more mixed; oriented primarily toward information or toward mutual support or toward an equal mixture of the two; limited to cancer patients or open to family and friends; open, with new participants continuing to join, or closed. There are also groups strictly for family members or friends. Some support groups have a particular focus, such as holistic treatment. Every group has a different personality, depending on its goals, members, and group leader.

It helps to have a facilitator who may or may not have had cancer but has experience in guiding groups. That way, members can explore painful feelings safely and freely, because they know there is a hand available to pull them out of any emotional quagmire. A trained leader also helps keep group members from taking on the feelings and burdens of others; thus, the group becomes an enriching rather than a depleting experience.

Any type of group can be helpful and effective—or not. A few are actively detrimental. I would promptly leave a group that induced strong guilt feelings in its members for having cancer or advised members to use alternative therapies instead of standard treatments for potentially curable cancers.

The local ACS unit usually has information about cancer support groups in the area. Women may hear about them from the oncologist, a nurse, or friends. ACS itself sponsors "I Can Cope," a series of eight education and support seminars for cancer patients and their families. One among several other possibilities is "The Wellness Community," listed in the Resources section at the back of this book.

Support groups, even when readily available and very good, are not for every woman. Some women take on every other woman's burdens and suffer for everyone; others feel extremely uncomfortable in a group setting. A potential difficulty for every woman is the possibility that she will have to cope with the premature death of one or more "sisters." For many women, however, a cancer support group is well worth checking out—or even starting.

INFORMATION SOURCES

Besides the specific information about her case that she receives from health professionals and any second opinion sources, a woman can learn a great deal about her type of cancer and about cancer in general from other sources. The American Cancer Society, which has units in most areas (phone number listed in the local phone book), can provide a wealth of information, including booklets and computer reports.

Trained personnel at the National Cancer Institute's Cancer Information Service answer general questions and will send free packets of information on almost any cancer topic. Physician Data Query (PDQ) of NCI offers up-to-the-minute treatment guidelines for anyone with access to a fax machine. Phone lines such as the Y-ME Breast Cancer Support Program, (800) 221-2141, or DES Action for women with cancers related to the drug DES, (510) 465-4011, are just two of several cancer hotlines that answer questions and provide emotional support.

The coming of the Internet and e-mail to personal computers has revolutionized the process of getting cancer information (and sometimes support) for many women. The woman who has access to a computer and a modem has at her fingertips information about state-of-the-art cancer thinking and therapy as well as cancer fundamentals. Internet sites include cancer survivor accounts and encouragement. Accessing one Internet address usually opens the way to many more. For women without Internet skills or access, several community cancer organizations offer help in getting started, including volunteer teachers and perhaps free access. A woman who has no interest in learning about computers herself can often find a family member or friend who would love to do some Internet cancer information hunting for her. Some women may wish to participate in a "chat room" or "bulletin board," where members exchange information and support by sending electronic mail messages to each other; they may prefer this to a face-to-face support group or use it along with a regular group.

Both fortunately and unfortunately, almost anyone can set up a website, which means that, although there is superb information and valuable support available, there is plenty of junk out there too. Most informed women would not want to pick their cancer therapy based on a story in a sensational tabloid at the grocery checkout counter—but many believe what they read on the Internet without applying a healthy dose of skepticism. Checking the credentials of any "experts" becomes crucial. (A sampling of addresses appears in the Resources section.)

THE HOSPITAL EXPERIENCE

Many women have never been patients in a hospital or have been there only for childbirth. It is foreign territory—and they would just as soon keep it that way. Many women with cancer never need hospitalization at all or stay in a same-day-care unit for only a few hours after a biopsy, for instance. Others enter the hospital for more extensive surgery, certain kinds of chemotherapy or radiation therapy, or for some complication.

What can a woman expect if she is hospitalized? For insurance reasons, most patients now stay in the hospital the shortest possible time. This means that anything that can be done before admission—blood work, imaging studies, physical examinations—may be done on an outpatient basis. It also means that hospitalized patients may be discharged from the hospital before they are fully recovered and may need more help at home than would be required after a longer hospital stay. Because patients are not hospitalized now unless they truly need acute care and because the number of hospital staff often does not reflect the high level of care needed, hospital personnel are often stretched—and stressed.

It makes sense to read and follow carefully any preadmission instructions from the hospital. Valuables, except for a few dollars, perhaps, and a wedding ring or watch, are best left home; if they are brought, the hospital staff will lock them up. It helps if people bring a list of any medications they are taking at home, including the name of the drug, the dosage, and the frequency, but not the pills themselves. Hospitals must follow strict fire safety regulations and may have special rules for small electrical appliances such as hair dryers.

Hospitals provide nightgowns and often slippers and robes. Women can bring their own, but may choose to wear hospital gowns part of the time because they are opaque, often easier to put on and take off, and can save the woman's nightwear from stains and soil after surgery. On the other hand, wearing one's own sleepwear helps preserve a bit of personal turf in unfamiliar territory. Likewise, many women bring a family photograph or something similar to put by their bedside to mark this as their spot and remind them of life beyond the hospital. This also tells health-care workers that this is a real person here and can serve as a conversation starter.

If she has surgery or other treatment in a teaching hospital, a woman may tell her story to, be examined by, and receive much of her everyday treatment from "house staff": residents and interns who have finished medical school and are licensed physicians, but are honing their clinical skills under the supervision of more experienced doctors. (Interns are not the same as internists, doctors who have received specialty training in internal medicine.) A woman will probably have "her" intern or resident, the person who has primary house-staff responsibility for her case. The house staff makes rounds once or twice a day, in a group, to examine her. When "her" intern is not available, another on-call intern will have information about her. Interns often rotate to another service every month or so while residents tend to stay longer in one department.

The surgeon or other cancer doctor acts as an attending doctor, supervising the house staff. The attending doctor may see each patient once or twice a day or has a covering doctor see her (on weekends, perhaps). If a problem requiring medical attention arises at another time, the nurse usually notifies the intern in a teaching hospital; if the intern or resident cannot resolve the problem, the attending doctor is notified.

Quite often now, a hospital or physician group will employ a *hospitalist,* a specialist doctor with extensive training and experience in the medical care of patients in the hospital. This doctor then "covers" hospitalized patients full-time for several attending doctors, providing much of the daily medical supervision while maintaining regular communication with the attending doctors. This scenario can work well for both the patient, who benefits from this care, and the doctor, who does not have to visit the hospital so often.

Hospitals have their own vocabulary, and it is always okay to ask what something means. Some common items include *p.r.n.,* an abbreviation for a Latin phrase meaning "as needed," referring to medicines or treatments given only at the patient's request; *NPO* for "nothing by mouth," meaning the patient is not supposed to eat or drink anything; and *void* for urinate. Many pain medications are ordered p.r.n.; if the woman does not specifically request them, they will not be given.

The woman in the hospital deserves considerate and respectful care, information about her diagnosis and treatment in words she can understand, and concern for her privacy. Her rights are further spelled out in the Patient's Bill of Rights, formulated by the American Hospital Association and often given to patients at admission or upon request.

On the other hand, consideration works both ways. That means, for example, using the nurse call bell when one needs help, but also asking oneself first: Is this a necessary request, something for which I need a nurse? Could I consolidate two or more requests?

There is a small but growing movement of hospitals that encourage interested patients to read and contribute information to their own medical charts. This practice reinforces the concept of patient and health-care workers as members of a team working together for the woman's health.

— *Kerry McGinn*

CHAPTER 7

Local Treatments for Cancer

Cancer is a thoroughly nasty disease—and the medical treatments for it will not win any popularity prizes. It is a trade-off: If we choose to undergo the discomfort of a cancer treatment now, it is because we think there is a good chance we will be better off in the long run. The therapies we have now for cancer are tolerable and may be worth enduring if they cure the disease or make it better.

Cancer therapy aims at one, or sometimes more, of three possible goals. Treatment can cure the cancer outright, dousing the fire completely so that the woman lives cancer-free for the rest of her days.

If cure is not possible, the backup goal is **control**, often for very long periods of time. Although cancer cells may linger, they cause the woman few, if any, complaints. Therapy may be able to keep cancer in this suspended mode for years and give a woman an extended disease-free interval. Another control scenario is the cancer that smolders most of the time, flaring up occasionally. Therapy puts out each small fire as it occurs, and the woman does quite well the rest of the time.

If neither cure nor control is possible, palliation almost always is. **Palliation** means relieving or reducing symptoms, making the person with advanced cancer comfortable, keeping the fire at bay. All three goals—cure, control, and palliation—are worthwhile.

WHAT LOCAL THERAPIES DO

The cancers discussed in this book are all solid tumors that begin in one location. Local therapies—surgery and radiation—are those that work for eradicating local disease. They are no help at all, however, in tracking down cancer cells that have left the immediate vicinity.

When the doctor says, "I recommend such-and-such therapy," a woman may wonder, "If I choose to do that, what am I letting myself in for?" This chapter provides an overview of the answers. Closer looks at specific treatments appear in the chapters about individual cancers.

SURGERY

Cancer surgery is usually considered elective rather than emergency surgery, which means that it usually does not have to be performed immediately. The woman waits anxiously, torn between "I don't want to do this" and "Let's get this over with—the cancer cells could be spreading right this minute!" But she is scarcely idle. Even if she will be hospitalized after surgery, she typically is not admitted until the morning of surgery. Before that, she undergoes any necessary tests and physical examinations as an outpatient, and may have a hospital preadmission interview to sign paperwork and to provide the hospital with insurance information.

Her gynecologist or surgeon tells her what she has to do to prepare for surgery. She may have to shower with a special bacteria-killing soap, take laxatives or enemas, or follow a certain diet. Unless she is having just a local (skin-numbing) anesthetic, she usually is instructed not to eat or drink anything for several hours before surgery, except perhaps for a few sips of water with any pills that she needs to take. The idea is to keep her stomach empty so that the stomach contents cannot back up when she is unconscious, possibly causing serious lung problems.

The traditional instruction has been "nothing to eat or drink after midnight." However, 1999 guidelines from the American Society of Anesthesiology call for a loosening of these restrictions for generally healthy adult patients: clear liquids, such as apple juice or chicken broth, permitted until two to four hours before surgery, with a light meal, such as a slice of toast and a clear liquid, permitted until about six hours before surgery. The evidence shows that following these timetables still leaves the stomach empty for surgery; in contrast, the guidelines recommend against fatty foods for at least eight hours before surgery because they exit the stomach more slowly. It may take years for the guidelines to be widely accepted, but it makes sense for a woman to ask about them.

On the morning of surgery, the woman goes to the presurgery area and is prepared for the operation. She signs the consent form for surgery if she has not done so already, and talks to the doctor or specially trained nurse who gives the anesthetic. She may also receive a sedative to relax her.

At some point, an intravenous (IV) line may be started. This is a tube, inserted into a vein, usually in a hand or arm, that makes it possible to administer fluids, medications, and blood if necessary, and to give the short-acting drug that induces, or begins, general anesthesia. Quite often, the woman receives a medicine through her vein that makes her forget the procedure completely, although she remains conscious and can follow directions; this "conscious sedation" can be given before general anesthesia or before some procedures that do not require general anesthesia.

In the operating room the woman is scrubbed and draped so that only the surgical area shows. This preparation helps protect the surgical area from contamination, as do the masks, gowns, and head coverings all the surgical personnel wear.

If the woman is scheduled for a "regional" anesthetic, which numbs the lower region of the body, she receives directions to curl up on the operating table. The anesthesia is begun through a narrow catheter (tube) carefully inserted through the previously numbed skin over the backbone into the space around the spinal nerves. When this takes effect, she will no longer be able to move or feel the area below the block. This cannot be done for breast surgery because a regional anesthetic to paralyze that area would also affect the lungs and heart. She may receive conscious sedation or other medication through her IV so that she dozes through the procedure or cannot remember it afterward.

Before a general anesthetic is started, the woman may have lots of small things placed on her, such as electrode patches to monitor her heart and a sensor placed around her finger to check that she is getting enough oxygen. If she is not already asleep from the sedative, the doctor or nurse giving anesthesia will tell her when the quick-acting general anesthetic is injected into her IV. Within a few seconds, she will be soundly, dreamlessly asleep. It may be hours before she wakes up, but it will seem like a second.

The IV anesthetic itself lasts only a short time, however. For a surgery lasting longer than a few minutes, a large tube is inserted through her mouth and down her throat after she is asleep. Through this, she receives a mixture of anesthetic gases and oxygen to keep her deeply unconscious but breathing well. The tube will usually be removed before she wakes up.

During the operation, the surgeon/gynecologist may use scalpels and scissors, an electrocautery wand to stop blood vessels from bleeding, or a laser. Even with a laser, the doctor still has to cut through the skin first.

After the operation, the woman is transferred to the postanesthesia recovery room where she wakes up gradually after a general anesthetic or regains feeling and movement below the waist after regional anesthetic. If she is scheduled to stay in the hospital, she is wheeled on a gurney to her hospital room where the nurses will help her transfer into bed. If she goes home directly from the recovery room, she receives written discharge instructions about medications, activities, precautions, and follow-up care.

Recovering from Surgery

Depending on the anesthetic and sedatives she received and how her body reacts to them, a woman may be instantly alert or remember almost nothing for the first day or so. But, sooner or later, she will notice tubes, bandages, and sensations.

TUBES A woman may temporarily feel that she has tubes dangling everywhere. She may still have her IV for fluids, antibiotics, and possibly pain medicine. If she does not need continuous IVs, the nurse detaches the IV bag and tubing and caps the end of the catheter near where it is inserted in the skin. The tubing is hooked up again only when necessary (for instance, for an antibiotic medicine that needs to be given every few hours). The rest of the time, the woman is free of the IV bag and tubing.

For a few days, tubes of some sort may drain extra blood or tissue fluid from the surgical area so it does not build up, cause discomfort, and strain the incision. A tube may provide a simple pathway or it may be connected to wall suction or a portable suction device. These devices are typically plastic containers (lemon-size bulbs or flat cylinders) that can be opened, emptied, and then compressed with the hands; as they gradually decompress, they create gentle suction.

The woman or the nurse can attach a dangling drain to the gown with tape or a rubber band and safety pin, taking care not to pierce or injure the drain. If the woman leaves the hospital with the drain(s) still in place, a nurse teaches her the very easy care needed. The doctor will pull out the drain when it is no longer needed. This is a peculiar sensation, rather like having a long worm removed from under the skin. It helps to take a deep breath first and then slowly exhale while the drain is being pulled. The tiny incision where the drain was inserted closes immediately.

A woman who has had chest surgery for lung cancer may have a special kind of tube inserted through the skin and the chest muscles into the space around the lungs; one or more chest tubes removes air or fluid from around the lungs so that the lungs can expand properly. The suction device for chest tubes will usually be larger and will rest on the floor at the bedside, but it is light enough for the woman to carry if she is walking.

After major surgery for a gynecologic or colorectal cancer, a woman can expect a Foley catheter, a tube inserted through the urethra (the opening to the bladder) to drain urine. Once the catheter is in the bladder, a small balloon in the catheter is inflated with water to keep the Foley from slipping out; when it is time to remove the catheter, the balloon is deflated and the catheter slips out. The Foley is connected to a portable drainage bag. This means that, for a day or more, the woman does not have to contend

Local Treatments for Cancer

with bedpans when she urinates because the urine drains out continuously. Some women complain of mild irritation from the catheter and may take a little while to relearn how to urinate normally after it is removed.

Sometimes, after abdominal surgery, the woman may have a narrow tube in her nose. This nasogastric (NG, or nose to stomach) tube may be attached to a suction source to remove gas and stomach juices until the digestive tract—pulled and pummeled by surgery—begins functioning again. Even without an NG, the woman may have to wait a few days before beginning liquids and then moving on to solid food.

BANDAGES AND SCARS The doctor ordinarily closes the surgical incision and either covers it with a bulky bandage at first or leaves the special tape strips or stitches open to the air. The tape strips fall off by themselves in about two weeks, and the doctor removes any stitches of the kind that are not absorbed by the body. Sometimes staples are used instead of stitches, and the doctor easily removes these with a staple remover about a week after surgery. Occasionally, the surgeon must leave the incision open to heal from the inside out, in which case it will need irrigation or special dressings.

Doctors and nurses will inspect the skin around the incision site to be sure that it is clean, retains normal skin color except for initial bruising, and is free of pus drainage. They look for signs of infection and for any large collection of tissue fluid or blood that may need to be drained. The woman continues to check the area after she goes home and seeks immediate medical help if anything looks or feels significantly different.

No matter how gorgeous an incision looks to the surgeon, it usually looks a lot less beautiful to its owner. In fact, the swelling will go down, the bruising will disappear, and the scar will fade. However, scars heal differently for every woman. Most of them get "uglier" with the normal healing process before they begin fading. Some scars eventually become almost invisible, while others—no matter how careful the doctor may have been—build up thick scar tissue, called **keloid**. While some women swear that rubbing vitamin E oil along the incision reduces scarring, many surgeons caution that doing this during the first several weeks after surgery slows the normal healing process. Although several scar creams and gels are available, the subject of scar healing needs much more research. The woman who forms keloids may want to talk with a plastic surgeon about new options.

SENSATIONS Studies indicate that nearly half of all people who get the kind of pain therapy routinely given after surgery—pain medicine p.r.n., or only when the patient requests it—still have moderate to severe pain. *P.r.n.*

pain therapy is often not enough. Most people expect to have pain after surgery, but studies have shown that pain can actually slow down the healing process and be a cause of postoperative problems. There are new methods and medications that can control postoperative pain.

For example, the doctor may order a patient-controlled analgesia (PCA) pump, which delivers IV pain medication directly into the vein when the woman presses a button. Following the doctor's orders, the nurse programs the pump to deliver a small continuous stream of medication and/or to give a set dose at certain intervals (1 mg of morphine no more often than every fifteen minutes, for instance). The woman does not have to wait for the nurse and often uses less medicine because she can always "stay ahead of the pain."

The pain medicine given in the first days after surgery may be a narcotic or a powerful nonnarcotic. Common routes for pain medicines are into the vein with an IV, under the skin or into the muscle with a shot, through a tiny tube into the space around the spine (an epidural), or by mouth. Using narcotics for a few days after surgery does not turn a woman into a drug addict. They do make some women feel woozy, however, and they slow down the intestinal tract, so constipation is possible. Nondrug treatments include massage, hot and cold packs, transcutaneous electrical nerve stimulation (TENS), relaxation, music or other distractions, and imagery.

Adequate pain control not only keeps the woman comfortable, but also helps her do what she needs to do to recover from surgery. It makes no sense for her to "tough it out" and refuse pain medicine—and then develop a blood clot or pneumonia because it hurts her too much to walk around, deep breathe, and cough.

Nausea is fairly common following surgery. One cause is anesthesia, which barely fazes some women but leaves others feeling nauseated for a day or longer. Pain medicine leads to nausea in some people. Women who have undergone surgery for gynecologic or colon cancers may feel nausea because of the digestive tract manipulation. In any case, there are some effective medicines for nausea—if the woman requests them.

Recovery "Do-It-Yourself"

There is a lot of "do-it-yourself" in recovering from surgery. General anesthesia insults the lungs and temporarily paralyzes the small hairs that line them and normally sweep out any impurities. In addition, when the woman lies on her back, common during and after surgery, the lungs have to expand against gravity. All this puts the lungs at risk for developing little collapsed areas, so they do not exchange oxygen and other gases—or cool the body—as effectively as they should. Any collapsed areas (atelectasis) can become a haven for lurking bacteria.

To prevent serious lung problems, the woman can breathe very deeply several times an hour while she is awake. If she is breathing correctly, filling her lungs to their depths, her diaphragm and abdomen will move out as she inhales and in when she exhales. She can check this movement by placing her hands flat on the abdomen, resting the thumbs on the bottom ribs on each side.

To help her breathe more effectively, a woman may be given a plastic gadget called an **incentive spirometer**. She inhales through a tube (rather like sucking on a large straw), which makes balls or some other device rise in a chamber so that she can gauge how deeply she is breathing. Seeing the concrete evidence of improvement inspires her to throw in an extra practice now and then—the "incentive" part.

Effective coughing moves any "junk" out of the lungs or at least keeps it from settling in and causing trouble. Holding a pillow or the hands firmly over the incision splints the area and makes it much more comfortable to cough. A woman can often trigger a cough by taking three slow, deep breaths in through the mouth and then holding the last breath.

Our bodies are built to move. They work much better when they do and get into trouble when they do not. At first, when the woman is still confined to bed, she can turn from side to side and exercise her legs and arms, moving them in small circles or contracting and relaxing them. This helps keep her blood moving so it does not pool and form a clot.

As soon as possible, however, she gets out of bed and begins walking—a few steps at first and then more. It gets easier quickly. Walking

+ helps expand the lungs

+ brings blood to the surgical site and begins gently stretching the tissues for prompt healing and greater comfort

+ keeps the blood from forming clots

+ helps get the digestive tract moving again (and is the best remedy around for the gas "cramps" that can make a person utterly miserable a few days after abdominal surgery)

+ protects the skin from bedsores

+ feels good

Once a woman is on her feet, it is not too difficult to walk; getting out of or into bed is the challenge. After enough surgeries to qualify me for "frequent-user upgrades," I know the secrets: It is much easier if one takes a deep breath beforehand and then moves while breathing out; this automatically relaxes the muscles so they do not tighten up and complain. The other technique is to move in one piece as much as possible. To help herself do this, the woman plans beforehand what she is going to do, and then uses her arms, the bed control, and the nurse as needed. A wheelchair, if one is available, makes a handy companion the first times out: Walking behind it holding on to the handles gives her a broad base to lean on—and a seat if she gets tired. An IV pole works well if it moves smoothly and does not tip easily.

RADIATION

Radiation therapy devices control the immense energy provided by atoms in transition and focus it to destroy local nests of cancer cells. Radiation can be used to destroy or shrink a primary tumor or to "sterilize" an area where a tumor was removed but that may still contain some stray cancer cells, such as the breast tissue remaining after lumpectomy surgery. It can also work well on a small metastasis made up of cells known to be sensitive to radiation, such as a bone "met." The radiation can come from a machine outside the body, as in **external radiation therapy,** or it can be delivered from an **internal radiation** source placed inside the body.

What is radiation, and how does it work? Every atom tries to be electrically stable, with the positive electrical charges at the core of the atom exactly balancing and holding in place the electrons, the negative charges orbiting outside the core. If there are too many negative charges to hold onto, these extra electrons (ions) rush away from the atom in a stream or ray of energy. This can happen because certain atoms are naturally unstable; certain variations (isotopes) of the elements uranium or cobalt, for example, are always in transition (radioactive) because their electrical charges are unbalanced. Or an ordinarily stable atom can purposely be made unstable in a specially designed machine.

If radiation rays reach the body, they collide with and disrupt the DNA in the body's cells and change the electrical balance in the molecules of the cells or the cell environment. The cells can die or can mutate; if they mutate but are still able to divide, they can pass along this mutation to daughter cells. If many cells get moderately damaged, the uncontrolled ionizing radiation can itself cause cancer (as occurred years after the atom bomb was dropped on Hiroshima).

In contrast, radiation therapy targets small local clusters of cancer cells for total destruction: The cancer cells either die immediately or are so damaged they can no longer divide. The rest of the body, which could not survive even a moderate dose of radiation given to the whole body, tolerates a very large dose given to a small area quite well (although radiation oncologists must work to protect the normal cells of the body).

However radiation therapy is delivered, there is some natural protection for the body. Because a cell's DNA is most exposed when the cell is dividing, the fast-dividing cancer cells are far more vulnerable to radiation than are most of the body's normal cells. Thus, while a lethal dose of rays will kill some normal cells in its path because they happen to be dividing, it will kill far more cancer cells.

External Radiation

External radiation machines either use a naturally occurring radioactive material (often a cobalt isotope) or, increasingly, make a stable isotope unstable and thus radioactive. In the machine, the electrons streaming from their source accelerate as they pass across some kind of high-energy field. The high-speed electrons then strike a positively charged target, which breaks them into even smaller "pieces" and focuses them in one direction: the radiation beam.

Depending on how fast they are moving, these packets of electrical energy can be made up of "pure energy," like X rays and gamma rays, or larger "particles" of energy, like electron, alpha, and beta rays.

The "pure energy" X rays and gamma rays can penetrate to the deeper tissues before releasing their payload of energy. Unable to penetrate so deeply, the lower-voltage "particle" rays work at skin level or just below. Most of the machines used now have an extremely high energy field and produce either X rays or gamma rays. However, the linear accelerator, a machine used frequently, can also be set with a lower energy field, producing an electron beam, if that is needed.

The radiation therapist selects the rays that work at the depth of the tumor. The beam is aimed to hit the cancer area while avoiding any vital organs near it. For instance, radiating a breast straight on could cause significant damage to the nearby lungs and heart, so the radiation is aimed at the breast "tangentially," from different angles. (Much of radiation oncology is physics—or maybe billiards!)

The total amount of radiation to be given is divided over daily doses, so that the normal cells that are in the way and cannot escape entirely (like the skin) have a chance to recover somewhat between doses. The amount of radiation is expressed in interchangeable units called rads or CentiGrays (cGy). For example, a woman might be scheduled to get a total of 4,500 rads, divided into doses of 150 rads every weekday for six weeks.

Still another strategy is to protect nearby areas with shields that block the radiation. These may be ready-made or custom-fit for the woman, and they are put in place every day before the treatment.

Healthy tissue resists radiation much better than weakened tissue does. Thus, the radiation therapy (RT) staff will encourage the woman to maintain very good nutrition. It is also important that she stay at a stable weight during therapy so that the treatment field does not change. She is also asked to keep the skin in the path of the radiation beam clean, gently dried, and lubricated with a product the RT department recommends.

Before external radiation treatment begins, the woman meets with the radiation oncologist at the hospital to learn about the therapy and undergo a full physical examination. She often undergoes imaging tests, such as CT or MRI, so that the radiation oncologist has all the necessary information about the tumor and the exact location of her vital organs before setting up the treatment field.

The radiation oncologist may then work with a radiation physicist or dosimetrist to discuss the most effective and safest angles and doses for the radiation beam. Together, they work out a radiation "prescription" for the woman.

The woman then comes to the hospital for **simulation**, a dry run of the treatment. No actual radiation is delivered during simulation, but the unfamiliar and often exceedingly "high-tech" machines can be unnerving. Simulation can be a lengthy process, as the radiation oncologist and technologists mark the skin to show the proposed field, assess angles, decide on and perhaps construct shields, take regular X rays to see if they have got it right, and so on.

Because it is crucial that the radiation machines treat exactly the same area each day, the technologists will mark the skin with either marking pens or tattoos to show the radiation field. The woman is told not to wash off any felt-tip pen markings, but they may need to be touched up frequently. They tend to sweat off or rub off on clothes, so clothes that need to be dry-cleaned should be avoided. They also make some women feel uncomfortably like marked beef at the butcher shop.

If tattooing is used, tiny purplish dots of dye are injected under the skin; it feels like pinpricks. Only a few tattoos are needed to mark the boundaries of the radiation field, but they are permanent, so that a doctor can always tell where radiation has been given. This is important because there are strict limits to how much total radiation can be given safely to one area.

Either the same day as the simulation or soon thereafter, the woman has her first actual treatment. This involves a few minutes of setting up, during which the technologist helps her get into exactly the right position, with, perhaps, foam pads placed under her head and knees, skin bared in the treatment field, and any shields put into place.

The technologist then goes to a computer console in an adjoining room from where he can still see the woman through a window. Alone in the room, the woman lies still but breathes normally during the minute or so the radiation is actually given. There is no pain or other physical sensation, although some women claim they feel warm or cool in the area of the radiation, which makes it easy for them to visualize the rays demolishing the cancer cells. After completion of the dose, the technologist returns and readjusts the woman and the machine if radiation is to be given from more than one angle. *The woman is not radioactive in any way at any time when she is undergoing radiation from an external machine.*

And that is all there is to the treatment, which may be repeated every day: usually some waiting, then a few minutes for setup, and a couple of minutes of radiation. The radiation oncologist will see the woman about once a week and may order periodic blood tests or imaging studies to keep track of her progress.

What are the common side effects? Severe (but temporary) fatigue is common—and surprising to many women. This occurs not only because the body has to work to repair the cellular damage from radiation, but also because of the wearying daily trips to and from the hospital. It is more severe if the woman is not eating well. Fatigue usually sets in a few weeks after treatment begins.

Temporary skin damage, like a sunburn, is common in the treatment field. This begins a few weeks after treatment starts: Radiation attacks the fast-dividing living cells beneath the surface skin layer of dead cells, and it takes a few weeks for the affected cells to reach the surface.

The deeper-penetrating X rays and gamma rays go through the skin without releasing much of their energy there, so skin damage is usually fairly mild; the shallower beta or electron rays cause more skin damage. The "sunburn" turns to tan and ordinarily fades within several weeks, although some people experience a permanent change in pigmentation. If damage is greater, the skin may become "weepy." Because weepy skin can be an entryway for germs and infection, radiation may be postponed for a few days or other treatment prescribed. Fair, sensitive skin is no more likely than other skin to be damaged. After radiation, the skin and the underlying tissues often feel thicker and firmer.

Each radiation therapy department has its own list of acceptable skin-care products. Some unacceptable products contain aluminum or other substances that might deflect radiation or intensify it.

Other possible side effects from external radiation depend on the area being treated, such as nausea or diarrhea if any of the intestinal tract is in the field of radiation. Specific side effects are discussed in the chapters on the individual cancers.

Internal Radiation

The other way to receive radiation treatment is from a radioactive source that is placed inside the body and continues to emit energy for a specified time. Each source is a radioactive isotope, which continues to decay—lose electrons and emit radiation at a certain known rate—until the oversupply of electrons is gone.

Occasionally, a radioactive isotope is injected into a woman's blood vessel and travels through her body while it continues to decay. These rays have not been accelerated and energized in a machine so they cannot go very far or escape through the skin. The woman can come and go as she wishes, and the radioactivity poses no risk to anyone else.

When a sealed source of radiation is placed inside the body, the treatment is called **brachytherapy**. The treatment plan for a gynecologic cancer might include inserting an empty applicator into a body cavity (such as the uterus) while the woman is in the operating room. Later, in the hospital room, the container is "afterloaded" with a sealed source of radioactive material that is brought to the room in a lead-lined box and inserted with special tongs.

The filled applicator is left in place to emit its rays for a certain number of days and is then removed. Because the body cavity is not closed completely on all sides, it is an inadequate barrier for the rays. Thus, the woman is considered radioactive the entire time the loaded applicator is in place, and she remains in her hospital room with a "Danger: Radioactive" sign on the door so that no one else is exposed unnecessarily. Visitors and health professionals follow very strict guidelines about how close they can be to her, and for how long, and they may use lead screens to shield themselves. Her body wastes are monitored for radioactive material and the nurses use special techniques to dispose of them.

Some of the same precautions apply when tiny radioactive seeds are afterloaded into minute tubes threaded through the skin and directly into the tumor area. The seeds and tubes are removed in thirty-six hours or so. As soon as any radioactive source is removed, the woman is no longer radioactive.

Typically, the woman hospitalized for brachytherapy feels very bored, quite isolated, emotionally strange (an "untouchable") and, depending on the applicator, somewhat physically uncomfortable. She may be on strict bedrest if there is any chance that the applicator could be dislodged with movement.

Occasionally, radioactive seeds are injected directly into the tumor and are allowed to decay naturally without ever having to be removed. Her radiation oncologist will tell the woman the precautions to use to protect other people.

However a woman receives radiation treatment, she will have many questions for her health-care professionals. Like every other woman undergoing local therapies for cancer, she has the right to answers—in words she understands.

— *Kerry McGinn*

CHAPTER **8**

SYSTEMIC TREATMENTS
FOR CANCER

Unlike the local therapies for cancer, the systemic therapies—chemotherapy, hormonal therapy, and biological therapy—work throughout the whole body, moving through the bloodstream and beyond to sniff out and destroy cancer cell "strays." They work on local tumors too, but usually not as effectively as the local treatments do.

CHEMOTHERAPY

". . . and so, of course, you'll need chemotherapy."

I don't cry easily but, as my surgeon said that to me over the phone, the tears started streaming down my face. I was scared because I had to acknowledge that there might be cancer cells loose in my body—and I was almost equally terrified by the whole prospect of "chemo."

That night I wrote the first poem I had written in years. Chemo became, for me, a "sky-wrenching" downpour that would flush any cancer cells out of my body. The last part of the poem went like this:

> *Umbrellas are not much use in a storm like this.*
> *It will be a long wet trudge home*
> *Until I am dry again.*

"Long trudge" says it fairly well for me. I won't try to pretend I loved chemotherapy, but I tolerated a few months of treatment to get "home" again to my goal of long-term good health. For me, in fact, chemo was not as bad as the horror stories and my imagination had painted it.

Chemotherapy is a different experience for every woman. How she responds to chemo depends not only on the regimen itself—there are all kinds and combinations of drugs and ways of receiving them—but also on how the woman's body and mind respond. Chemo hits some women pretty hard and barely fazes others, while many women are somewhere in the middle, with at least some tiredness and a sprinkling of other symptoms.

In the last few years many chemo "courses" have become shorter. Effective new medications, products, and techniques help relieve side effects. All of this makes the process easier. As scary as it is to wait for that first chemo dose, it makes sense to adopt a "wait and see" approach.

Why Use Chemotherapy?

Cancer chemotherapy is the use of drugs to kill cancer cells throughout the body. The doctor may recommend it for one of several reasons:

- ✦ If it is *known* that cancer cells have spread from the organ where they originated. In case of known distant metastasis, chemotherapy can often relieve current symptoms or prevent or postpone future ones.

- ✦ If it is *reasonably suspected* that cancer cells might have strayed. **Adjuvant,** or assisting, chemotherapy means cancer drugs given in addition to surgery and/or radiation to kill any microscopic metastases that *might* be lingering in the body after all the known cancer has been removed.

- ✦ To decrease the size of a solid tumor so that it can be treated with a local therapy, or as control or palliation if local treatment is not possible.

Obviously, if there is no detectable disease to start with, as with adjuvant chemotherapy, doctors cannot see immediate results from chemotherapy. In general, however, they hope for **complete remission,** in which no more disease can be detected in the body, whether for a brief time or for long enough to be considered a cure. There can be **partial remission,** in which the detectable disease (such as the size of a tumor) decreases by at least 50 percent. Even **stabilization** of a cancer at a level where it is not causing major symptoms can significantly improve the overall quality of a woman's life.

Oncologists usually prescribe chemotherapy drugs by looking at how *groups* of people with a similar diagnosis have fared on specific drugs or drug combinations. But *individual* tumors in *individual* people react in *individual* ways. This means that, especially when the oncologist is prescribing adjuvant chemotherapy and cannot see immediate results, a patient might not get the chemotherapy that would work best against her cancer, or she might get chemotherapy with little chance to benefit her.

In theory, at least, a laboratory test that looks at how pieces of an individual tumor respond to different drugs or drug combinations *in vitro* (in the test tube) could give valuable information about which drugs have the best chance of working *in vivo* (in the woman's body). That is the idea behind cell culture drug resistance testing and chemosensitivity assays, several of which have become commercially available or are currently being developed to test which chemotherapy drugs a specific tumor is "resistant" or "sensitive" to. The most accurate of these assays correctly predict resistance (what does not work in the body) over 90 percent of the time and sensitivity (what does work) over 75 percent of the time. Plainly, though, what happens in the test tube does not always happen in just the same way in the body.

The biggest problem with getting an assay is that it requires planning *before* surgery so that the surgeon or pathologist has the special container and mailing package available to send fresh (not frozen) tumor to the company. Getting an assay also requires a tumor specimen that is large enough for the pathologist to get necessary diagnostic information and still have some tumor to send; the more tissue available, the more drugs or combinations that can be tested. An assay typically takes a week or longer and costs about $1,000.

Early assays were so inaccurate that they did not offer much help, and many doctors are not aware that they have improved significantly. Often, assays are neither necessary nor useful, but it may be worth asking about them—before surgery—if chemotherapy is likely. Both doctors and women can find out more from cancer journals or from the Internet; useful Internet search terms include *chemosensitivity*, *cell culture drug resistance testing*, or *Weisenthal Cancer Group*.

How Chemotherapy Works

Because cancer cells divide more often than most normal cells do, they are more vulnerable to drugs that interrupt the cell cycle. The side effects of drugs occur because the other body cells, especially those that normally divide often, are not immune. However, healthy normal cells bounce back much better than dysfunctional cancer cells do. The science (and art) of giving chemotherapy lies in killing as many cancer cells as possible without permanently damaging too many healthy ones.

Most of the traditional chemo drugs fall into one of four classifications, often called "the four As," with each classification working differently. **Antimetabolites** attack as the cell is dividing and starve it by giving it a fake nutrient. **Alkylating agents** bind with the cell's DNA during any phase of the cell cycle to prevent the cell from dividing. **Antitumor antibiotics** (not to be confused with the kind of antibiotics used for infections) infiltrate the DNA so that the cell cannot grow. **Vinca alkaloids** interfere with the formation of the chromosomal "spindles" necessary for cell division. During the last few years, new chemo drugs have been produced that work by different mechanisms and do not fit into the four As (such as Taxol, which is from the yew tree and has received considerable publicity).

Many chemotherapy regimens combine two or more drugs on a certain schedule to maximize the effectiveness of each agent. This fighting on all fronts combines noncycle-specific drugs, which attack at any time during the cycle, with cycle-specific agents. This combination approach can also "confuse" the cancer cells so that they do not develop a resistance to the individual drugs.

A course of chemotherapy usually consists of the same cycle of drugs repeated two or more times. The course may last from two to twelve months, depending on the type of cancer and the treatment protocol. Typically, each cycle lasts a few weeks and includes time for giving the drugs, waiting for them to work, and then allowing the body to recover and rest somewhat before the next cycle starts.

The oncologist planning the cycle considers the strengths and weaknesses of each drug to decide what to give when. For instance, if drug A, given on day one of the cycle, is known to take eight days to "set up" the cancer cells so that they are at their most vulnerable to drug B, then drug B would be given on day eight.

Each chemotherapy cycle is expected to kill a percentage of cancer cells everywhere in the body. Between cycles, the cancer cells that are not killed continue to divide, but before they recover too many of their numbers, the next cycle attacks. Thus, if one cycle kills 75 out of every 100 cancer cells, 25 will still be left. The remaining cells may rebuild to 27 before the next cycle of chemo destroys 75 percent of the remainder, leaving 7 cells to face the next onslaught. The idea is to get the cancer cells down to a number that the body's own defenses can handle.

Chemotherapy drugs are strong medicine, and there is a fairly narrow line between the amount that kills cancer cells and the amount that can kill the person. However, doctors need to give doses that are strong enough to be effective. This means that any chemotherapy must be prescribed by someone—usually a medical oncologist—who knows the drugs, their toxicities, and their side effects thoroughly. The oncologist either administers the chemotherapy directly or oversees specially trained chemotherapy nurses who perform the actual administration.

Receiving Chemotherapy

The first appointment includes a history, a physical examination, and plenty of discussion—but usually no chemotherapy. The oncologist talks about the goal of therapy, the potential benefits, the course and cycle being recommended, the drugs and what they do, and the risks and side effects. The course advised depends on the history and the results of the physical exam, the records from pathology and any surgery or radiation therapy, laboratory and imaging tests, and the statistical chances that chemotherapy can make the specific situation better. Then the woman goes home to think about it.

If she chooses to go ahead with chemo and will be receiving treatment in the doctor's office or a hospital "infusion center," it makes sense for her to bring someone with her the first time to see how she reacts to the medicines—and just to hold her hand. Ordinarily, however, even if she does experience side effects, they will not appear until several hours later.

What might a chemo appointment be like? The woman has a "complete blood count" drawn, either beforehand or in the doctor's office. She may take a prescription antinausea pill and may see the oncologist, often once per cycle, for a brief physical exam and to talk about how treatment is going.

The oncologist or oncology nurse inserts an IV catheter into a hand or arm vein and either "pushes" (injects with a syringe) or drips one or more chemo agents from an IV bag. When this is finished, the IV catheter is removed, the woman sits in the office for a few minutes to be sure she does not develop a reaction to the drugs, and then she goes home.

A cycle for one common regimen for breast cancer has the woman receiving two drugs injected through a vein, a process that takes a few minutes, on the first and eighth day of her twenty-eight-day chemotherapy cycle. She also takes a specified number of chemotherapy pills at home every day from the first day through day fourteen, and then spends the last two weeks of the cycle recovering.

Another woman, who has ovarian cancer, also might have a twenty-eight-day chemotherapy cycle, but she spends the first four days of each cycle in the hospital receiving continuous IV chemotherapy, and then goes home to recover for twenty-four days until the next cycle starts.

Still another woman, with metastatic cancer, may get a continuous, tiny infusion of one chemotherapy drug dispensed by a small pump she carries with her at all times and brings to the oncologist's office to be refilled. The idea behind this technique, used most often with metastatic cancer when other therapies have not worked, is to use small, constant "zaps" without giving the cancer cells time to recover.

Systemic Treatments for Cancer

103

Chemotherapy Routes

Chemotherapy drugs can be swallowed as pills or in another oral form, injected under the skin or into the muscle, given directly into a vein or artery, or infused into a body cavity. Depending on the most effective **route** for each drug—how it needs to be given to work best and most predictably—it can be given in the hospital or the doctor's office, or it can be taken by the woman at home.

A common route is through the vein. This gives the drug immediate access to the circulatory system where cancer cells can hide, and the drugs can go anywhere in the body that the circulatory system reaches. It is also worth noting that some chemotherapy drugs are deactivated if they are taken by mouth and have to travel through the digestive tract, and it is uncertain how well and quickly some drugs will be absorbed.

Some women have large veins in their arms and have no problems receiving drugs intravenously. Other women have veins that make it difficult to start and keep IV access. Others may be receiving a chemotherapy agent that is especially rough on the veins or can cause major local damage if it reaches the tissues surrounding the vein. Even a woman with "good" veins may be at risk when receiving the most damaging of these, the **vesicants**.

The woman who either has "poor" arm veins or is scheduled to receive a vesicant or similar drug may need longer-lasting access to a large central vein in the chest. There are all sorts of access devices that can last for several weeks, months, or even years. They can be used to give IV medications and to draw blood for blood tests (see the chart on page 105).

Occasionally, the oncologist wants the chemotherapy to target an organ that is connected to a large artery. For a liver metastasis, for instance, chemo might be infused into an artery and go directly to the liver. This kind **of intra-arterial chemotherapy** is given with a special pump to overcome the blood pressure in the artery. In this case, chemotherapy is being used more as a local treatment than a systemic one.

Intraperitoneal chemotherapy, which is sometimes used in ovarian cancer, infuses the chemo into the abdominal cavity through a special access chamber on the abdomen or chest. Since the chemo stays in one place, bathing the organs in the abdomen, the side effects are confined to that area and the drug can be given in very high doses.

Side Effects of Chemotherapy

Each chemotherapy drug follows its own pattern of which kinds of fast-dividing normal cells it attacks, but the cells most often affected are those

Devices used to Access a Central Vein

Peripherally inserted central catheter (PICC): long catheter inserted into arm vein, threaded up through arm to central vein.

> *Advantages:* easy insertion by specially trained nurse; requires no surgery to insert or remove. Easy to access: remove cap and begin therapy.

> *Disadvantages:* not appropriate for long-term therapy (over six weeks or so): catheter must be flushed every few days and site dressing changed; catheter visible on arm.

> *Most useful:* if woman's arm veins "give out" near end of chemo.

Nontunneled central catheter: catheter inserted directly into central vein near collarbone.

> *Advantages:* no surgery to insert. Can have two or three separate "lumens" (channels) if needed. Easy to access.

> *Disadvantages:* not appropriate for long-term therapy (more than a month): catheter must be flushed and site dressing changed; catheter visible on upper chest.

> *Most useful:* if woman's arm veins "give out" near end of therapy and she needs multiple IV access.

Tunneled central catheter (Hickman, Groshong, etc.): catheter inserted in skin and then tunneled through tissue for several inches before it enters central vein.

> *Advantages:* can be used indefinitely. Can have several lumens. Easy to access.

> *Disadvantages:* minor surgical procedure to insert. Catheter must be flushed regularly and site care given. Catheter visible on chest.

> *Most useful:* long-term use for woman who needs frequent IV access for therapy and for blood tests.

Implanted port (portaCath, LifePort, PASport, etc.): small metal or plastic port, stitched into place under skin, connected to catheter. Some ports rest under the chest or abdominal skin with the catheter inserted directly into a central vein.

> *Advantages:* can be used indefinitely. Port is under skin so that, except when port is being used, no catheter shows above the skin and no skin care is necessary. A few larger ports have more than one lumen.

> *Disadvantages:* minor surgical procedures when port is implanted and removed. More difficult access: needle stick, using special technique and supplies necessary to access port through the skin; must be done each time the port is used and to flush port once a month or so when it isn't being used. Small scars from insertion and removal. Port can show as round bump under skin.

> *Most useful:* woman undergoing long-term therapy who needs IV access only once or twice a month. There are also several small ambulatory ("carry around") or implanted pumps to deliver continuous small doses of chemo.

Possible complications with any central line include infection, vein irritation, or a blood clot.

in the bone marrow, which make blood cells for the body; in the hair follicles; along the digestive tract; and in the ovaries. Almost everyone who undergoes chemotherapy also suffers some degree of fatigue.

There is no correlation between the number and severity of side effects a woman experiences and how well the chemo is working. Therapy can be completely effective for the woman who sails through treatment. And attitude definitely matters: If a woman thinks of chemotherapy as powerful and effective medicine, she will probably tolerate any side effects better (and may even have fewer) than the woman who looks at the treatment as terrible poison.

FATIGUE   "I don't have much energy" is probably the most common general complaint of people who receive chemotherapy. Fatigue is the broad term for many connected symptoms: tiredness, lack of energy, exhaustion, weakness, inability to concentrate, sleepiness, no "get up and go," lack of interest in doing things. The fatigue from chemo ranges from "just a little tired once in a while" to "so tired I can't move." The fatigue tends to follow the chemo cycle and gets better during the recovery phase, but it also tends to get somewhat worse with later cycles. Because many people feel "wiped out" for at least a day after IV chemo, it makes sense for a woman to schedule treatment so that she can have a couple of days of downtime afterward (such as Friday afternoon appointments for a working woman, so that she can rest over the weekend before going back to work). Another common fatigue time occurs several days to two weeks after the drugs are given, at a predictable time when the blood cells in the body are at their lowest point from the chemotherapy before they start building up again.

No one is absolutely sure why there is fatigue (although fatigue with cancer and its treatment has become a very popular research topic in the last few years, which may mean more answers soon). It could be because the whole body is working overtime to dispose of dead cancer cells and rebuild healthy cells. Also, the psyche is struggling to cope with the changes cancer is making—more hard work. The woman is often not eating or sleeping well and may not be getting much exercise. During the later cycles she may be somewhat anemic, if chemotherapy affects her red blood cells. If she is tired, she may have to decrease her activities, which may leave her feeling bored and useless, which, in turn, increases her tiredness—a vicious cycle. Depression, insomnia, pain, and fatigue all feed upon each other; for instance, the woman who is fatigued may feel depressed because of her limitations, which, in turn, saps her energy more.

My favorite general fatigue-fighting recommendations for the woman beginning a course of chemo are these:

1. Be very kind to yourself and listen to your body (take a nap, do not drag yourself to an event).

2. Schedule a treat for yourself during the recovery period in each cycle to serve as your carrot on a stick (a simple overnight trip, perhaps).

3. Get some kind of exercise as often as possible. Amazingly enough, a program of walking and other mild exercise often makes women feel more energetic.

MORE ON EXERCISE Some women who were ardent exercisers before a cancer diagnosis continue their regimes with little change. Among other benefits, a reasonable exercise program decreases stress, increases appetite, and promotes sleep and digestion—and just makes people feel better. One caution: Many doctors do not want patients to exercise vigorously for a day or so before any blood test because exercise temporarily increases blood cell counts toward normal, a benefit most of the time but not when the doctor wants "real" blood test results.

Many women find that fighting fatigue is counterproductive and that it works better to relax more (some use relaxation training), ignore anything that does not absolutely have to be done, and pace their activities.

If chemotherapy leads to major anemia, the woman may need more than iron pills and healthful eating to improve her energy level (see the following section on bone marrow side effects).

BONE MARROW SIDE EFFECTS How chemotherapy affects the marrow in the large bones of the body is the side effect that worries doctors most. The **bone marrow** produces the white blood cells that protect the body, the platelets that help blood to clot, and the red blood cells that deliver oxygen everywhere in the body. The white blood cells and platelets turn over very quickly in the body, lasting only a few hours to a few days, and thus are especially vulnerable to chemotherapy. The red cells, on the other hand, divide every several months—so that their numbers usually dip significantly only after a few months of chemotherapy (or very high doses of specific drugs).

Each chemotherapy drug has a known **nadir,** the number of days after it is administered before the white blood count and the platelets reach their lowest point and start rebounding. Different drugs and dosages affect the bone marrow differently, and that is one of the factors oncologists balance when they are combining chemo drugs.

The oncologist usually orders a complete blood count at the beginning of each cycle and sometimes at the nadir to see what is happening. The woman will probably be told to report quickly any signs of infection or bleeding, especially at nadir. Other than that, she ordinarily will not need to pay much attention to what is occurring in her bone marrow, because the body normally maintains a wide safety margin in its total number of white blood cells and platelets. For many women receiving standard doses of many chemotherapy drugs, blood cell changes do not pose any major problems.

However, if a woman has an extreme drop in **neutrophils,** a specific kind of white blood cell that protects the body against infection, she is considered **neutropenic**. This means that she is at definite risk of infection. Some of the normal signs of infection, such as redness, heat, and swelling, happen as a direct result of the white blood cells' battle against bacteria or other causes of infection—but without enough white blood cells these usual signs may not occur. What a woman needs to watch for especially are fever (a quite reliable sign), shaking chills, pain when urinating, coughing, chest pain, shortness of breath, sore throat, severe headache or stiff neck, and pain at an IV site.

If a woman is due to have chemotherapy but her blood test shows that the number of white blood cells has fallen below a certain level, even with no signs of infection the doctor will usually postpone chemo for a week and recheck the blood work. Some doctors will prescribe "just-in-case" antibiotics until her white blood cell count climbs to a safer level. At the first sign of any infection, she may be hospitalized to receive IV antibiotics. (Unfortunately, there are no safe white blood cell transfusions.)

When doctors prescribe a chemo regimen that usually makes people severely neutropenic, they may also prescribe a daily "shot" of a blood cell growth factor for a few days, starting at least twenty-four hours after the chemotherapy is given. **Granulocyte colony stimulating factor** (G-CSF, filgrastim, Neupogen) is a biological agent, a type of protein that stimulates the bone marrow to produce more neutrophils faster so there is a lesser and shorter dip. When doctors give huge doses of chemotherapy for a stem cell or bone marrow transplant, they may use **granulocyte-macrophage colony stimulating factor** (GM-CSF, sargramostim, Leukine) to speed up production of both neutrophils and the white blood cells called **macrophages**. Neither G-CSF nor GM-CSF prevents neutropenia, but they make it milder and shorter so there is much less chance of serious infection. These growth factors are very expensive, which is why they are used only in situations where there is high risk of infection. They also require daily injections under the skin; the woman or a family member often learns to give these.

An extreme drop in platelets (**thrombocytopenia**) puts a woman at risk for bleeding. She may never have any bleeding, but she may notice nosebleeds, bleeding gums, pink or red urine, bloody or tarry black stools, unexplained bruises, or several tiny, flat, round, purplish-red spots on the skin. The basic problems are bleeding longer than normal after an injury or bleeding after activities that would not usually cause a problem. Severe thrombocytopenia is often treated with platelet transfusions until the woman's own platelets bounce back. Clinical trials of biological agents such as **recombinant human interleukin-11** are currently, if slowly, underway to see if they effectively and safely reduce the need for platelet transfusions.

The woman who knows her platelet count is very low needs to brush her teeth very gently and avoid flossing if it makes her gums bleed, keep her bowel movements soft so constipation does not cause bleeding, use sanitary napkins rather than tampons if she has menstrual periods so that the vagina does not get irritated and bleed, and avoid taking aspirin or similar drugs that can increase bleeding. Sometimes she will receive hormone treatment to stop her periods temporarily while she is receiving chemotherapy. If skin or gum bleeding occurs, she can apply gentle pressure for at least five minutes.

In contrast, the red blood cell life cycle is rather leisurely, so that it takes the red cell count longer to dip, but also longer to recover on its own. After a few months of treatment, severe anemia may occur because of decreased red cells, and the woman may feel extremely tired or short of breath. Severe anemia is usually treated with blood transfusions. To prevent or treat some kinds of serious anemia, the doctor may prescribe epoetin alfa (erythropoietin, Epogen, Procrit). This biologic agent, which mimics a hormone produced by the kidneys, speeds up production of red blood cells in the bone marrow. Like the growth factors for white blood cell production, epoetin alfa is expensive and requires injections, often three times a week for several weeks.

Moving a proposed new medicine from development through clinical trials into clinical use takes many years, a frustrating process for any woman waiting impatiently for treatment, although probably necessary in terms of judging drug safety and effectiveness. One website for checking the progress of new drugs against these blood problems (and other chemotherapy and biological therapies) is www.phrma.org/searchcures/newmeds/webdb.

HAIR LOSS While doctors worry about the effects of chemotherapy on bone marrow, most women are more concerned about the possibility of losing their hair. Not every chemo drug targets the fast-dividing hair cells, but plenty of them cause some women to lose some hair, and a few cause almost every woman to lose all or most of her hair. The oncologist should inform the woman about how the specific drugs she will receive are likely to affect her hair.

This temporary **alopecia** (hair loss) may affect not only the scalp, but also the eyebrows and eyelashes, pubic hair, and underarm hair. The hair may start regrowing near the end of chemo or soon afterward—and the silver lining to this cloud is that even normally straight, limp hair often regrows as thick, lustrous, and curly. This lasts for about two years, and then the hair reverts to its former texture. Many a woman, asked about her gorgeous hair several months after chemo ends, has had to give primary credit to her oncologist!

With the drugs that cause major alopecia, the scalp tends to become tingly and "strange feeling" two to three weeks after the drug is first given. The hair begins falling out, a little at first and then in large clumps. Almost no woman is really prepared for the loss.

If a woman knows she is going to receive one of these drugs, it is smart to get her hair cut as short as possible beforehand; that way the handfuls of hair on her pillow or in the shower are smaller and a little less devastating. Some women put a strip of tape across a strip of hair before it is cut, and then tape or sew across the strip to make bangs to wear under a scarf or turban.

Washing her hair very gently, combing it without pulling it, avoiding harsh hair products, and using a satin pillowcase to avoid friction on the scalp may postpone hair loss. If their hair starts falling out, many women wear a cotton scarf or turban in bed to collect the hair, or may consider shaving the scalp.

It is easier for the woman who plans to wear a wig to begin shopping for one while the salesperson can see her natural hair color and style. Some shops specialize in hairpieces for people undergoing chemotherapy; addresses should be in the telephone book or available from the oncologist, the local American Cancer Society unit, or support groups. Other women prefer scarves (cotton ones are usually the most comfortable and stay on the best), a wig in a totally different style, turbans, hats—or going proudly bald. The American Cancer Society produces a free catalog of flattering, reasonably priced hats, scarves, turbans, and hairpieces (not wigs). The catalog, called *tlc,* or *Tender Loving Care,* is available on request by calling (800) 850-9445.

Some chemo drugs are unpredictable. Standard doses of cyclophosphamide (Cytoxan) for breast cancer, for instance, cause a few women to lose all their hair, a larger group to experience considerable thinning, and another fairly large group to be minimally affected.

If there is almost no chance of the cancer spreading to the scalp, the oncologist may allow the woman to wear a "cold cap" over her scalp for a few minutes before the drug is given, and for about forty-five minutes afterward. The theory is that the cap, which cools the scalp dramatically (this feels decidedly strange), discourages the chemotherapy drug from settling there. Getting an effective cold cap can present problems, but some clinical trials have shown good results with the Penguin Cold Cap Therapy System (made in Britain) for many women, even those undergoing chemotherapy that usually causes major hair loss. Cold cap use requires a high degree of commitment, some discomfort, and probably some expense. For Internet users, browsing "chemotherapy alopecia" brings information on cold caps as well as on investigations into certain chemical or biologic agents, such as cyclin-dependent kinases, that may decrease hair loss.

Many women who do not lose their hair still favor a short haircut to disguise hair thinning, and they treat their hair very gently. Others find they can cover patchy hair loss well with a longer hair style.

COMPLEXION CHANGES Along with hair loss and changes in hair texture, some women experience temporary complexion changes. For women undergoing cancer treatment who have beauty questions, the American Cancer Society; the Cosmetic, Toiletry, and Fragrance Association Foundation; and the National Cosmetology Association jointly sponsor a nationwide program called "Look Good, Feel Better." Every participant receives a large packet of skin care and makeup products at no charge. Then, depending on the local program, she may get an individual makeover or a group session. Information is available from the local ACS unit.

I am always happy to recommend "Look Good, Feel Better." When I was nearing the end of a grueling experience with several surgeries, months of chemotherapy, plus radiation, I saw a small notice in the newspaper about this new program in San Francisco. I signed up as one of the first participants—and finished my makeover less than an hour before the San Francisco earthquake of 1989. We were all quaking, along with our city, but as neighbors gathered for mutual support, I received several compliments on how well I looked, all of it due to "Look Good, Feel Better"! Years later, I helped set up "Look Good, Feel Better" group sessions at the cancer center where I worked, and I thoroughly enjoyed the fun everyone had with individual makeovers with volunteer cosmetologists, wig stylings, scarf- and turban-styling tips, and simple refreshments. Information is available from the local ACS unit.

THE DIGESTIVE TRACT The cells lining the digestive tract from mouth to anus turn over about once a week—which makes them prime targets for several chemotherapy agents. Women undergoing chemo may have no problem at all or may experience anything from occasional mild queasiness to days of nonstop vomiting, often beginning several hours after receiving IV chemo. It is fairly common, too, for women to complain of a funny taste in the mouth, loss of appetite, food aversions (just the thought of a particular food turns the stomach), and mouth sores. Either diarrhea or constipation is also possible.

Although they sometimes occur together, nausea and vomiting are two very different experiences. Nausea is the distressing feeling that vomiting may occur, but vomiting may or may not actually happen. Nausea and vomiting have different patterns, and control of one may not improve the other.

To complicate the situation, there are three different time patterns of nausea and vomiting that can occur with chemotherapy, and a person can experience one or more. The **acute** type occurs within several hours of chemotherapy and goes away within a day or so. The **delayed** type starts after twenty-four hours and usually peaks about three days after chemotherapy. While it is usually milder than the acute type, it may last up to a week, which can make it quite distressing. The third type, **anticipatory** nausea (and occasionally vomiting), occurs after the woman has become nauseated or vomited after at least one dose of chemotherapy. With later doses she may feel nauseated *before* the chemotherapy or even months *after* her last dose if something reminds her of the experience—including encountering her chemotherapy nurse at the grocery store a year later!

Chemotherapy drugs are classified into categories by their **emetogenic potential**, or how likely they are to cause vomiting (emesis), so the oncologist and the woman have some information when they plan her treatment. But the other factor is how the individual woman will react, and that, of course, is difficult to know beforehand.

Great advances have been made in treating the acute nausea and vomiting that almost always occur with highly emetogenic chemotherapy drugs, the ones that cause vomiting for almost everyone. The early 1990s saw the introduction of a new class of drugs that block the action of the chemical serotonin in the area of the brain that controls vomiting. These **5-HT3 antagonists**—ondansetron (Zofran) and granisetron (Kytril) are the most common—revolutionized the treatment of severe nausea and vomiting from chemotherapy. These drugs can be given through the vein a few minutes before the dose of chemotherapy and then every several hours afterward for the first day or two. Even one dose given in the doctor's office may curtail or eliminate vomiting. Pill forms are not as powerful, but they are convenient for home use and may relieve delayed nausea and vomiting.

The 5-HT3 antagonists are quite expensive. Women receiving less emetogenic chemotherapy may need nothing at all, or may fare well with less costly medicines or other treatments for either acute or delayed nausea and vomiting.

Common antinausea medicines available as pills, suppositories, and even injections include prochlorperazine (Compazine) and metoclopramide (Reglan). Some women find the antianxiety drug lorazepam (Ativan) helpful: "I was nauseated and vomiting—but I didn't care." Many oncologists at least mention marijuana, or the legal version, Marinol, as a possible treatment. Some women use the "seasickness bands" found over the counter at most pharmacies or travel stores; a more high-tech possibility, reputed to be more effective for chemotherapy nausea, is a ReliefBand (Woodside Biomedical), a wristband with a miniature battery-operated nerve stimulation unit that works on acupuncture principles and is available by prescription only.

It is currently easier to prevent severe nausea than the mild queasiness that affects some women taking chemo pills for two weeks out of every four. Besides the therapies mentioned above, women swear by various personal remedies, such as herbal teas, acupuncture or acupressure, distraction, exercise, motion sickness wristbands, self-hypnosis, relaxation or visualization, or simply keeping something—carrot sticks, ginger snaps, sour hard candy—in the stomach all the time. Eating small frequent meals, avoiding concentrated fatty foods, and having someone else prepare meals are also useful strategies. Because fatigue and nausea build on each other, anything that relieves fatigue may also help the nausea.

One of the key principles in treating nausea or vomiting is to attempt to prevent it with effective therapy beforehand rather than trying to "catch up" afterward. Aside from increasing the woman's comfort, this greatly reduces the chances of anticipatory nausea. If severe anticipatory nausea does occur and does not improve with drugs or simple treatment, **systematic desensitization**, or **counterconditioning,** works by teaching the woman to relax completely and then slowly bringing in parts of the chemo experience until the stimulus (the prospect of having chemo) no longer brings about the automatic response of nausea.

Besides the distress they cause, severe nausea or vomiting can lead to dehydration and malnutrition if the woman cannot take in and retain enough fluids and nourishment. Weight loss of more than five pounds, dry mouth, and loose skin are danger signals to report immediately. Women sometimes find it helpful to suck on a hard candy to mask the "taste" of intravenous chemo.

Since it is crucial to stay as well nourished as possible during chemo so that the body can do its share of the work, women may have to use considerable ingenuity to stay on a balanced diet. Blender drinks were my ace in the hole, but there are also some cancer treatment recipe books available, including a free pamphlet, *Eating Hints: Recipes and Hints for Better Nutrition During Cancer Treatment,* available from the Cancer Information Service at (800) 4-CANCER (422-6237). Even if she does not experience nausea or vomiting, many a woman develops a real aversion to any food she eats the evening of a chemo day. It makes sense for her to avoid eating her favorite foods at that time, at least until she finds out whether this is a pattern for her. Something light, like broth and crackers, often works best.

Mucositis and **stomatitis** are two names for inflammation and sores in the mouth that can be a serious side effect of a few chemotherapy drugs. These tend to begin when the white blood cell count drops and improve when the count rises again.

Women first notice a slight burning sensation and some redness. If it gets worse, the membranes of the mouth and lips develop white patches, swelling, and small open sores or even large bleeding sores or throat problems. Of course, this makes it hard to eat and swallow and makes it easy to get an infection.

To help prevent problems, women can rinse their mouths frequently with warm water and baking soda (about one-quarter teaspoon soda to one glass of water); the oncologist may recommend another type of rinse. One nursing research study suggests holding ice chips in the mouth while getting IV chemo that can be given over a few minutes, on the same principle as the cold cap for the scalp. If the mouth does become inflamed, there are several special mouthwashes available, which typically contain a combination of ingredients to numb, protect, and heal the membranes; research continues into which is the most effective rinse. The oncologist may also prescribe pain medicine or antibiotics as needed. It is an excellent idea to see a dentist for teeth cleaning and repair *before* starting chemo and to practice careful dental hygiene during the course. Any other dental care during chemo should be coordinated with the oncologist. Dental problems can increase bad tastes in the mouth and the risk of stomatitis; they can also be the source of serious infection when the white blood count is low. (My dentist recommended that I rinse with Listerine twice a day. Thank you, no! As I discovered quickly, alcohol-based mouthwashes are excruciatingly painful on a mouth that is even slightly raw, and they just dry it out more.)

The woman may develop changes in bowel habits from the chemotherapy drugs, other medications she is taking, or changes in her activity and diet. For constipation, she can increase fluid intake, dietary fiber, and activity. All medication for either constipation or diarrhea needs to be approved by the oncologist.

THE REPRODUCTIVE TRACT   A few chemotherapy drugs commonly used in treating women's cancers attack the fast-dividing cells in the ovaries of premenopausal women. This is a side effect but, in the case of the cancers influenced by female hormones, it may be medically desirable too.

That is no reason for the woman to be thrilled, however. It is common for her to stop menstruating a few months after treatment begins, and to experience menopausal symptoms such as hot flashes, night sweats, and vaginal dryness. Women not too far past menopause and postmenopausal women who have stopped taking hormone therapy before starting chemotherapy may experience some of these symptoms too.

Sometimes the woman begins menstruating again after treatment ends—often with a very irregular pattern at first—but the closer she is to the normal age of menopause, the more likely it is that the changes are permanent. She is usually discouraged from taking hormone replacement therapy for fear of nourishing stray cancer cells, although research is reexamining this advice. (See "Menopause—Without Hormone Therapy" in Chapter 25 for information on both hormone replacement therapy after hormone dependent cancers and effective non-hormone treatment of menopausal symptoms.)

OTHER SIDE EFFECTS Every chemotherapy drug has its individual fingerprint of known side effects. One drug zeros in on the heart, while another may cause tingling in the feet. Some of these occur only at a dosage—either one-time or cumulative—that is too high for the woman's body and is considered toxic; others can happen with any dosage. Some toxicities can be prevented if the woman follows directions exactly (like drinking lots of fluids to protect the bladder with the drug Cytoxan). New drugs are appearing that can be given with a specific chemotherapy medicine to block a certain kind of damage, such as dexrazoxane (Zinecard), which can decrease heart damage when larger-than-normal doses of the drug Adriamycin are prescribed. Many side effects—but not all—go away after chemo finishes, or even between doses.

The woman needs to find out from her oncologist the most common and serious side effects of any chemotherapy drug she is taking and if there is anything she can do to minimize them. The website www.oncochat.org has a current list of commonly used chemotherapy agents and their side effects—along with all sorts of other information.

HORMONAL THERAPY

Some women's cancers depend on a supply of female hormones in the right balance so that they grow and thrive. The idea behind hormone therapy is to change the hormonal environment of cancer cells anywhere in the body so that they starve.

Doctors are trying strategies—sometimes with considerable success—that include manipulations with female hormones, weakened female hormones that fool the cancer cells, "antihormones" that block female hormones, and male hormones. These involve not only medicines but sometimes surgery or radiation to remove or destroy hormone-rich glands such as the ovaries. Because breast cancer is the only women's cancer in which hormonal therapy is used with any frequency, this treatment is discussed more thoroughly in Part Two, in the chapters on breast cancer.

Of course, these hormone manipulations can and do cause symptoms. Women who are premenopausal, recently postmenopausal, or newly off hormone replacement therapy, appear to be more susceptible because their own hormones are more active. Different hormone medications can cause PMS-like symptoms, menopausal changes, or masculinizing changes such as a deeper voice, acne, and facial hair.

BIOLOGICAL THERAPY

Biological therapy (biologic response modifiers) is a relative newcomer in cancer treatment. It is not new at all in the treatment of diseases, however, since every vaccination against measles and polio follows one basic biological therapy strategy: teaching the body's own immune system to attack something that should not be there.

Biological therapy can use highly purified proteins to wake up the body's defenses or make them work together better. Other biological therapies try to increase the numbers of defender cells, make the individual cells more effective, or mark the cancer cells more clearly as targets. Interferon and interleukin, for instance, are two proteins that occur naturally in the body and can be grown in large quantities in the laboratory. They are being investigated in clinical trials against some forms of cancer, but have not shown much promise yet in women's cancers.

Researchers are currently experimenting with **monoclonal antibodies,** laboratory copies of the normal antibodies that attack specific kinds of cancer cells. These monoclonal antibodies are beginning to be harnessed to carry chemotherapy or radioactive compounds directly to the target cells: "smart bombs" on the cellular level. But there are problems. Monoclonal antibodies can attack the wrong cells, for instance, or the body can start seeing the biological therapy proteins as foreign and attack them. As with chemotherapy, side effects can make the patient miserable or even be life threatening.

Everything that researchers learn about how genes promote or suppress cell growth, how cells receive hormone signals from the body, how cells become abnormal, and how cancer cells invade other tissues or build blood vessels to nourish themselves or spread through the bloodstream might someday become part of a biological therapy. The hope is that someday we will be able to prevent cells from becoming abnormal enough to become cancer or find some way to coax them to becoming normal, functioning, contributing cells again.

Successes are appearing already. The biological agents used to push the white blood cells or red blood cells to recover faster after chemotherapy are examples of biological response modifiers that are saving lives or making them better now. The monoclonal antibody trastuzumab (Herceptin) is commonly used now for women whose breast cancers "overexpress" the HER2/neu protein. Oncologists frequently prescribe the biological agent levamisole (Ergamisol) along with chemotherapy for colorectal cancer. Although biological therapy is still more promise than delivery in women's cancers, many oncologists and cancer researchers remain firmly convinced that it will be the major source of tomorrow's cancer victories.

CLINICAL TRIALS

A **clinical trial** is a study done under stringent conditions to evaluate a new therapy. The new treatment is tried because there is reasonable hope that it will be more effective than current therapy. Clinical trials, done after extensive animal studies, can be the source of treatment breakthroughs—or can show that a therapy is a blind end.

The most believable clinical trials randomly assign patients to either a group receiving the experimental treatment or to a second **control** (comparison) group receiving the standard treatment or a placebo. Until the study is over, no one—patient, doctor, or researcher—knows who received what. If there is no standard therapy available for a particular condition, the treatment group is compared with people who received no treatment.

Cancer clinical trials are carried out in three phases. A Phase I trial tests the experimental treatment in a few patients to find out how to give the therapy most effectively, how much can be given safely, and whether there are side effects that have not shown up in animal studies. Since less is known about the treatment at this early stage, a Phase I trial is the riskiest. Usually the only patients allowed in this phase are those with metastatic cancer who do not have other treatment options.

Phase II studies build on the Phase I information to look at how the proposed therapy works in different kinds of cancer. Finally, Phase III studies involve patients in all stages of cancer to compare the experimental treatment with standard therapy to see which is more effective, and to try variations in dosage and timing.

Patient expenses in clinical trials vary widely, but it is common for women in Phase I and II trials to be treated without charge. Phase III trials may or may not make experimental drugs available free of charge, but the woman and/or her insurance must often pay for any standard treatments, such as routine surgery, blood tests, or doctor visits. Insurance companies often balk at paying for "experimental" treatments, so it is smart to check out costs and insurance coverage beforehand.

Phase I trials are ordinarily carried out at major cancer centers with hospitalized patients. By the time the treatment reaches Phase III trials, however, the researchers know a great deal more about the treatment. Thus, Phase III trials may be carried out at a cancer center or out in the community through the Community Clinical Oncology Program (CCOP) of the National Cancer Institute. CCOP, with clinical trials in many states, gives researchers a much larger pool of potential participants. In addition, it allows many more cancer patients to be part of a study if they so wish, and it moves research findings more quickly and smoothly into standard practice.

Historically, most cancer patients have not participated in clinical trials. For many women, however, doing this can be a way to help not only themselves but generations of women to come. Every successful anticancer agent we have now came out of clinical trials, and finding out that something *does not* work is equally important information.

PAYING FOR CANCER TREATMENT

Cancer treatment is expensive. In addition, many a working woman must take time off work for surgery or other therapy and may lose salary. How does she cope?

For the woman in a hospital, the social worker, discharge planner, or financial counselor can provide information about available financial aid and help her make her way through the insurance thicket. In the doctor's office, one of the office staff should have basic information. In the United States, health insurance, Medicare, or Medicaid/Medi-Cal usually pays many or all of the medical bills, but the woman needs to read and ask questions about her particular policy.

If available, sick leave benefits from work or disability insurance (private or state) can help with living expenses. U.S. Federal Government disability payments come through the Social Security Administration for those who are totally disabled or expect to be totally disabled for at least one year; many women with cancer will be back at work long before then.

It is vitally important to fill in and file any insurance paperwork as promptly as possible. The woman who either does not find out what she needs to do or—in the midst of everything else going on after a cancer diagnosis—forgets to do it may miss out on coverage she could have received.

A pamphlet, *Cancer Treatments Your Insurance Should Cover,* is currently out of print but can be read online at www.accc-cancer.org/publications/ patientbrochure.asp. The American Cancer Society may also have information about financial resources for cancer treatment.

Women who are "medically indigent" because they have little money and are either not insured or underinsured may be able to obtain cancer therapy through a county hospital—and many county hospital cancer programs are superb.

Several drug companies provide certain cancer drugs at reduced rates or even free for those who cannot otherwise afford them. The American Cancer Society has information for oncologists; websites with lists of drug companies who offer such assistance include www.accc-cancer.org/publications/hotlines.asp and www.cancersupportivecare.com/drug_assistance.html. The free audio program, *The Cancer Toolbox,* contains a section on paying for cancer treatment (see pp. 73–74 and Resources). Certain clinical trials that pay the cost of all or some treatment may also be an option.

Many people in the United States are unhappy with the current state of health insurance but, for now anyway, changes appear to be happening slowly and gradually. Thanks to the 1996 Kassebaum-Kennedy legislation, more people with serious health problems can get health insurance or transfer it to a new job. Nevertheless, major problems remain, and until they are solved, one of the best sources of information about insurance for the woman with cancer is the National Coalition for Cancer Survivorship, 1010 Wayne Avenue 5th Floor, Silver Spring MD 20910; (301) 585-2616 or www.cansearch.org/canserch/canserch.html.

— *Kerry McGinn*

CHAPTER 9

COMPLEMENTARY AND ALTERNATIVE THERAPIES FOR CANCER

Neither physical recovery nor life extension is the test of the value of spiritual approaches to cancer. The test is the effect they have on the living experience of the person involved.

— *Michael Lerner*

Complementary and alternative therapies, or complementary and alternative medicine (CAM), is also sometimes called *integrative* medicine. CAM includes a wide variety of healing philosophies, approaches, and therapies. Nearly 90 percent of all people with cancer combine complementary therapies—many using several of these modalities—with prescribed anticancer therapies. People with cancer spend more for these nontraditional treatments than is spent for nontraditional treatments for all other conditions combined. There is growing acceptance of the view that complementary therapies play a positive role in improving the quality of life for people facing cancer and cancer treatment: These forms of treatment work with traditional cancer treatment and are useful in relieving some of the side effects of chemotherapy, radiation therapy, and surgery, and in boosting the immune system and relieving stress. Savvy health-care marketing experts, doctors, nurses, and other health-care providers have figured out that integrating these therapies into traditional oncology practice is both good practice *and* a profitable addition to the services offered in the practice.

The White House Commission on Complementary and Alternative Medicine Policy, a commission appointed by President Clinton in 2000, issued its final report in March 2002, recommending several steps to improve the accuracy and reliability of information on these modalities and to encourage use of safe, effective complementary and alternative medicine practices. The Commission's recommendations include mandating that these therapies and their practitioners be held to an appropriate level of accountability—implying that research be conducted to help health-care professionals and health-care consumers make informed choices about complementary and/or alternative therapies. Other recommendations include asking states to require that all providers disclose their training as well as establish requirements on licensure and certification of CAM practitioners. Additional federal funding suggested by the Commission would underwrite research of CAM therapies. Finally, Commission recommendations urge health insurance and managed care companies to cover safe and effective CAM therapies. More information on the Commission and its proceedings are available on its website: www.whccamp.hhs.gov.

Amidst growing acceptance, there is lingering fear that patients and families will be swindled by unscrupulous practitioners using unproven and, in some cases, harmful treatments. More than a few people seeking miracle cures dangerously delay conventional treatment for what might be curable cancers. For people who have cancers that don't have a high cure rate, unproven therapies might seem to offer hope for a better and longer life, but critics see unproven treatments as cruel and costly hoaxes, particularly when an unproven therapy is touted as a cure. Not one of the therapies described here—or any that has been reported in other lay or professional literature—has been scientifically proven to cure cancer.

Most people who use some type of unconventional therapy do not reveal this information to their doctors or nurses—a secret that can be dangerous if the treatment has side effects. It's not that these people are devious, it's just that many experience disapproval or even ridicule from doctors and nurses who lack knowledge about the use of complementary therapies. Many people use an unconventional cancer treatment *before* getting conventional cancer therapy. For these people, the delay could decrease the chance that treatment will succeed.

Some CAM therapies are helpful as *complements* to conventional cancer treatment. Women need to choose wisely from among complementary and unproven therapies. Many comprehensive books, websites, community lecture programs, and other resources can help consumers learn and make informed decisions about the use of alternative and complementary therapies throughout the cancer experience. This chapter is intended only as a brief introduction to point readers in the direction of factual and useful information.

To keep things simple, the terms and how they are used here reflect those agreed to in the U.S. Congressional Report *Unconventional Cancer Treatments* (1990). **Mainstream** and **conventional treatments** refer to those that are widely used in major American cancer centers. Surgery, radiation therapy, chemotherapy, hormonal therapy, and biological therapy are conventional treatments for cancer. **Unconventional approaches** are those that fall outside mainstream cancer care. As time goes on, more of the so-called unconventional approaches slide into mainstream use as supplements to conventional therapy. **Complementary therapies** add to, or *complement,* conventional therapy and include mind/body techniques and herbal remedies all aimed at symptom control and improving the quality of life. **Alternative therapies** refer to treatments that are further outside the mainstream and are sometimes seen as another way—an alternate way—of treating the cancer. **Adjunctive therapies** are closer to mainstream and include emotional and behavioral activities such as support groups, psychotherapy, imagery, and hypnosis.

There are at least a hundred known unconventional treatments, and variations exist within each major category. Unconventional treatments can be simple or complex and range from slight to drastic changes in a person's lifestyle.

The best unconventional treatments are those that improve quality of life, promote general health, and engage the person in helpful ways. The worst unconventional treatments exist only for the financial gain of the practitioner. Many of the unconventional treatment plans have good and bad elements—which makes the situation confusing for laypeople and health-care professionals alike.

Therapies can be open or closed. **Open therapies** are those in which the nature of the treatment—how it works, its theory—is openly revealed. In **closed therapies,** a major part of the therapy plan is not revealed to the person being treated. Closed therapies increase suspicion about the practitioners' motives.

Practitioners of unconventional treatments vary in their level of competence and the care given during the treatment. A specific treatment can be open and ethical, but the practitioner may not be qualified to give the care.

Typically, treatment plans last just over a year. Some cost as much as $20,000 annually, but most cost far less. Insurance and managed care plans may cover some forms of unconventional therapy in part or in full, but a woman would be wise to check her insurance plan before assuming any form of unconventional therapy will be covered.

WHO USES THESE FORMS OF TREATMENT?

Contrary to popular belief, it is *not* the uneducated, poor person who gets duped into trying unconventional cancer treatments. Generally, people who use complementary and alternative therapies are among the more educated, informed, and well-to-do health-care consumers.

People don't need to travel to Mexico or the Bahamas to find and get complementary and alternative treatment. Medical establishments in Europe, Japan, and China are quite open to unconventional therapies, so they are easier to find there. Even so, only about 2 percent of all U.S. citizens who use unconventional therapy leave the United States to find it.

There has been a backlash against the slow-moving Food and Drug Administration's drug approval processes—evidenced in demonstrations by AIDS activists urging, and getting, a speedier approval process for new AIDS drugs. Another reason for the interest in complementary and alternative therapies in the United States is that cancer is treated much more aggressively in this country than in European and Asian countries. An article in *Civilization* (April/May 1997) points out that the "assaultive nature of high-tech medicine helps explain the appeal" of the "no-tech" approaches to cancer care. This is particularly important for women. In France, for example, more emphasis is placed on preserving sexual organs. French doctors advocated lumpectomies and partial mastectomies much sooner than did U.S. doctors. Many Latin doctors share the same concerns. An American woman is more likely to have a hysterectomy than a woman with a similar diagnosis in England, France, or Germany. This preference for gentler cancer therapies leads the French to greater acceptance of therapies such as homeopathy.

In Germany, people with cancer have more choices of therapies than in any other modern country. Popular choices there include naturopathic, herbal, homeopathic, spiritual, and conventional cancer treatments.

In Great Britain, a woman's choices are influenced by the British health-care system and ease of access to unconventional therapies. When conventional therapy is used, it is likely to be much less aggressive than would be recommended in the United States.

Homeopathy, which treats diseases with very dilute doses (anywhere from 100 to 10,000 dilutions) of substances that would produce symptoms like the disease in a healthy person, was a leading treatment form in the mid-1800s. Homeopathy fell out of favor in the early 1900s, but now has an increasing base of support. There are approximately three thousand homeopathic practitioners in the United States, about one-third of them medical doctors or osteopathic doctors. While conventional cancer treatment produces numerous destructive side effects, homeopathy produces none. Homeopathic remedies can be found on the shelves of local supermarkets, and Americans spent over $200 million on homeopathic remedies alone in 1996.

Spending for all alternative medicine services in the United States exceeds $21 billion annually, and an additional $27 billion is spent on therapies, with at least $12.2 billion being paid directly by consumers (as opposed to being paid for by insurance companies or other third-party payers). Fear, or the wish to avoid the unpleasant side effects of conventional cancer therapy, may well send patients looking for care somewhere other than a conventional treatment center.

American medicine is rarely "user friendly," and it seems to be growing more unfriendly all the time. Many women really want to be actively involved in getting well, and in the United States at least, patients are all too often the last to be consulted about treatment plans. An office visit with a doctor in the United States, even when the doctor is seeing a woman with a new cancer, lasts an average of sixteen minutes. Doctors spend, on an average, from one to three minutes giving information (though most doctors believe they spend seven times that long). The "patient" spends about eight seconds asking questions. This is in great contrast with the generous amounts of personal attention given by many practitioners of unconventional therapies. A homeopathic doctor, for example, may spend up to two hours with a new patient. During this first visit, the doctor will try to gauge how the woman's symptoms have affected her life. The physician and the woman will devise a remedy that exactly fits her symptoms.

Unproven or unorthodox complementary treatment methods are not for every person who has cancer—or at least, not every form of therapy is right for every person with cancer. I cannot imagine my father using imagery or relaxation techniques even though he suffered from pain, nausea, and vomiting during his battle with lung cancer. I wish he could have found relief through some of these methods, but for him such ideas were just "too far out."

On the other hand, many people have shared remarkable stories of how just plain hope, alternative belief systems, and various unorthodox therapies have improved both the quality and quantity of their lives. I have watched men and women survive against all odds—or at least survive long enough to achieve some hoped-for goal. For some, the quality of their survival was most important. My father survived much longer than the statistics gave him, and he didn't use anything special like imagery or nutritional therapy. He always said he was "too stubborn to just give up and die." And he had things he wanted to finish before he died.

Lorraine faced a cancer of unknown origin that was widespread even when it was diagnosed. I gave her the Simontons' book *Getting Well Again,* and she found a group that helped her develop skills in guided imagery. She lived for five years, at least four and a half years longer than the statistics gave her—much of that time without symptoms or problems from her cancer. During that time, she worked as a docent at a local art museum, was involved in several charity organizations, and helped found a cancer support group in a community hospital.

Jane had late-stage ovarian cancer at diagnosis. She was a young, ambitious, determined woman. Despite the prediction that she had less than six months, she lived more than three years, married, and helped other women deal with the side effects of cancer. I fondly recall the attractive and creative things Jane could do with silk scarves to cover her bald head as she went through several rounds of chemotherapy. Jane continued to work at her job, enjoyed friendships, and lived beyond anyone's predictions.

Alex, a young man with lymphoma, had a tough time coping with the side effects of radiation and chemotherapy. He had every chance for cure, but the treatment bordered on more than he could—or wanted to—handle. He joined Lorraine's support group and discovered artistic talent he did not know he had, which gave him a new kind of fulfillment. He has since celebrated nearly twenty years of being cancer-free, has married, and has hosted several one-man shows of his art.

Ascella had metastatic breast cancer, but she wanted to see her daughter graduate from high school. She went through aggressive conventional therapy, but she also traveled to a health spa in Lourdes, France. She did see her daughter graduate.

My college roommate and friend, Cindy, had malignant melanoma, and her prognosis was dismal even when she was first diagnosed. Five years after her initial diagnosis, the melanoma returned. Cindy found a clinical trial program that gave her extra months, during which time she spent valuable time with her teenage daughter, resolved some issues in her marriage, and found a dream job that offered her artistic fulfillment and the chance to prove herself.

These are just a few personal stories of people who wanted to live. Adding up the evidence from these and many other women's experiences, it would be foolish to deny the impact of the interaction between the mind, body, and spirit on the body's ability to fight disease and heal itself.

WHAT IS UNCONVENTIONAL CANCER THERAPY?

In 1990, the U.S. House of Representatives asked the Office of Technology Assessment (OTA) to develop a clinical trial to study the effect and safety of Immuno-Augmentative Therapy (IAT). This resulted in the creation of a panel—and funding of $2 million to develop criteria to assess unconventional cancer treatments. 1992 saw the creation of the Office of Alternative Medicine (OAM) within the National Institutes of Health (NIH), primarily to encourage alternative or complementary medicine practitioners to submit their therapies to scientific scrutiny. It was initially funded at $7.5 million; in 1997, the funding was $12 million. In 1998, OAM became the National Center for Complementary and Alternative Medicine, with a budget of $50 million, and in 2000, the budget was close to $90 million. An amendment to the NIH budget gives its director the authority to permit research on unconventional therapies by licensed doctors. In October 1998, the Office of Cancer Complementary and Alternative Medicine (OCCAM) was established to coordinate the National Cancer Institute's (NCI) CAM research activities. The NCI offers assistance to unconventional practitioners who wish to document the effectiveness of their therapies for cancer. Interest in alternative and complementary therapies is clearly growing.

Over the years, the NCI has tested many unconventional agents including laetrile, antineoplastons, and hydrazine sulphate. Respected American universities, including Duke, Johns Hopkins, and UCLA, are increasingly involved in researching complementary therapies, and results are being put into practice at some of our most renowned cancer centers. The National Institutes of Health continues to fund studies in CAM therapies, with a good deal of interest focussed on combining these therapies with conventional anticancer treatment. There are some currently accepted cancer treatments that were once considered quackery. Some of the modalities getting a great deal of attention include electro-acupuncture, maitake mushrooms, Chinese herbs, and vitamin C. Most CAM therapies used by women with cancer fall into the following categories:

- metabolic and dietary

- herbal

- megavitamin

- psychological/psychosocial

- physical

- traditional or folk medicine

- spiritual healing

- pharmacological (using drugs or special preparations)

Different practitioners advocate variations and sometimes combinations from these categories, which are discussed in more detail below.

Exposure to traditional Chinese medicine is still new to most Americans and Europeans. Even health-care professionals who practice in or near the many "Chinatowns" in Europe and the United States are mystified by the belief systems and practices that make up traditional Chinese medicine. Chinese pharmacies, whether in a Beijing hospital or San Francisco's Chinatown, carry a wide assortment of animal, plant, and mineral products. The numerous shelves in these pharmacies contain these products, in delicate vials and bottles, arranged in some sort of order known only to the practitioner.

In Beijing's Sino-Japanese Friendship Hospital, each patient receives a specially prescribed and mixed herbal preparation twice daily as a complement to chemotherapy and radiation treatment. After discharge from the hospital, patients continue with the herbal preparation at home. According to Chinese nurses, patients seem to feel less tired or fatigued as they go through cancer treatment, and other side effects like nausea and vomiting seem *not* to be as difficult for these patients as for their counterparts in America and Europe. It is worth noting that in America and Europe more people are becoming interested in using the herbs and potions of traditional Chinese medicine in the treatment and management of cancer and its symptoms.

Chinese medicine contends that changes in seasons and the weather, including wind, cold, heat, moisture, dryness, and internal heat, affect the human body. The interaction between external disease-causing factors and emotions creates imbalance, resulting in disease. Treatment plans and prescriptions are designed to restore balance in the person. It is said that the "object of Chinese medicine is the person, not just the illness."

Acupressure and Acupuncture

Acupressure, an Asian healing technique, includes **reflexology** and its Japanese form, called **shiatsu.** Acupressure is a form of massage that uses **acupoints,** or *tsubos,* thought to be points of decreased electrical resistance that follow the body's **meridians** (energy channels). Stimulation of the tsubo, the meridian, or a portion of one or more meridians can improve energy flow, in turn affecting organs distant from the area being stimulated. This energy flow can have a positive impact on physical health, stress level, and the emotions and can be useful in pain and stress management.

Shiatsu and acupressure address mind, body, and spirit and, like other Asian healing therapies, imply a significant role for the mind/body relationship in the development of disease. According to shiatsu theory, no one

*Comple-
mentary
and
Alternative
Therapies
for Cancer*

127

meridian is affected in isolation. A change in one can cause a number of other changes in the quality of others. Shiatsu is especially useful as a means of relieving stress and anxiety. It involves the serial application of firm but gentle pressure by the fingertips, with pressure being held for two to five minutes throughout a session that usually takes about one hour. Shiatsu and acupressure can be effective as disease prevention; because disease refers to stress-related issues, health promotion can come from the practice of these stress-relieving measures. Acupressure techniques provide the mechanism for the use of Reliefband™, a band worn like a wristwatch to decrease nausea—whether it is caused by motion sickness or is a side effect of cancer therapy. (See www.reliefband.com.)

The five-thousand-year-old science of **acupuncture**, which evolved from acupressure, uses needle insertion to open energy flow and relieve pain. Acupuncture is performed by licensed practitioners, while acupressure can be done by laypersons. Both were derived from the Chinese *Nei Jing*, the oldest written medical text (dated about 300 B.C.), which is now being consulted by practitioners of Western medicine. The basic goal of Chinese healing is to strengthen the flow of "*ki*"(sometimes also referred to as *chi* or *qi)*—the life force—which in turn balances energy flow to create well-being. The meridians are the channels that carry ki through the body. The chakra system employed in Reiki and Native American healing (see pages 153 and 156), and the meridians used in acupressure, acupuncture, reflexology, and shiatsu, are similar in that they are all energy channels.

Research shows that endorphins are produced when acupoints are pressed, warmed, or needled. It is probable that acupressure causes hormonal changes and stimulates the immune system. A researcher at the University of Maryland has used the electronic version of acupuncture, "electro-acupuncture"—applying low-level electric current through the acupuncture needles—and has found it useful in decreasing the nausea and vomiting that is a common problem for people taking chemotherapy.

METABOLIC AND DIETARY THERAPY

Cancer treatment is generally much more effective if the person is well nourished, so diet is tremendously important during cancer treatment and recovery. While scientific evidence on optimal cancer diets is incomplete, health-care professionals generally recommend a balanced diet, often with multivitamin supplements—which include vitamins C, E, and A and some minerals such as zinc—to enhance cell renewal and healing. Many women find that consulting with a dietitian who is an expert in cancer is very helpful.

The majority of people with cancer use some form of metabolic or dietary therapy, with or without conventional cancer treatment. The theory behind metabolic therapy is the belief that body toxins and wastes interfere with healing, and this therapy focuses on removing toxins from the body. Practitioners believe cancer results from degeneration of the liver and pancreas as well as the immune system in general. The interaction of the lungs and blood vessels—the body functions that provide oxygen to all body cells—is also disrupted. By clearing the system of the toxic end products of chemicals we take in and by avoiding taking in new ones, the body's cells receive more of the nutrients needed for health.

Dietary therapies focus on the nutrients a person takes into her body. Most dietary cancer therapies are vegetarian. Treatments usually require that the patient's diet include specific foods. Some of the more common diets involve grapes, raw foods, and wheatgrass extract. Some dietary and metabolic regimens include detoxification. Mainstream medicine does not recognize detoxification at all, but it is a vital component of many alternative and complementary programs.

Regimens vary from one practitioner to another. Typical metabolic therapy plans include special diets, detoxification by colonic cleansing (enemas or high colonics), and regular doses of vitamins, minerals, and enzymes. Coffee enemas and high colonic irrigations using wheatgrass or other substances are used to "detoxify" the liver. Though most clinics offering metabolic therapy are in Mexico, there are a few in the United States, Europe, and Canada. In 1991, American actor Michael Landon used metabolic and nutritional therapy as a primary treatment for his cancer of the pancreas and described his treatment in detail, including coffee enemas and carrot juice supplements, on "The Tonight Show" a few weeks before he died.

Metabolic therapy was first advocated by Max Gerson in Germany in the 1920s; his diet was the best known nutritional therapy until the introduction of macrobiotics. The **Gerson diet,** derived from a combination of Gerson's research and European folk medicine, begins with a raw, vegetarian diet modified with some cooked foods and later with animal products. The patient drinks vegetable and fruit juices every hour, has several types of enemas, and drinks several glasses of fresh calf's liver juice or carrot juice daily. Gerson brought his treatment to the United States and continued using it there until his death in 1959. A modified version is promoted by his daughter at the Gerson Institute in Bonita, California, and at the Gerson Clinic in Tijuana, Mexico.

In 1980, American actor Steve McQueen drew media attention when he opted to go to the Kelley Clinic at Plaza Santa Maria (south of Tijuana) for treatment. The Kelley theory is that cancer is caused by a pancreatic enzyme deficiency. Dr. Kelley, a dentist, developed the Kelley Enzyme Test and the Kelley Index of Malignancy—questionnaires used to analyze tumors and prognosis. The **Kelley regimen** is a nutritional program based on vitamin and enzyme supplements and computerized metabolic typing. Kelley no longer practices, but his plan is still used in several forms by his followers.

Macrobiotics is probably the most widely used nutritional approach to cancer in the United States. Its proponents offer both preventive and curative claims. Macrobiotic therapy is based on the traditional Eastern concepts of balance and harmony—the balance of opposite and complementary energies, yin and yang, which in healing strategies extend to body functions. According to macrobiotic theory, there is a "mother red blood cell" in the intestine from which all body cells and organs derive. Intake of foods balanced in yin and yang qualities promotes health and counteracts disease. Deeper reflections on the yin-yang balance also bring in the spiritual aspect of life. Macrobiotic diets, derived from a traditional Japanese diet, are largely low-fat, complex carbohydrate, vegetarian diets—including only whole grains, some specially cooked vegetables, and miso, a soybean product believed to prevent cancer development. The major hazard of macrobiotic therapy is, strangely enough, malnutrition.

The Nobel Prize winner Dr. Linus Pauling coined the term **orthomolecular medicine,** sometimes called **orthomolecular nutrition** or **megavitamin therapy,** to express his belief that disease could be cured by giving the body the right molecules of nutrients through good nutrition. The word *orthomolecular* comes from combining *ortho,* a Greek work for "right" or "correct," with the word *molecule,* defined as the most simple structure of any compound. So, **orthomolecular** literally means "the right molecule."

According to orthomolecular thinking, physical and psychological disorders can be reversed by correcting or normalizing the body's balance of vitamins, minerals, amino acids, and other normal body substances. Those who adhere to orthomolecular therapy make every effort to eat nutritious foods in a diet that is high in fiber and low in fat. Vitamin, mineral, and other nutrient supplements are prescribed depending on the condition being treated. Orthomolecular practitioners believe that the government's recommended daily allowance (RDA) of vitamins and minerals may prevent diseases related to severe deficiencies, but that these levels do not promote optimal health—that some people may need much more than the RDA levels.

Dr. Pauling advocated vitamin C as a complement to conventional therapy to support the patient's natural defenses in the treatment and palliation of cancer. While the RDA for vitamin C is 45 milligrams (0.045 grams) per day, Dr. Pauling and others recommend doses up to 10 grams per day, oral or intravenous, in the treatment of cancer. The oral dose starts at 1 to 2 grams per day and gradually increases to around 10 grams. Proponents of this approach admit they do not know the best dose. Researchers are looking at the role of vitamin C in preventing cancer and preventing its spread once it has developed.

Overuse of vitamins can be harmful. Some vitamins interfere with the action of conventional chemotherapy and radiation therapy. Vitamin C, for example, is taken up by cells in an oxidized form that could counteract the effects of chemotherapy and radiation. When taken in the high doses used in orthomolecular regimens, vitamin C may cause diarrhea, causing problems in fluid and electrolyte balance for frail cancer patients. For these reasons, it is important for a woman to talk to the doctor and nurse involved in her overall treatment plan before using megavitamin therapy during cancer treatment.

The program advocated by Dr. Virginia Livingston and used at the Livingston-Wheeler Medical Clinic in San Diego integrates diet, nutritional supplements, and immunotherapy. Treatment includes immune-enhancing vaccines (bacille Calmette-Guerin), a vegetarian diet, and coffee enemas. Dr. Livingston claimed to have discovered a microbe that causes cancer and a vaccine to counteract it. The **Livingston diet** evolved from the Gerson diet and can include megavitamin therapy. However, the Livingston-Wheeler therapy has been totally dismissed by mainstream practitioners. A recent study found that survival rates did not differ between people going through the Livingston-Wheeler program and people receiving conventional cancer therapy in a university cancer center. Actually, people getting conventional therapy maintained better quality of life throughout the study period, while more Livingston-Wheeler patients had such negative side effects as decreased appetite, pain, and breathing problems.

Metabolic regimens can cause major problems for the people following them because of the risks that come along with colonic cleansing. Colonic cleansing involves the use of enemas, with enema solutions composed of a variety of liquids, including water, salt water, and coffee. The colon (bowel) may be punctured or otherwise damaged by the enema tube during the procedure, resulting in irritation or infection. The bowel tissue may be overloaded with fluid, cutting off blood flow to these tissues. Enemas can pull important electrolytes (potassium, for example) out of the body. The resulting deficit of electrolytes can cause heart irregularities and death.

Dr. Keith Block, of the University of Illinois School of Medicine, advocates a middle-ground approach of combining unconventional and conventional cancer treatments. While his specialty is internal medicine, he has done advanced research into the nutritional and behavioral aspects of cancer and has developed an approach to cancer care and treatment based on a philosophy of compassionate caring for others. Dr. Block was a member of

NCI's Unconventional Cancer Treatments Advisory Panel, and his work is widely followed—though not necessarily promoted—in the mainstream medical community.

The Block model of care has six basic elements: biomedical, psychosocial, biochemical, biomechanical, medical gradualism, and the use of diagnostic and therapeutic tools that are minimally invasive. He uses the most effective and least invasive procedures first, and more aggressive tools only later, if and when they become necessary. He uses laboratory evaluations to show the activity and aggressiveness of cancers; antagonists, which combat the side effects from conventional therapy; and agonists, treatments or specially developed drugs that increase the effects of conventional cancer treatments. Dr. Block claims to design treatment plans that use conventional and unconventional therapies specific to each patient. He promotes self-care to the greatest extent that an individual is capable of, urging patients to consider what they need, how they respond to challenges, what they experience as stress, and how they learn. These elements of each person's psyche are considered in the entire treatment plan.

Other important parts of the Block regimen are physical conditioning and diet. The nutritional component of the program has evolved from macrobiotics. The dietary recommendations are similar to the low-fat preventive diets endorsed by the American Heart Association, the American Cancer Society, and the National Cancer Institute. The major difference is that this "preventive" diet is continued after the diagnosis of cancer. The diet draws 50 to 60 percent of its nutrients from complex carbohydrates. Fat intake, mostly from vegetable sources, ranges from 12 to 25 percent, and the rest of the daily caloric intake comes from protein sources. The diet uses exchange lists similar to diabetic exchange lists, based on whole-grain cereals, fruits, nuts and seeds, vegetables, legumes, and limited amounts of certain fish and poultry. Megavitamin supplements are not emphasized, though vitamin supplements are encouraged where there is evidence that they are helpful. Specific nutrients like vitamins A and E and trace minerals are used to bolster immune functions impaired by malnutrition, the effects of conventional treatment, or the cancer itself. Block also uses some natural supplements like echinacea and garlic to boost immune function and counter the side effects of treatment.

HERBAL THERAPY

Herbal medicine is one of the world's oldest therapeutic practices. More than three thousand different plants have been used worldwide throughout history in the treatment of diseases, including cancer. It wasn't until the

1920s and 1930s that herbal preparations gave way to manufactured drugs. Within the past decade, herbal therapies have made a comeback; books and articles describing their use now often appear in medical libraries as well as in lay bookstores, professional journals, and popular magazines. Herbal therapy is used to help the body restore and maintain balance. Since the Dietary Supplement Health and Education Act of 1994 classified herbs as nutritional supplements, herbs do not need U.S. Food and Drug Administration (FDA) approval. However, before the passage of this law, six herbs did get FDA approval: capsicum, when used as a topical analgesic; witch hazel, used as an astringent; and aloe, cascara, psyllium, and senna, all used as laxatives.

Traditional herbal practices use a whole plant or crude extracts of the plant. Traditional Chinese healing practices that combine herbs with acupuncture and other techniques are used by people in the United States for pain management, to control side effects, and to improve the quality of life. Chemicals from some fungi—especially edible and inedible mushrooms—are known to affect tumor growth and stimulate immune activity. Medicinal mushrooms including the shitake, maitake, Ganoderma, and *Cordyceps sinensis* varieties are being studied with results indicating that some of the mushrooms' properties stimulate the immune system, increasing the body's ability to kill or inactivate cancer cells. A mixture of eight Chinese herbs called PC-SPES is being bought in large quantities over the Internet and used by many men with prostate cancer. A few studies that show some decrease in metastatic disease has generated interest among mainstream cancer researchers.

Many of these "natural" herbal products are active agents—they might be helpful, and they might *not* be harmless or safe. Several reports in the medical literature tell of severe liver and kidney damage caused by a few of the herbs. In addition, many herbs negate or increase the effect of prescription medicines used for heart problems or bleeding disorders. Some herbal products or mixtures are contaminated with products not mentioned on the labels, and different batches of the same product may vary. In short, herbal therapies can relieve symptoms, promote well-being, and improve the quality of life for people with cancer. They must, however, be used wisely. See the table starting on the next page for an overview of commonly used herbs.

Chaparral tea has been used as a folk remedy for leukemia and cancers of the kidney, liver, lung, and stomach. Native Americans in the southwestern United States use chaparral for many illnesses, including cancer. Tea is made from tiny leaves and twigs or the bark of the creosote bush that is found in the Southwestern desert. Chemicals derived from the creosote bush have been found to have some antioxidant properties, which may

*Comple-
mentary
and
Alternative
Therapies
for Cancer*

133

Herbs Useful in Cancer Care

Herb	Form taken	Uses and actions	Considerations and warnings
Acidophilus *Lactobacillus acidophilus* Bacid, Lactinex, Probiotic	Tablets, powder granules, capsules 10 billion organisms/day in divided doses	To balance normal flora in the gastrointestinal tract, to treat or prevent vaginal and urinary tract infections when using antibiotics As a treatment for *Clostridium difficile* Being tested for use with bladder and breast cancer	Acidophilus is a bacteria, but is considered an herbal supplement by some Not recommended for people with lactose intolerance
Agrimony *Agrimonia eupatoria, Philanthrops agrimonia eupatoria* Sticklewort, Cocklebur, Liverwort	Tea, tablets, gargle Take orally, 3–6 g daily As a poultice, apply several times daily	Used in China as a cancer therapy For diarrhea, for inflammation of skin, mouth, pharynx, and intestine as tea or gargle Used as an astringent to treat cuts and scrapes	Avoid during pregnancy and lactation It contains tannins, causing digestive upset in large doses
Alfalfa *Medicago sativa* Lucerne, Purple medick, Purple medicle, Buffalo herb	Tablets, capsules, liquid extract from leaves, flour in food, infusion, sprouts, poultice, seeds No standard dose has been determined	Saponin acts on the heart, vascular, nervous, and digestive systems Poultice of seeds are used for boils and insect bites Has been used as a diuretic	May increase blood clotting time if taken with the drug warfarin May cause decrease in white and red blood cells, and platelets
Aloe *Aloe barbadensis* *Aloe carpensis* Aloe vera, Burn plant, Elephant's gall, Lily of the desert, Medicine plant	Extract, powder, jelly, cream, shampoo Topical: apply as needed Oral: Extract, 20–30 mg at bedtime 0.05 g aloe powder as a single dose in evening As *aloe carpensis*, 0.1 g in evening	Used topically for minor burns, sunburn, cuts, abrasions, acne Used orally as a laxative Depresses transmission of nervous impulses, resulting in pain-relieving and anti-inflammatory effects	Avoid during pregnancy and lactation Increases effects of some heart medications, diuretics, and steroids Avoid long-term use as a laxative Stop using if abdominal cramps occur after the first dose Avoid in intestinal block, inflammatory conditions of the colon, appendicitis, and undiagnosed abdominal pain

Herbs Useful in Cancer Care

Herb	Form taken	Uses and actions	Considerations and warnings
Angelica *Angelica Archangelica* Nature's answer, Angelica root liquid, European angelica, Angel's wort, Garden angelica Angelica sinesis Dong Quai, Dan Qui, Tang Kuei	Liquid extract, tincture, essential oil, whole herb Dose of drug: 4.5 g Liquid extract: 0.5–3.0 g Tincture: 1.5 g Essential oil: 10–20 drops Two capsules 2–3 times daily	Loss of appetite, mild gastro-intestinal tract spasms, gas, and feelings of fullness Sedative, mild laxative effects Has been used for coughs, bronchitis, loss of appetite, indigestion, fever Estrogen-like effects, has been used for premenstrual symptoms	Avoid during pregnancy and lactation May cause photosensitivity (increased sensitivity to sunlight) Improves blood clotting May cause hypotension
Anise *Pimpinella aniseum* *Illicium verum*	Oral daily dose is 3 grams Tea: drink one cup in the morning or evening as an expectorant One small spoon daily for stomach complaints—single dose 0.5–1 gram before meals	Used for cough, bronchitis, fevers, colds, inflammation of mouth and throat, indigestion, loss of appetite In folk medicine, used for gas, menstrual problems, liver disease, and as a digestive aid	Avoid during pregnancy or lactation Interferes with MAO inhibitors used to treat some mental health problems Interferes with hormone therapy High doses and limited fluid intake can cause bowel obstruction
Arnica *Arnica montana* Arnica flowers, Arnica root, Leopard's bark, Mountain tobacco, Wolfsbane	Tincture (3x–10x dilutions with water) As a poultice, use daily Ointments of 15% oil or 10–25% tincture in a neutral base daily As a mouthwash, tincture in 10x dilution daily	Used for fever, colds, skin inflammation, bronchitis, inflammation of mouth and throat, blunt injury and tendency to infection Used as a topical analgesic and antiseptic	Overdose can lead to poisoning and heart muscle problems Adds to effects of warfarin Avoid if allergic to arnica, chrysanthemums, sunflowers

(Adapted from: Decker, G.M., & Myers, J. "Commonly Used Herbs: Implications for clinical practice." Clinical Journal of Oncology Nursing, 5(2) special pullout insert, 2001; and Decker, G.M. (ed.). An Introduction to Complementary and Alternative Therapies. Pittsburgh, Oncology Nursing Press, 1999.)

Herbs Useful in Cancer Care

Herb	Form taken	Uses and actions	Considerations and warnings
Astragalus *Astragalus membranaceus* Beg Kei, Bei Qu, Membranous milk vetch, Astragali, Tragacanth	Capsules: 400–500 mg, eight to nine times daily Tincture: 15–30 drops of 1:5 dilution twice daily	Used for colds and upper respiratory infections Stimulates immune system Increases red blood cells Antioxidant, diuretic Strengthens intestinal movement	Avoid use with immunosuppressant drugs Avoid during pregnancy and lactation, and during acute infection Additive antiviral effects with the drug acyclovir Used with other anticoagulants, may increase risk of bleeding High doses may affect nerve function because of selenium content
Bearberry *Arctostaphylosuva-ursi* Foxberry, Manzanita, Mountain box, Bear's grape	In powder form: 10 g of drug in a single dose Dry extract: 0.4 g in a single dose As an infusion or cold compress: 3 g to 150cc water up to four times daily As a homeopathic: 5–10 drops one to three times daily	Used for urinary tract infections Used as an antimicrobial, diuretic, and anti-inflammatory	Avoid during pregnancy and lactation Use with caution with electrolyte imbalance, kidney disease, stomach problems, and bowel irritation Liver damage with long-term use
Black Cohosh *Cimicifuga racemosa* Black smoke root, Black cohosh powder, Rattleroot, Rattleweed, Bugbane	Capsules: 60–545 mg Tablets: 60 mg and 120 mg Alcohol-aqueous extracts (40–60%) or isopropanolic-aqueous (40%), corresponding to 40 mg drug daily for no more than 6 months	Used for menopausal symptoms, PMS Sometimes combined with St. John's wort for depression and moods associated with PMS and menopause Reports about estrogen-like effects are conflicting Thought to relax the uterus	Avoid during pregnancy or lactation Some stomach/bowel side effects have been reported Can increase effects of blood pressure medicines, causing hypotension (low blood pressure) High dose may cause vomiting, headache, dizziness, hypotension, pain in arms and legs Therapy should not exceed 6 months Extracts contain alcohol and should not be used by people with history of substance abuse

Herbs Useful in Cancer Care

Herb	Form taken	Uses and actions	Considerations and warnings
Blessed thistle *Cnicus benedictus* *Holy thistle*	Tea or mild decoction (an extraction created by boiling)	Used for nausea, diarrhea, loss of appetite, and relief of menstrual symptoms Used to improve memory	May interfere with antacids and H_2 blockers Contact dermatitis, nausea, and vomiting are more common with high doses
Capsicum peppers *Capsicum* Cayenne, Zanzibar peppers, Capsaicin, Chili pepper, Red pepper, Mexican chilies, Tabasco pepper	Externally: Cream (0.25% and 0.75% capsaicin) applied not more than 3–4 times daily Internally: Decoction, two cups daily Zostrix: 0.025% or 0.075% capsaicin for post-herpetic neuralgia	Used to relieve muscular tension and rheumatism Has been used topically to treat peripheral neuropathy, muscle spasms, postmastectomy pain, post-herpetic (herpes zoster) pain	Avoid during pregnancy and lactation There is no agreement on therapeutic dose and determination of side effects Taken internally, increases bowel motility and causes gastrointestinal irritation Topical use may cause blisters and/or skin ulcers May cause increased clot formation in the blood Causes irritation if used in open wounds or near the eyes Interacts with and may negate benefits of aspirin
Chamomile *Matricaria recutita* *Matricariae flos* Pin heads, German chamomile, Chamomilla, Hungarian chamomile, Single chamomile, Wild or genuine chamomile	Liquid and solid preparations are available for external and internal use Internally: single daily dose, about 3 g as an infusion; liquid extract: 1–4 ml or one cup of fresh tea three to four times daily External: bath additive, wash, or gargle, several times daily	Used topically as an anti-inflammatory agent for skin irritations, inflammation of the mouth and throat, wounds and burns Used internally to relax muscles, for cough, bronchitis, fevers and colds	Can cause contact dermatitis and severe allergic reaction (anaphylaxis) in people who are allergic to ragweed, asters, chrysanthemums, and anyone with hay fever and asthma caused by pollens Contraindicated in people allergic to *Compositae* family (arnica, yarrow, feverfew, tansy, artemesia) Not to be used with acute gastrointestinal symptoms (vomiting, abdominal pain, cramping, diarrhea) May mask other disorders

Herbs Useful in Cancer Care

Herb	Form taken	Uses and actions	Considerations and warnings
Condurango Condurangarinade *Marsdenia condurango*	Aqueous extract: 0.2–0.5 g daily Tincture: 2.5 g; infusion: one cup 30 minutes before meals; liquid extract: 2–4 g Must be kept in sealed container and protected from light	Used as appetite stimulant or to treat indigestion Stimulates production and secretion of saliva and gastric juices In the late 1800s there were claims it cured early cancers Used by the indigenous people of South America for syphilis	Avoid use with the drugs carbamazepine, paroxetine, ritonavir, sertaline, digoxin, atropine, scopolamine May stimulate the central nervous system, cause visual changes and seizures
Cranberry	Two to four glasses of juice daily	Used to treat urinary tract infections Reduces calcium in the urine Reduces formation of kidney stones	No known contraindications Drink adequate amounts of water Avoid cranberry juice with sugar
Echinacea *Echinacea angustifolia* Black sampson, Rudbeckia, Purple coneflower, Hedgehog, Red sunflower	Capsule, liquid preparations, semisolid external preparation Tincture: 30–60 drops three times daily; Liquid preparation: 6–9 cc of juice IV	Used to prevent and treat flu, colds, bronchitis Has anti-inflammatory and immune stimulation effects Used internally for headaches, stomach aches, muscle aches	People with autoimmune problems, HIV/AIDS, and TB should avoid all forms of Echinacea Avoid during pregnancy and lactation May alter effects of immunosuppressant drugs May cause allergic reactions in people with allergies to daisies and chrysanthemums Side effects might include nausea and other gastrointestinal problems

Herbs Useful in Cancer Care

Herb	Form taken	Uses and actions	Considerations and warnings
Evening primrose oil *Oenothera biennis* Fever plant, King's cureall, Night willow herb, Scabish, Sun drop	Capsule and oil For ectopic eczema: 6–8 g daily in divided doses For mastalgia (breast pain): 3–4 g daily in divided doses	Used for atopic eczema Used for asthma, whooping cough, eczema, breast pain, PMS, MS, RA, Raynaud's disease Used as a linoleic acid supplement Used to treat diabetic neuropathy	May cause seizures in people using phenothiazine medications Side effects include headache, inflammation, thromboses Immunosuppression is possible if used for more than a year
Feverfew *Tanacetum parthenium* Featherfoil, Midsummer daisy	Available in capsules Doses: 200–250 mg daily in divided doses	Decreases inflammatory response Used for fevers and headaches	Avoid during pregnancy and lactation Avoid use with anticoagulants Avoid if allergic to anything in the *Asteracae* family May cause nervousness and mild gastrointestinal upsets Rebound headaches, insomnia, fatigue, and nervousness can occur when its use is stopped
Flax seed *Linum usitatissimum* Bio-flax, Flaxseed Oil, New Energy, Lint Bells, Winterlein	Daily dose for constipation: one dessert spoon of whole or bruised seed with 150 ml of liquid 2–3 times daily To lower cholesterol: 35–50 g daily of crushed seed For decreased clotting: 1–2 tablespoons flax seed daily Absorption is better when taken with food Keep in a sealed container and protected from light Refrigerate oil and protect from light	Used for chronic constipation Used to reverse laxative abuse Used to treat irritable bowel Used to relieve menopausal hot flashes Used to treat skin inflammation Used to decrease cholesterol	Avoid in ileus Avoid in conditions where fluid intake is limited If used without enough fluid intake, ileus (blockage of the small bowel) can occur Immature seed pods are poisonous Overdose can cause mild to severe symptoms ranging from shortness of breath, weakness, rapid and ineffective heart beat, unstable gait to paralysis and seizure

Herbs Useful in Cancer Care

Herb	Form taken	Uses and actions	Considerations and warnings
Garlic *Allium sativum* Allium, common garlic, Stinking rose, Poor man's treacle	Average oral dose: 4 g fresh garlic or 8 mg of essential oil daily or one fresh clove one to two times daily. For arteriosclerosis: 600–800 mg daily of powder or dried garlic To lower cholesterol: 600–900 mg daily of garlic powder For high blood pressure: 200–300 mg garlic powder three times daily Topical use: Fresh garlic applied to the skin no more than a few hours	Lowers cholesterol and triglycerides Reduces blood clot formation Possibly stimulates immune sysem Has antimicrobial and antiviral effects Externally used for corns, calluses, muscle pain, neuralgia, arthritis, sciatica, and joint pain	May cause headache May increase muscle pain and weakness, fatigue, and dizziness Garlic powder may cause abdominal pain, nausea, vomiting, diarrhea, and decreased oxygen-carrying capacity in the blood Increased risk of bleeding when used with anticoagulant medications Interferes with platelet (blood clotting) function May cause body odor and halitosis Frequent contact may cause allergic reaction Extended topical use may cause burns Anticancer claims are unproven
Ginger *Zingeber officinale* Ginger root, Ginger kid, Ginger powder, Quanterra Stomach Comfort	Capsules/powder Daily dose for anti-vomiting and nausea: 0.5–2 g Store in cool place and protect from light Do not store in plastic	Used for loss of appetite, motion sickness, and upset stomach Stimulates digestion Increases gastric motility In Chinese medicine, is used to treat colds, nausea, vomiting, and shortness of breath Blocks blood clot formation	Avoid use with gallstone conditions Overdose can cause changes in the central nervous system, depression, and irregular heart beat

Herbs Useful in Cancer Care

Herb	Form taken	Uses and actions	Considerations and warnings
Ginkgo *Ginkgo biloba* Maiden hair tree	Should contain 24% flavone and 6% terpene lactones 120 mg daily	Used to relieve symptoms of brain function changes, dementia, vascular changes, dizziness and tinnitus Has been used for memory loss and to improve concentration	Can cause mild gastrointestinal problems Can cause changes in blood pressure Has adverse effects on oocytes (unreleased eggs in the ovaries) Can cause bleeding problems, including intracranial hemorrhage Avoid using with medicines known to increase risk of seizures
Ginseng *Panax ginseng* Five-Fingers redberry, American Ginseng, Chinese Ginseng, Korean Ginseng, Oriental Ginseng	Main ingredient consists of ginsenosides Daily dose: 1–2 g of the root Infusions: 3–4 times daily for 3–4 weeks To improve cognitive function: 400 mg daily oral dose To decrease blood sugar: 100–200 mg daily To treat erectile dysfunction: Korean red ginseng: 600 mg 3 times daily	Used for fatigue and to improve stamina Used to improve concentration In folk medicine, used for loss of appetite, anxiety, impotence, and neuralgias Has antioxidant and lipid decreasing properties Reduces blood glucose levels Some activity shown in reducing growth of lung cancer cells (adenocarcinoma) that are resistant to cisplatin	Avoid during pregnancy and lactation Use with caution with heart disease and diabetes Estrogenic: avoid using with estrogen-responsive tumors May cause hypertension (high blood pressure) Overdose can cause ginseng abuse syndrome that includes hypertension, sleeplessness, edema, and nervousness May cause breast pain (mastalgia) May negatively interact with antidiabetic drugs, insulin, warfarin, NSAIDs, antiplatelet agents, monoamine oidase inhibitors, and some diruetics
Goldenseal	Tincture: 5–30 drops Tea: 1 teaspoon of the root in 1 cup water	Often found in "immune boosting" herbal preparations	Avoid use with anticoagulants May cause hypoglycemia

Herbs Useful in Cancer Care

Herb	Form taken	Uses and actions	Considerations and warnings
Green tea *Camellia sinensis* Black tea, Chinese tea	Administration by infusion or capsule Daily dose: 300–400 mg of polyphenols (the active ingredient); three cups of tea = 250–320 mg of polyphenols	May be beneficial as a cancer preventative Has immune stimulant properties Used to treat diarrhea Used for stomach disorders, migraine headache, fatigue, vomiting, diarrhea, and to increase performance Mouthwash inhibits dental caries Caffeine has a stimulating and antidepressant effect	Avoid use with cardiac disease, kidney disease, hyperthyroidism, and psychiatric disorders Overdose (more than 300 mg caffeine or 5 cups daily) can cause restlessness and tremors Vomiting and abdominal spasm are signs of overdose Can interact with antacids, carafate, many heart medications, theophylline, warfarin, and monoamine oxidase inhibitors
Kava kava *Piper methysticum* Ava, Ava pepper, Intoxicating pepper, Kawa kawa pepper, Tonga, Kew	Capsules: 150–300 mg of root extract (50–240 mg of kava pyrones) daily Tincture: 30 drops with water three times daily Infusion: one half cup twice daily, with food	Used for nervousness, stress, insomnia, and anxiety Has muscle relaxing and antispasmodic effects In folk medicine, used as a sedative	Contraindicated during pregnancy and lactation Contraindicated for certain types of depression Increased risk of suicide Contraindicated with alcohol, sedative medicines, and anti-anxiety drugs
Maté *Ilex paraguariensis* Mateblatter, Yerba maté, Jesuit's tea, Paraguay tea, Bartholemew's tea	Herb for infusions, powder for internal use. Also available as a single tea or in tea combinations. One teaspoon of tea = 2 grams Average daily dose = 3 grams	Used to increase stamina Used to treat mental and physical fatigue Externally used as a poultice for ulcers and inflammation Stimulant	Associated with cancer of the esophagus and liver disease Excretion might be delayed if used with the drugs cimetidine, ciprofloxan, verapamil May negate effects of benzodiazepines and other central nervous system stimulants

Herbs Useful in Cancer Care

Herb	Form taken	Uses and actions	Considerations and warnings
St. John's wort *Hypericum perforatum* Hardhay, Umber, Goatweed, Klamath weed, Tipton weed	For depression: 300 mg (of dried herb) three times daily Tea: 2–3 g of dried herb in boiling water Standardized extract (0.2%), capsules: 250 mg 3–4 times daily or 500 mg two times daily As 0.3% extract: 300 mg capsule three times daily	Used for anxiety and depression Used for skin inflammation, blunt injury, wounds, and burns Has been used to treat anxiety, bronchitis, asthma, gall-bladder disease, indigestion, and weakness	Interacts or interferes with action of many prescription and over-the-counter drugs, including digoxin, cyclosporine, and etoposide Avoid with monoamine oxidase inhibitors May cause constipation, abdominal cramps, dry mouth, fatigue, photosensitivity, dizziness, insomnia, and restlessness
Red clover *Trifolium pratense* Purple clover, Trefoil, Wild clover, Cow clover, Meadow clover	Oral: liquid extract: 1:1 1–3 ml 3 times daily; Infusion: 4 g up to three times daily Topical: as a liquid extract	Used as an antispasmodic, expectorant Used to increase immune functions Used topically for psoriasis and eczema Has been reported to inhibit cancer-causing cell changes	Avoid during pregnancy and lactation May interfere with antiestrogens (tamoxifen) Do not use with oral contraceptives, estrogen, progesterone, aspirin Should not be used by those with a history of breast cancer
Valerian *Valeriana officinalis, Valerianae radix* Valerian root, All-heal, Amantilla, Setwall, Vandal root, Setewale, Garden heliotrope	Expressed juice, tincture, extracts, tablets, and capsules for internal use: Extract: 100–1,800 mg daily; Root powder: 15 grams daily internal dose; tincture: 0.5–1 teaspoon (1–3 ml) one to two times daily Externally: use as a bath additive	Used for restlessness and sleeping disorders caused by nervous conditions, mental strain Used to improve concentration, reduce stress, headache, anxiety	Avoid during pregnancy and lactation Avoid operating machinery or driving Side effects include gastrointestinal problems headache, restless states, sleeplessness, and changes in heart function May increase effects of depressants Has additive effects when used with barbiturates and benzodiazepines Avoid use with alcohol Should not be confused with valium

promote healing. A study of chaparral tea was completed in 1970 at the University of Utah. In a few patients it seemed to produce a slight antitumor response, but the methods used in the study were not described well and its results have not been duplicated in other studies. Chaparral tea is not without risks: It has been linked to liver failure requiring liver transplantation.

Essiac is an herbal preparation developed in Canada based on a Native American folk recipe. Rene Caisse, a nurse, was the sole proprietor of Essiac from 1920 to 1970. The story goes that Nurse Caisse obtained the recipe from a Native American woman and began to use it on a family member who had cancer. She found it was effective and began to make it available to others, calling it "essiac," her name spelled backward. Before she died in 1978, Caisse gave the formula and marketing rights to the Resperin Corporation of Ontario. Resperin provides Essiac to people with cancer through a special agreement with the Canadian Federal Health Offices.

Essiac supposedly contains four ingredients: Indian rhubarb, sheepshead sorrel, slippery elm, and burdock root. The proportions are not publicly known. NCI's Natural Products Branch reports that breakdown products from each ingredient are known to show some antitumor activity. The mixture, as supplied by Resperin, was tested in two trials at the Memorial Sloan-Kettering Cancer Center in New York and found to have no effect on tumors and to be toxic in high doses. The Canadian health system reviewed the results of Essiac treatment on eighty-six patients. Only one of the eighty-six felt better after Essiac therapy, and four had an objective, measurable response. Four more were stable, and the rest had no benefit, could not be evaluated, or had died.

Currently, Essiac is not approved for marketing in Canada, but it is available to certain patients in certain conditions—primarily when no other treatment is available. Practitioners using Essiac discourage the use of conventional therapy (radiation, chemotherapy) while the preparation is being used.

Hoxsey therapy was developed when Harry Hoxsey's grandfather noticed that his horse's tumor disappeared after the horse had grazed in a field filled with herbal wildflowers. Grandfather Hoxsey used a preparation made from the wildflowers on a family member who had a tumor and believed that the tumor vanished. Harry Hoxsey received the original recipe from his father and opened the first clinic in Dallas in the 1920s. By 1950, the Hoxsey clinic was one of the largest private cancer centers in the world, with branches in seventeen states. After multiple clashes with the FDA, the Dallas clinic closed in the late 1950s. A Tijuana clinic, under the direction of Hoxsey's nurse, has continued to use variations of the Hoxsey remedy since 1963.

According to Harry Hoxsey, chemical imbalances cause mutations that eventually result in a "vicariously competent cell" that is cancer. Normalization of body fluids creates an unfavorable environment for these cells, and they eventually die. His remedy corrects the abnormal blood chemistry and normalizes cell metabolism. Hoxsey's regimen can be used internally (taken as a pill or tonic) or topically (applied to the skin). Nutritional supplements and dietary restrictions are also part of the overall treatment plan, but the herbal preparation is the best-known part of the regimen. The regimen involves one of two formulas. One contains potassium iodide, licorice, red clover, buckthorn bark, burdock, stillingia, berberis, pokeweed root, cascara amarga, and prickly bark. The second formula contains potassium iodide and elixir lactate of pepsin, which is a protein-digesting enzyme.

Although no clinical trials have demonstrated its usefulness against cancer, Hoxey's formula has a long history of use in Native American cultures. Some of its ingredients show strong anti-flammatory effects, and anticancer actions have been noted in some cancer cells studied in the laboratory. Canadian studies currently being conducted may yield information about whether there is any basis for continuing to explore the usefulness of Hoxey's formula.

Mistletoe preparations are available in several forms. They have been mainly used in Switzerland, Germany, and other European countries, and less commonly in the United States. Trade names include Plenosol and Iscador; both are fermented extracts combined with metals like silver, copper, and mercury. Iscador is currently available in Switzerland, Germany, the Netherlands, the United Kingdom, Austria, and Sweden. It is not approved for sale in the United States, but American doctors can order it from European manufacturers. The Lukas Klinik in Switzerland uses Iscador with a regimen of conventional therapy, homeopathic preparations, a vegetarian diet, artistic activities, light exercise, baths, oils, and massage.

Crude mistletoe extracts and Iscador have been studied with mixed results. Some antitumor effects have been noted in some animal studies. There seems to be some increase in immune functions related to Iscador, but that could be caused by normal reactions to bacteria and other components in the preparation. Supporters claim that Iscador increases both the length of survival and the quality of life, stabilizes disease, causes tumor regression, and improves a patient's general condition.

A nurse tells me that she has been following a woman for several months who receives chemotherapy and also uses a ground mistletoe preparation. The woman's blood counts are more stable than would normally be expected, and she has no problems with nausea and vomiting. As an experiment, the nurses in the clinic asked this woman to stay off the mistletoe for

Complementary and Alternative Therapies for Cancer

just one cycle of chemotherapy. Sure enough, her white blood cell count dropped much more than usual, and she had nausea and vomiting that she had not experienced when she was on the mistletoe. Needless to say, the woman continues to use her extract! It must be said, though, that mistletoe preparations can be quite toxic, increasing blood pressure and heart rate. Mistletoe should not be used by anyone taking monoamine oxidase inhibitor antidepressants. Therefore, one's use of mistletoe should be made known to doctors and nurses involved in cancer therapy and the management of other medical and emotional conditions.

Pau d'arco, an herb available in health food stores, is marketed by American companies in capsule, tea, and powder forms. Pau d'arco is also called *taheebo, lapacho, ipes, ipe roxo,* and *trumpet bush.* It is grown in South America and is a popular folk remedy for various forms of cancer and other diseases, including malaria. It is reported to be a "strengthening and cleansing agent." Research studies have focused on one of the chemicals derived from it: lapachol. Proponents cite an unpublished study as evidence of its antitumor effect and its ability to enhance the immune system. Its major danger is its ability to cause blood clotting at the doses given for cancer treatment.

PSYCHOLOGICAL APPROACHES

Mental imagery, or **visualization,** is useful in the management of cancer. During "gentle imagery" a woman focuses on imagining peaceful, pleasant scenes. Gentle imagery is often used with relaxation, meditation, and hypnosis. In "guided imagery" a woman visualizes the symbolic destruction of cancer cells. Imagery can be used to reduce pain and stress, and maybe even to change the course of disease. It is a major component of the total program described by the Simontons in *Getting Well Again.*

Imagery in healing can be traced to ancient cultures. Historical records from Babylon, Assyria, and Greece document the use of imagery to chase disease from sick people. Imagery is also a part of Freudian psychoanalysis, and some kinds of imagery are used in biofeedback, Gestalt, and desensitization therapies. Imagery is useful in changing bodily processes, emotional status, self-image, physical performance, and behavior.

Imagery is a mental picture of a reality or a fantasy. It can include all five senses—sight, touch, hearing, smell, and taste. In guided imagery, a person intentionally creates an image that she chooses, and through this image, she communicates with her body processes. Some sort of relaxation exercise is usually the first part of guided imagery, followed by action imagery and end-result imagery—imagining what the desired end result will be.

Guided imagery used by a woman with cancer might go like this: The woman uses a simple relaxation exercise, such as silently repeating the word *relax,* to release muscle tension. When she is relaxed, she pictures her cancer in any way it appears to her and then images her form of treatment. For example, she might see chemotherapy spreading itself through her blood and being picked up by the cancer cells. (My friend Lorraine imaged the chemotherapy as piranhas eating up the cancer cells.) The woman then images her cancer shrinking or being destroyed, and her white blood cells removing dead cancer cells from her body. Lastly, she sees herself healthy and her body free of disease.

Meditation is any activity that keeps attention pleasantly focused in the present moment, clearing the mind of daily events and problems. Its purpose is to raise self-awareness, a first step in regaining control of the mind. Self-awareness and mental control are important tools in self-healing. There are different approaches to meditation; most attempt to achieve a state of suspension of logical thought and emotional processes. People who advocate meditation believe it recharges the immune system and helps it to function more effectively. In their book, *Meditation as Medicine,* authors Dharma Singh Khalsa, M.D., and Cameron Stauth gather and describe a good deal of scientific evidence for the healing forces of meditation. They contend that meditation helps maintain physical and emotional well-being, promotes spiritual growth, and eases many of the symptoms so common to people with cancer. There are many forms of meditation, but a large number of studies focusing on transcendental meditation (TM), the form made popular by the Beatles, reveals that the relaxation response that occurs during TM can affect hormone levels that relate to stress, blood pressure, pain, and many other physical and emotional states.

Hypnosis, another form of tapping into mental processes, is becoming more accepted as a complement to conventional therapy for relaxation and pain control.

The study of **psychoneuroimmunology** (PNI) by the medical establishment has given legitimacy to these complementary therapies. But it was quite a different story in 1978 when the Simontons were ridiculed for their belief in imagery techniques. This is a perfect example of turnaround in conventional wisdom regarding unconventional cancer therapies. Evidence that mental imagery works is only recently becoming accepted. Growing scientific exploration in psychoneuroimmunology examines the connection between the mind and the body—particularly the effects of mental processes on hormone production and the nervous and immune systems.

Many people with cancer find that mental training, including visualization and relaxation, helps them cope with the side effects of cancer and cancer treatment. Nurses often teach and use relaxation, imagery, and

*Comple-
mentary
and
Alternative
Therapies
for Cancer*

147

music therapy to help people decrease the nausea and vomiting caused by some chemotherapy drugs. Even when these techniques cannot increase the quantity of life, they contribute to the quality of life.

Diversional activities might be considered a sort of cousin to imagery and relaxation therapies. Humor therapy, leisure activities, recreational therapy, and music and art therapies are used in various settings to help people cope with cancer and its treatment. Cancer treatment can cause long hospital stays and social isolation. As the woman is physically and emotionally separated from friends and family, she may have decreased physical and emotional motivation to take part in leisure pastimes. All of these things take their toll.

Music has been used for teaching, celebration, and self-expression. It has also been used to summon and encourage soldiers in battle. During World War II, music was used to calm shell-shocked soldiers. (Some women with cancer feel shell-shocked too!) Since that time, the use of music as a therapy has steadily grown.

Ever since the invention of the phonograph in the 1800s, music has been used in hospitals to induce sleep. There is a relationship between the tempo of music and responses of the human nervous system; relaxing music with a repeating rhythm reduces anxiety. Music has a positive effect on the sensory and emotional reaction to cancer pain—possibly because it stimulates the release of endorphins, the body's natural painkillers. It can reduce anxiety during medical procedures. As a universal form of communication, it bridges age, culture, language, and education. Some women enjoy playing musical instruments, which can be a satisfying way to fill time or a wonderful gift to share with others. For information about music therapy, how to find a music therapist, and other related information, contact the American Music Therapy Association, 8455 Colesville Road, Suite 1000, Silver Spring, MD 20910 (website: www.musictherapy.org).

Laughter and **humor** are recognized as important parts of the coping and healing processes. There is a relationship between humor and increased immune system activity that seems to help prevent infections. Norman Cousins described his use of humor to relieve pain and other distressing problems in his book *Head First: The Biology of Hope*. People who enjoy humor also have better morale and an increased sense of well-being. Not only does humor help relieve anger, anxiety, and tension, it can actually be of physical benefit. It improves breathing, heart and blood vessel functions, muscle and bone structure and function, hormonal production, and immune function.

Art therapy and other forms of creative expression are being used to help adults and children cope with cancer. These creative activities can help women understand themselves better, make changes in their behavior, and express their feelings in a safe, nonthreatening way. Art can provide diversion and relaxation and support self-esteem.

PHYSICAL APPROACHES

Physical treatments have an accepted, supportive role in conventional cancer treatment. Exercise and mobility are key components in a holistic cancer care program. Rehabilitation concepts, including physical and occupational health, are at last considered crucial in comprehensive cancer care. Programs like the American Cancer Society's "We Can Weekend" combine physical exertion—hiking, climbing, swimming, canoeing—with group work, peer support, and counseling.

Exercise

Exercise is important. Very often, people with cancer are advised to "take it easy" and "get plenty of rest." Certainly, fatigue is a common cause of decreased quality of life for many people living with cancer and cancer treatment, but unnecessary bedrest and prolonged immobility result in a *loss* of energy and function. Our bodies work on a "use it or lose it" principle. Unless muscle groups are stimulated and used, they waste away and the woman gets weaker and weaker.

In several studies, many people started exercising while going through cancer therapy or after therapy. Women using exercise during chemotherapy for breast cancer found an increased sense of control and an increase in their functional abilities. Women who exercise have less tension, anxiety, depression, and fatigue, and actually have increased feelings of well-being. Exercise can also help control the nausea caused by chemotherapy and radiation. My friend with ovarian cancer makes it a point to walk her dogs a couple of times each day. The only bad result is that she looks so good and so healthy that her doctors have trouble believing she is in pain! But, she says, without her walks she would have more pain and, more importantly, would lose the companionship she enjoys with her dogs.

T'ai chi is a gentle exercise program that has been used for centuries by the Chinese in which slow motions mimic animal movement. Many fitness and community centers offer t'ai chi classes, but the techniques are also described in books, videos and websites. T'ai chi has been shown to lift mood, improve body balance, reduce falls, and increase physical strength.

Qi gong (qigong) (pronounced "chee gong"), literally meaning "working with energy," is another ancient Chinese form of exercise that blends breathing exercises, movement, and meditation. You can perform Qigong while sitting, standing, or lying down. Some forms of Qigong may also use self-massage, arm, leg, and stretching and circular body movements. Although scientific evidence is lacking, supporters credit Qigong with reducing stress and fatigue and improving circulation, disease resistance, and physical strength. Some suggest that Qigong can improve immune function and prolong survival in people with cancer and HIV/AIDS.

Yoga is another self-care measure that many use as a relaxation technique. Yoga originated in India more than five thousand years ago and is based on ancient Vedic teachings. Its traditional goal is to attain good health, including a simple diet, outdoor exercise, a tranquil mind, and an awareness of the relationship with one's creator. Yoga has a physiologic effect on circulation and muscle tone and is used for relief of symptoms including back pain, stress, fatigue, anxiety, muscle tension, and many of the symptoms that often afflict people who are dealing with cancer. It is getting easier to find yoga instructors even in small communities. It might be more difficult to find a yoga instructor who also is aware of special cautions that women with cancer should use. People with bone metastases can use yoga, but they must take special precautions to avoid placing stress on weakened bones.

Be aware that there can be risks associated with any form of exercise. For this reason, a woman should start an exercise program only after appropriate screening, a medical checkup, and a review of the non-cancer-related health factors such as heart, blood pressure, and orthopedic problems (knees, ankles, back, and so on). Symptoms that need to be considered and assessed before a woman starts any new exercise program include the following:

+ known cancer spread or metastases to bones

+ bone marrow depression or suppression

+ an irregular pulse or a resting pulse of more than 100 beats per minute

+ frequent leg pain or cramps

+ chest pain

+ rapid onset of nausea during exercise

+ dizziness, blurred vision, feeling faint

+ bone, back, or neck pain that is new

+ fever

+ shortness of breath

A walking program is the simplest—and perhaps the best—exercise. Shoes should be designed for walking or jogging, with a cushioned midsole and skid-proof outer sole. They should lace up and have smooth, soft areas inside that will not cause blisters or sores. Clothing should be comfortable. In winter, a hat or hood will prevent heat loss. Other expensive equipment is not needed. The pulse rate is the best indicator of the amount of work the body is doing. When walking, count the pulse for six seconds and add a zero to get the beats per minute. To benefit from exercise, the pulse should be increased to the "training range" and kept there for ten to twenty minutes.

Training pulse range

Age in years	Suggested training pulse rate/minute	Pulse, 6 seconds
<20	140–150	14 or 15
20–30	130–140	13 or 14
30–40	120–130	12 or 13
40–50	110–120	11 or 12
50–60	100–110	10 or 11
60+	90–100	9 or 10

(Winningham, 1991)

Touch

Touch is the most sensitive of our five senses. We all have it, and we can all use it to improve the quality of our lives. During illness, touch is sometimes forgotten or neglected. Historically, the fear of contagious diseases prevented people from the benefit of touching another person. We have all seen pictures of the study in which sad little monkeys cling to a cloth-wrapped metal substitute in an effort to touch something resembling their own species. Unfortunately, many people with cancer have been denied the physical comfort that can be provided by touch. Today, people with AIDS are very aware of the need for, and their frequent lack of, the physical touch of another person.

   Massage has been described as a therapy for illness since the fifth century B.C. It offers nurturing and relaxation that can be a special complement to other cancer therapies. While there is no evidence that massage cures disease, massage does ease muscle tension, increase joint flexibility, and increase blood flow to specific body parts. Most massage techniques involve combinations and variations of kneading, manipulation, or the application of methodical pressure and friction to the body. Massage therapists or "bodyworkers" commonly use the following strokes:

1. *Effleurage:* superficial or deep gliding, long, rhythmic strokes that warm the muscles; the whole hand moves over the body toward the heart

2. *Petrissage:* kneading with the fingers and thumb of each hand in C-shaped motions to stimulate the muscle

3. *Friction:* circular movements with thumbs, fingers, or heel of the hand to penetrate deeper muscle layers or work around joints

4. *Tapotement:* quick, vigorous, rhythmic strokes like tapping, cupping, slapping, or pummeling to stimulate muscles

5. *Vibration:* shaking movements with fingers or the hand to stimulate or relax muscles

There is some confusion about the use of massage with cancer patients. Some formal massage therapy schools turn cancer patients away, leaving practitioners with a phobia about touching people with cancer. Fear that massage techniques may cause cancer cells to break away and spread is common. In reality, there is no evidence that gentle massage of the body causes cancer to spread.

Use of massage with cancer patients is gaining acceptance among the established medical community, and studies are being conducted by nurse scientists to explore its usefulness more fully. Do note, though, that cancer experts do caution against using deep bodywork and massage directly over a tumor, and massage should be avoided in areas affected by lymphedema, in the presence of deep vein thrombosis, in areas in which lesions or sores are present, or near incision sites and obvious tumor sites.

Massage can indeed be an important addition to an overall cancer management plan, but it is important that the massage therapist understand the cancer status—such as the site of the cancer, any known metastatic sites, and the location of medical devices such as central lines and vascular access ports. Treatment history will also be important information to share with the therapist since skin changes, increased sensitivity, edema, and the risk of bruising and bleeding should be considered when planning the form of massage that can be offered....

The effects of one human touching another, with care and concern, offer both the caregiver and the patient a truly meaningful experience. The benefits derived from massage include relaxation, reduced swelling, decreased stress, relief of fatigue, improved sleep, and decreased pain. The book *Medicine Hands: Massage Therapy for People with Cancer* by Gayle MacDonald is a good source of in-depth information.

In **therapeutic touch**, the practitioner doesn't really touch at all, but rather holds her hands inches away from the patient's body and, in so doing, stimulates electrical activity in the aura that surrounds the patient. Touch healing is described in the *New Testament*, and women healers have used it for centuries; some believe its origins rest with survivors of Atlantis. Native Americans use forms of therapeutic touch that amazingly resemble those found in Tibet, South America, and Africa. Today this technique involves a systematic protocol pioneered in America by Dolores Krieger, professor of nursing at New York University, and now taught at more than eighty colleges in North America. It is used at many American hospitals as a supplement to conventional therapies. Krieger's methods assume that the human being is an open system and that illness represents an imbalance in a person's energy systems. The healer is charged with rebalancing these systems.

The three phases in the therapeutic touch process are *centering, assessing,* and *rebalancing.* During centering, the therapist/healer meditates so that her thoughts are opened to input from her client. During the assessment phase, she tunes in to imbalances in the energy fields around the client's body. Finally, during rebalancing, the energy fields surrounding the body are smoothed out and redirected. The process usually takes no longer than twenty minutes.

Therapeutic touch has been effective in relieving postoperative and generalized pain, improving red blood cell levels, lowering blood pressure, and decreasing anxiety, stress, and headaches in many people. Practitioners claim that therapeutic touch can correct anemia and swelling (edema) and aid in the healing of bone fractures.

Reiki (pronounced "ray kee") is a formalized laying on of hands in which "master" status is given to only a few practitioners; it is expensive to achieve. Reiki can be a beautiful addition to other healing processes. It originated in ancient Tibet, traveled to China and Japan, and was brought to the United States in 1938. In Reiki, formal physical positions are used in a sequence for applying energy over specific energy centers (**chakras**) of the body. Reiki is learned and mastered through a series of three stages, or degrees. The beginning degree opens the healer's ability to channel her energy and teaches her the healing positions. The second degree involves learning Reiki as a distance healing process. The third degree allows the healer to be known as a "Reiki Master" and to teach others.

Laying on of hands is a way of applying energy to relieve pain, speed healing, regenerate energy, and calm nerves. It can be useful in helping women cope with the distressing symptoms of cancer and its treatment. It can be done by the woman herself; she does not necessarily have to find a healer, though the human-to-human bond and sharing process is a meaningful component of the healing process. The energy transferred by the laying on of hands can be completely positive and beneficial, and harms no one. Anyone can do this type of healing to help herself or others.

Reflexology, like acupressure, is based on the idea that pressure placed on nerve reflex points can stimulate the healing powers of these areas. Reflexology techniques applied to the feet, hands, and ears may contribute to the management of symptoms such as headache and nausea.

Therapeutic touch, Reiki healing, and reflexology can seem a little spooky. But skilled, intelligent healers, many of them nurse colleagues, use and enthusiastically endorse these healing techniques. A group of nurses at the University of Iowa College of Nursing has established a network of nurse healers. Their stories are amazing and wonderful. Patients with illnesses or problems that seemed impossible to control benefited from these healing forces. Pain, nausea, and vomiting problems were allayed, making a tremendous difference in the quality of life. Many practitioners are looking for ways to document the effects of these techniques. Some believe that the energy exchange activates parts of the immune system, allowing the body to fight cancer, infection, and other stressors more effectively.

SPIRITUAL APPROACHES

Spirituality and **religion** are words and ideas that get used interchangeably, but they can be very different things. Not all people who have a sense of spirituality consider themselves religious. Spirit and spirituality relate the essence of a person to her world and give meaning to existence. Spirituality and health have been intertwined from early times, when priests and shamans were the first healers. Spiritual well-being can be the cornerstone of health, integrating one's inner resources—the physical body, rational mind, emotional psyche, and intuitive spirit. A 1971 White House Conference on Aging defined spirituality as "the human belief system that pertains to humankind's innermost concerns and values, which ultimately affects behavior, relationship to the world, and relationship to God—however the individual defines the order of the universe."

The days and months after a diagnosis of cancer are a time filled with concerns about life and death. People try to find the meaning of their eventual death, the meaning of the cancer experience, and the meaning of the life remaining to them. Very early, people come to realize that facing cancer and cancer treatment is going to be a huge challenge. To meet the challenge and put out the effort needed, it is natural for people to look for meaning in what faces them. In an especially interesting study, six major themes evolved that relate to how a person interprets the meaning of the cancer experience and which activities, life experiences, relationships, values, beliefs, and philosophies people look to for meaning:

+ seeking an understanding of the personal significance of the cancer diagnosis—"Why me?"

+ looking at the possible outcomes of the cancer diagnosis

+ reviewing one's life

+ changing one's outlook toward self, life, and others

+ living with cancer

+ rekindling hope

Support during the search for meaning comes most often from personal faith and social support. Social support involves relationships with others that are expressed as care and love. Faith helps people cope through renewal of an inspirational contact with their religion and/or God or a deeper aspect of themselves. In turn, hope develops as a result of renewed faith. For many, formal religion is not important in this process, but most people say that their idea or feeling about God has always affected their lives. This idea of God represents a person's spirituality. It includes religion, but is not limited to religion.

There are countless spiritual approaches to healing. They generally share a common precept that the healer must gain access to a hidden reality in order to share the power and wisdom of the universe with others in need. For example, a healer in India maintains that she communicates with the universe through a link provided by a Hindu saint. In a tribal culture, a healer might make a different but similar spiritual link; it could involve a sacred plant, a rock, or quartz crystals. Sometimes, spiritual healing is referred to as **shamanism** and its practitioners as shamans. In shamanism, conflict, pain, and suffering are part of ordinary reality. The goal of shamanism is to attain an experience of nonordinary reality (shamanic ecstasy)—that is, moving beyond time and becoming one with the universe. The shaman helps people to move between ordinary and nonordinary reality and, in doing so, to experience deeper harmony within themselves and to heal pain.

The practice of laying on of stones and crystals is fascinating. Quartz crystal and gemstones are used for healing in Native American cultures, South America, Africa, Europe, Egypt, and India. Legend has it that people on the lost continent of Atlantis used clear quartz crystals as their major source of energy, and healing was powered by crystals and gemstones.

Native American shamans and medicine women in several tribes use crystals and turquoise on various parts of the body to tap into wisdom. Today, crystal work and the laying on of stones are being used to release physical disease and work with the emotional sources of physical illness. Healers work to change the electrical field, or aura, that surrounds the body. The aura is believed to be made of eight levels of energy or light and four bodies that surround the body. The etheric double is the first of the four bodies and is closest to the physical. Moving outward from the skin, other levels are the emotional body, the mental body, and the spiritual body. Gemstones of different colors are coordinated with the different energy levels. The chakras, or energy centers, are activated by laying on stones. Each chakra has unique characteristics and healing uses. Even though individual chakras can be targeted, laying on of stones is most often done to bring the whole woman into balance.

A central part of all spiritual healing processes is helping the woman accept and love herself. Louise Hay believes that illnesses, which she calls "dis-eases," are the result of emotional and mental stresses. Cancer, Hay says, is "probably" caused by deep hurt and long-standing resentment, deep secrets or grief that eats away at the self, and carrying hatreds. Hay believes that "dis-ease" can be cured by reversing mental patterns. She describes metaphysical causation, "the power in words and thoughts that create experiences," as crucial in creating and healing dis-ease. The mental work of releasing and forgiving are healing processes. Old thought patterns should be replaced by healing affirmations. For cancer, Hay suggests this affirmation: *I lovingly forgive and release all of the past. I choose to fill my world with joy. I love and approve of myself.*

Some people interpret Hay's message to mean that the person with cancer is to blame for causing the cancer or, if she does not get well, she is to blame for the failure. The confusion may rest with a lack of universal interpretation or definition of being "well" or being "healthy."

Healers, from the ancient shamans and medicine men and women to the healers of today—people like Dolores Krieger, O. Carl Simonton, Stanley Krippner, Rachel Naomi Remen, and Jeanne Achterberg, who has done work with women's healing—have a definition of wellness different from the conventional medical one. Wellness and health are not necessarily the same as absence of disease, and getting well does not necessarily mean getting cured of the cancer. On the contrary, healing can mean finding a balance among the physical, emotional, intellectual, and spiritual dimensions of one's condition, and one's life.

PHARMACOLOGIC AGENTS:
DRUGS AND SPECIAL PREPARATIONS

Antineoplastons, chemicals formed from substances found in urine, are being developed and promoted by Stanislaw Burzynski, M.D., at the Burzynski Research Institute near Houston, Texas. At least ten types of antineoplastons, available only at Burzynski's clinic, are given orally or intravenously, mostly orally. The clinic charges from $135 to $685 for a day's therapy, in addition to room, board, diagnostic tests, catheters, and pumps used for IV therapy. An initial deposit of $5,000 is required, and treatment costs can run to tens of thousands of dollars per year. Patients must travel to Burzynski's clinic to get this treatment.

Dr. Burzynski claims that antineoplastons are a "totally new class of compounds," urinary peptides that reprogram cancer cells. In other words, they are substances normally made by the body as part of the body's natural defense system. According to Dr. Burzynski, when the body fails to produce enough antineoplastons, cancers are allowed to develop and grow; giving antineoplastons helps to restore the normal defense system.

In 1991, the National Cancer Institute assessed the responses of a group of patients treated at Burzynski's clinic. Dr. Burzynski was invited to select patients from his clinical experience. The NCI reviewers saw evidence of antitumor activity in the antineoplastons and proposed that a formal clinical trial be done to provide a clear and unbiased evaluation of the response rate and toxicity of antineoplastons given to adults with brain tumors.

The study began in 1993 at the Memorial Sloan-Kettering Cancer Center in New York City, the Mayo Clinic in Rochester, New York, and the NIH Clinical Center in Bethesda, Maryland. However, only nine patients volunteered to take part in the study, and the NCI and Dr. Burzynski could not agree on ways to increase the number of patients to be included. Such a small "sample population" would never allow sound conclusions to be drawn, and the studies were shut down before they were completed. Although the NCI claims to continue to look for ways to determine the value of antineoplastons, no form of antineoplaston has come to the FDA for approval.

In Burzynski's clinic, most patients begin with small doses of antineoplastons that eventually increase to an optimal level—which is not clearly defined. Some patients also get low-dose chemotherapy. So far the treatment seems to be nontoxic, but a small percentage of people have reported some side effects. There are no reports of serious side effects in the literature; however, articles about antineoplastons have appeared only in lay

Complementary and Alternative Therapies for Cancer

157

magazines and nonscientific, non-peer-reviewed literature. One magazine article claimed that 46 percent of people taking antineoplastons for colon cancer had a total remission. Most successes are reported to be in the treatment of cancers involving the bladder, brain, breast, prostate, and bone. They may also be effective for ovarian cancer. Dr. Burzynski says clearly that antineoplastons are not effective for all cancers and asserts that most people taking his treatment have a positive response. On the other hand, two early NCI trials completed in 1983 and 1985 showed no increase in survival rates and no apparent effect on tumors associated with two antineoplastons.

In 1997, Dr. Burzynski was in a federal courtroom facing charges that he allowed antineoplastons to be shipped out of Texas. The trial was reported daily in newspapers and evening television news broadcasts across the state. Emotional pleas from patients charged the government with the "ongoing persecution of Dr. Burzynski," saying that we risk losing "the most important breakthrough in cancer therapy of this century." There were accusations that other scientists are withholding information about the value of antineoplastons in fighting cancer (Dr. Julian Whitaker's *Health and Healing*, mid-February supplement, 1996). The trial was not about whether antineoplastons do or don't work. Many believe that Dr. Burzynski is under attack because he has developed his treatment outside of the established medical system. At any rate, the trial ended in a hung jury—no verdict and no decision. Dr. Burzynski continues his practice in Houston.

Coenzyme Q_{10} (also called CoQ_{10}, Q_{10}, vitamin Q_{10}, ubiquinone, or ubidecarenon) is a natural substance made in our bodies. It was first identified in 1957, and interest in it as a possible cancer treatment started in 1961 when deficiencies were noticed among people with some forms of cancer. Coenzyme Q_{10} is normally found in most body tissues, but levels decline as we age. The highest tissue levels are found in the heart, liver, kidneys, and pancreas, with the lowest levels found in the lungs. It functions as part of a process that speeds up chemical reactions in the body and is used by cells to produce the energy needed to maintain cells and help them grow. Our bodies use coenzyme Q_{10} as an antioxidant—one of the substances that protect cells from the highly reactive and damaging effects of chemicals called free radicals—a process that most experts believe plays a role in the development of cancer.

Studies on coenzyme Q_{10} have been done to describe its chemical structure and functions. In animal studies, coenzyme Q_{10} seems to stimulate the immune system and protect heart tissues from the damaging effects of the drug doxorubicin, a drug contained in a great many chemotherapy regimens. A similar protective effect has been observed in early clinical trials on a very small number of human patients. Other studies have been done to test the value of this enzyme given as a supplemental adjuvant therapy for cancer, but results have so far been mixed. There is concern from some scientists that the antioxidant properties of coenzyme Q_{10} might actually interfere with the action of cancer therapies that depend on the formation of free radicals—the main anticancer action of some types of chemotherapy and radiation therapy. Overall, there is encouragement among the scientific community to continue making an investment in testing the potential benefits and risks of coenzyme Q_{10} used on its own or in combination with other forms of therapy.

Coenzyme Q_{10} is usually given orally, as a pill or capsule, but it can be injected into a vein. Although no serious side effects have been reported, some people who use coenzyme Q_{10} do experience some sleep problems or insomnia, skin rash, nausea, dizziness, headache, heartburn, fatigue, increases in liver enzymes, and upper abdominal pain. It might interfere with the action of some prescription drugs, including those that lower cholesterol, medications used to treat diabetes, and warfarin, which is used to prevent development of blood clots.

The U.S. Food and Drug Administration has not approved coenzyme Q_{10}, but since it is distributed as a dietary supplement, FDA approval is not required and it is distributed by several companies. Since dietary supplements are not regulated, manufacturing composition may vary from one brand to another and even from one batch to another.

Cancell, Entelev, Sheridan's Formula, Jim's Juice, Crocinic Acid, JS-114, JS-101, 126-F, and **Cantron** are all different names for the same substance: a liquid that has been produced and distributed as a treatment for cancer and other diseases since the late 1930s. According to the FDA, its ingredients include the chemicals inositol, nitric acid, sodium sulfite, potassium hydroxide, sulfuric acid, and catechol, but the exact composition is not public knowledge. None of these ingredients is known to be an effective treatment for any form of cancer.

This formula has an interesting history. It was first developed by a chemist named Entelev and given free to people with cancer. Production was taken over by another manufacturer, the formula was renamed "Cancell," and it was once again distributed free of charge to people with cancer, AIDS, and other illnesses.

The two manufacturers explain that Cancell/Entelev works in a way that compares to the way the body wards off infection and other foreign bodies. According to one theory, the product alters cancer cells so that the body recognizes them as foreign and sets up processes that destroy the seemingly foreign bodies. A second theory involves cellular changes in which the cells self-digest and are replaced by normal cells.

*Comple-
mentary
and
Alternative
Therapies
for Cancer*

159

Cancell/Entelev is taken by mouth, inserted into the rectum, or applied to skin at the wrist or foot. While taking Cancell/Entelev, people are usually advised to take the digestive aid "bromelain" and avoid high doses of vitamins C and E. The most common side effects include fatigue during the initial weeks of treatment and nausea.

Even though the manufacturers of Cancell/Entelev claim that a number of successful animal studies demonstrate its value, none of these studies have been published in scientific journals. Instead, claims for the product rely primarily on individual claims and testimonials. The NCI authorized studies testing the anticancer value of Cancell/Entelev, which were completed between 1978 and 1991. The findings indicated that it has no effect on cancer. Consequently, the NCI determined that no additional study on this substance is needed. Information about its effectiveness has not been submitted to the FDA, it is not approved for use in the United States, and manufacturers have been prohibited from distributing the mixture since 1989.

Hydrazine sulfate was popularized as an antitumor drug in the 1970s. A few studies demonstrated some tumor response, and some patients reported they felt better. The major effect seemed to be improved nutritional status. It has since been proposed as a treatment to prevent the weight loss and muscle wasting that occur with many forms of cancer. In early studies, hydrazine sulfate was also associated with an increase in survival time. Based on these studies, it is being tested for its effects on nutritional status and the effects of nutritional status on the progress of various forms of cancer.

Dimethyl sulfoxide (DMSO), a chemical solvent, is sometimes combined with other agents—particularly vitamin C and laetrile—to treat cancer. DMSO is not believed to be able to kill cancer cells. Its promoters claim that it dissolves the protein shell around cancer cells and thereby restores the abnormal cell to normal. Health food store literature promotes DMSO in the management of symptoms of tuberculosis, herpes, and arthritis. One form of DMSO has been approved by the FDA for the treatment of bladder inflammation (cystitis).

Cellular treatments, also called **live cell therapy, cellular therapy, cellular suspensions, glandular therapy,** and **fresh cell therapy,** involve injecting or swallowing processed tissue from animal fetuses (usually sheep, cow, or shark). The type of cells given correspond to the organ or tissue that is affected by the cancer. Its users claim that the injected cells travel to similar organs and stimulate that organ's function. The known side effects and dangers result from allergic reactions and infection. Cellular therapy is not widely practiced in the United States. It was developed and popularized in

Switzerland in the 1930s and moved to Tijuana in the late 1970s. It is now available in perhaps five clinics.

Laetrile is the best known unconventional cancer treatment development over the last twenty years. By the mid-1970s at least seventy thousand people were using it for cancer prevention, cancer treatment, and pain control. By 1977, twenty-two states had legalized its use. It has lost some appeal since studies at the Mayo Clinic disproved any positive effect, but it is still available at cancer clinics in Mexico.

Amygdalin, laetrile, Laetrile (brand name), sarcarcinase, nitriloside, and vitamin B-17 are all chemically similar substances used for laetrile treatment. The active ingredient is found in the pits of apricots and other fruits, and its use is based on two theories about the cause of cancer. According to one theory, cancer is caused by **trophoblastic cells**—cells normally present during pregnancy to protect the fertilized egg from being rejected by the mother's body, which for some reason are present in the body of the person with cancer. Another theory is that cancer is a disease caused by a vitamin deficiency—a lack of the vitamin laetrile. Proponents of laetrile believe that it kills cells selectively, affecting only cancer cells and leaving normal cells alone. Claims made in the 1970s reported that laetrile had antitumor effects. Now most practitioners use laetrile as a part of a regimen that may include other agents such as DMSO, vitamins, minerals, amino acids, enzymes, oxygen, and cellular therapy.

Laetrile naturally contains at least 6 percent cyanide and is toxic in large doses. Combining it with some other foods actually causes the release of more cyanide. There are also wide variations found in the potency of sampled laetrile containers, and some bottles have been found to be contaminated by bacteria and viruses.

Immuno-Augmentative Therapy (IAT) was developed in the 1970s by zoologist Lawrence Burton, Ph.D., who practiced out of a clinic in New York State. In 1977, he founded the Immunology Researching Centre in the Bahamas. In 1987, a clinic opened in West Germany and another in Mexico in 1989.

IAT is based on the theory that restoring optimal immune function allows the immune system to find and destroy cancer cells. These immune functions then serve as a natural weapon to control carcinogenesis. Advocates of IAT claim that it can control or stabilize most cancers and cause others to regress. Dr. Burton also claims that IAT is effective against multiple sclerosis and AIDS. However, although Dr. Burton has described his success in newspapers, magazines, and television interviews, he has not allowed his work to be reviewed through objective scientific standards nor has he published descriptions of his work in scientific journals. In 1984, five patients returning from Dr. Burton's Bahaman clinic gave samples of the IAT to NCI scientists for analysis. The materials being called IAT were identified as simple blood proteins with no immune or antitumor activity at all. For these reasons, the medical community continues to view IAT as having unproven value.

To further complicate the picture, all the samples were contaminated with germs and viral hepatitis. Since then, another seventy samples have been analyzed by the Centers for Disease Control, the NCI, and other independent laboratories, with similar findings. The viruses responsible for causing AIDS (HIV) and hepatitis B were found in the IAT materials, giving the IAT material the ability to transmit AIDS and hepatitis B to patients being treated with IAT. In 1986, the Food and Drug Administration issued an import alert that allows U.S. customs and the U.S. Postal Service to seize all biological agents brought into the United States. The clinic was closed in July 1985 by the Bahaman government, but allowed to reopen several months later with Dr. Burton's promise to maintain quality control and sterile conditions. IAT material samples tested in 1987 were determined to be free of the HIV and hepatitis viruses.

Treatment consists of daily self-injections of processed blood products, to be administered for the rest of the person's life. The complete regimen can include other drugs, especially steroids. Practitioners suggest that large tumors be removed surgically before the start of IAT, but they discourage chemotherapy and radiation therapy.

In conflicting reports of the same study, one group of researchers determined that the study was evidence for the efficacy of IAT, while a second group analyzing the same data decided that no valid deductions could be made about the effect of IAT. This is typical of the differences between mainstream and unconventional practitioners. Negotiations to arrange a clinical trial for IAT have fallen through several times. Dr. Burton died in 1993, but the Immunology Researching Centre in the Commonwealth of the Bahamas remains open under the direction of Dr. R. J. Clement. There are currently no clinical trials planned.

Oxymedicine uses hydrogen peroxide and ozone to destroy tumors. These oxygen treatments are not widespread in the United States, but there are clinics in Mexico and Germany. Oxygen treatments are usually used to complement other therapies. For example, the Gerson Clinic in Tijuana added ozone enemas to its regimen. Oxymedicine is based on the idea that a buildup of manmade toxins from foods, food additives, and environmental pollution is the major cause of degenerative diseases, including cancer. Therefore, the appropriate treatment is to detoxify the body and reverse the disease with dietary changes. A second premise is that tumors thrive *without* oxygen and are killed by substances that increase oxygen to the tumor site.

Ozone, a gas, is administered by direct infusion into the rectum or muscle—often in an infusion of blood. In most regimens a pint of blood is removed from the patient, treated with oxygen, and then returned to the patient. Hydrogen peroxide in dilute forms is given by mouth, through the rectum or vagina, into the veins, or added to baths. Advocates believe that the peroxide oxidizes toxins, kills bacteria and viruses, and stimulates immunity.

Shark cartilage is the basis of a relatively recent development in cancer treatment. On a trip to my hometown in Iowa, I visited a friend's mother who had been dealing with ovarian cancer for several years. Even though she lives in a small town and does not travel much, she had, like many people dealing with cancer, discovered several sources of information about alternative therapies for cancer. She asked my opinion of shark cartilage pills.

The rationale for shark cartilage, according to its proponents, is that "sharks rarely develop cancer, either in clear open waters or in water highly polluted with carcinogenic chemicals. The key to their resistance seems to lie in their boneless skeleton."

It turns out that the fact that sharks seem somewhat more immune to cancer than humans has been of interest to researchers at the NCI for several years. But even though sharks do develop cancers, a 1983 study showed that shark cartilage contains a substance that interferes with the development of blood vessels that feed tumors (*antiangiogenesis*), which in turn limits tumor growth. The questions have not been fully explored, but even without definitive study, shark cartilage continues to be promoted as a means to prevent the development of cancer or to slow its progress after it has developed. The process of antiangiogenesis has, however, been the source of great excitement and intense study over the past several years, and may ultimately become an important cancer treatment strategy.

Shark cartilage is available in health food stores and from mail-order outlets as pills or capsules. While it is supposed to be nontoxic, the woman who first told me about its use had to stop using it. She said the pills made her "sick to her stomach," with cramps, nausea, and vomiting. As soon as she stopped taking the pills, the symptoms ceased. *Sharks Don't Get Cancer* by Lane and Comac (1992) and the newer edition *Sharks Still Don't Get Cancer* (1996) review events and research that led the authors to believe shark cartilage may be useful in the treatment of cancer and other chronic diseases.

Krebiozen is a substance that originally came from the serum of horses injected with a fungus. Later it was developed from mineral oil and creatinine, a substance that is normally made and excreted by the body. Despite the fact that neither of these substances is known to have any antitumor activity, Krebiozen gained a following during the 1950s and early 1960s. The U.S. government assessed Krebiozen therapy in 1963 in a review of the cases of more than 500 patients who were reported to have been helped by the treatment. The review committee concluded that Krebiozen had no therapeutic effects in people with cancer.

Hariton-Tzannis Alivizatos, or the **Greek Cancer Cure,** was developed by Greek microbiologist Dr. Hariton-Tzannis Alivizatos, who used a series of serum injections to treat people with cancer. He never published his therapy's results or allowed scientists to review his work before he died in 1991.

PROGRAMS USING COMPLEMENTARY THERAPIES

Many complementary therapy programs use combinations of therapies and work toward helping people achieve their unique goals for recovery and healing. Social or peer support, emotional and spiritual interventions, dietary changes, massage and therapeutic touch, and guided imagery are key components of several formalized cancer support programs. The Wellness Community—started in Santa Monica, California, in 1982 and promoted by Gilda Radner—now has centers in many cities across the United States. It offers mutual aid groups that focus on positive emotions and mental activities, and self-help skills that increase the possibilities of recovery. Some programs offer one-to-one sessions with a psychotherapist and other varied group activities. Services are free and programs are supported through community and corporate donations.

Dr. Bernie Siegel, author of *Love, Medicine, and Miracles,* founded a program called Exceptional Cancer Patients (ECaP) in New Haven, Connecticut, in 1978. The program is based on Siegel's belief that attitude influences survival time, and it includes individual and group support and uses dreams, drawings, and images to increase awareness of each person's healing potential. Psychotherapy is available, as are books and video and audio recordings. There is only one center, but training sessions have allowed people to develop ECaP-like groups in other locations. Patients are charged for all sessions. Critics of the ECaP program charge that Dr. Siegel implies that cancer results from poor emotional patterns, a theory that has not at all been supported by scientific data.

Commonweal was established in 1976 by Michael Lerner, Ph.D. It is located on sixty acres of the Pacific coast near Bolinas, California, north of San Francisco. It is a nonprofit corporation supported by foundations and public agencies as well as individuals. Commonweal offers several different educational and healing experiences, including retreats and workshops planned to help people "explore issues, choices, feelings and concerns that people with cancer often have, in the company of others, with an experienced and concerned staff." According to its website (www.commonweal.org), the Commonweal Cancer Help Program (CCHP) is "dedicated to helping people seek physical, emotional, and spiritual healing in the face of cancer." An all-inclusive workshop fee is approximately $2,000 per person, and enrollment is open to partners and other close support people. Limited financial assistance is available to those for whom the enrollment fee would prevent their participation. Commonweal has spawned similar programs, including Ting-Sha Institute Cancer Help Retreats in Pt. Reyes, California (www.tingsha.org); Hawaii Cancer Help Retreats in Kamuela, Hawaii (phone: [808] 885-0995); Callanish Healing Retreats in Vancouver, British Columbia (info@callanish.org); The Center for Spirituality, Healing and Wellness in Clarkesville, Georgia (info@centerhealing.org); and Tapestry Retreat in Calgary, Alberta (helenmac@cancerboard.ab.ca). More information and links to other retreat centers are available from the Commonweal website, the address for which is listed above.

An increasing number of local facilities provide a range of services and programs designed to promote healing specifically for people with cancer. The services and programs reflect the unique setting, the skills of available providers, and the needs of the people the program is designed to help. Cancer survivors who have participated in such programs frequently refer to them as "cancer camps for adults"(referring, of course, to the many camps that are available to kids with cancer). There are many of these facilities—too many to report here. The outdoor sporting goods chain Orvis supports a recovery program designed for breast cancer survivors called "Casting for Recovery," using fly fishing as an enjoyable and restorative activity. American Cancer Society units throughout the country hold weekend retreat programs for survivors, and sometimes entire families, called "We Can Weekends." The oncology practice management company US Oncology has established an ongoing program called "Life Beyond Cancer"—an annual weekend retreat for women survivors (most of whom have been or are being treated in US Oncology practices) that is planned around sessions to help women become more effective advocates for their own needs and the needs of other survivors, and to allow them to experience many complementary modalities. A unique and central goal of this program, however, is that women take the ideas home and become involved in finding ways to use similar ideas in their own communities.

As yet, there is no central listing for all such programs, but the interested woman can use Internet search engines to locate the programs, using

*Comple-
mentary
and
Alternative
Therapies
for Cancer*

165

"keywords" like "cancer retreat," "cancer support," "cancer education," or "cancer survivors." With the growing realization that the mind/body/spirit approach is what people want and expect, we can look forward to an ever growing and exciting array of programs…and the increasing likelihood that every woman will be able to find a program that meets her needs and expectations.

A Sample of Local Facilities

Harmony Hill is a nonprofit wellness retreat center in Union, Washington, a rural setting with a view of the Olympic Mountains. It provides programs for people dealing with the challenges of living with cancer, their caregivers, and health-care providers. The facility offers cancer retreats—three-day programs for people living with cancer and their companions. The center is available for health-care professional renewal retreats too.

Sunstone Healing Center in Tucson, Arizona, is the culmination of a broad-based community effort. Sunstone's development is the result of a partnership with Arizona Oncology Associates, the University of Arizona College of Medicine's Cancer Center and Program in Integrative Medicine, and Canyon Ranch. A number of smaller business entities, students, cancer survivors, and cancer-care professionals contributed to making structural renovations, additions, and program and services planning. It too is a small, intimate facility, offering a range of services such as massage, Reiki, counseling, and support groups for people living in the Tucson area. With ten two-bed rooms, it can also accommodate guests from outside Tucson and offers a serene setting for small retreats. Complete information is available on Sunstone's website: www.sunstonehealingcenter.org.

Big Sky Cancer Recovery and Resource Center, located in the Bozeman, Montana area, is an example of how the partnership of survivors, caregivers, and health-care professionals can initiate change in a community. During initial planning stages, when cancer survivors and caregivers identified a need for wise professional guidance, the center's board approved and designated a professional role they call "the navigator." The navigator's tasks are these: to help cancer patients find objective information about treatment options; to assist with decision-making, planning, and problem-solving; to help devise long-term wellness plans; and to give guidance in finding and using community resources. The center also offers a cancer resource library, support groups, and immersion retreats for men and women with cancer and for cancer-care professionals. For more information, check The Big Sky Cancer Recovery and Resource Center's website at www.bigskycancerresource.org or e-mail info@bigskycancerresource.org.

Most women want help finding legitimate, acceptable ways to improve their health, however each individual defines it. But the fear generated by a cancer diagnosis and the attendant feelings of helplessness can make a woman easy prey for anyone promising a cure. How can a woman, faced with so many decisions, find and integrate the best unconventional therapies with her conventional cancer care? How can a woman find rational, responsible complements to her treatment plan?

Conventional therapies go through heavy scrutiny in order to pass two crucial tests: (1) have they been proven safe when provided by a competent practitioner? and (2) have they proven effective? Women trying to separate facts from fantasy for all cancer therapies need a similar healthy dose of skepticism. Keep in mind the following:

✦ No single test done once can definitively diagnose cancer.

✦ There is no agency that approves or verifies claims made in advertisements before they are printed. Authorities can take action only after they are alerted to an advertisement that is in print.

Beware of testimonials that sound too good to be true because they probably are. Common characteristics of quack advertisements are the following:

✦ the product or treatment is said to offer a quick and painless cure

✦ the formula for sale is described as "special," "secret," "ancient," or "foreign" and/or is available only through the mail or from one supplier

✦ the only "proof" offered that the product works comes from testimonials or case histories from satisfied users

✦ the product or treatment is touted as a scientific "breakthrough" or "miracle cure" that has been held back or overlooked by the conventional medical community

Before buying or signing up for a product or program, check it out with

✦ your doctor, pharmacist, nurse, or another health-care professional

✦ the Better Business Bureau

✦ local offices for consumer complaints

✦ the state's attorney general

*Comple-
mentary
and
Alternative
Therapies
for Cancer*

167

- the Federal Trade Commission

- the Food and Drug Administration

- the postmaster or the Postal Inspection Service (HHS Publication No. 85-4200)

The National Cancer Institute recommends that patients and families consider the following questions when making decisions about cancer treatment:

- Has the treatment been evaluated in clinical trials? (A reference librarian can help patients interested in a particular treatment find out whether it has been reported in reputable scientific journals.)

- Do the practitioners of an approach claim that the medical community is trying to keep their cure from the public? (No one genuinely committed to finding better ways to treat a disease would knowingly keep an effective treatment a secret or try to suppress such a treatment.)

- Does the treatment rely on nutritional or diet therapy as its main focus? (At this time, there is no known dietary cure for cancer. In other words, there is no evidence that diet alone can get rid of cancerous cells in the body.)

- Do those who endorse the treatment claim that it is harmless and painless and that it produces no unpleasant side effects? (Because treatments for cancer must be very powerful, they frequently have unpleasant side effects.)

- Does the treatment have a "secret formula" that only a small group of practitioners can use? (Scientists who believe they have developed an effective treatment routinely publish their results in reputable journals so they can be evaluated by other researchers.)

For the time being, decisions to use or not use complementary or alternative therapies are not clear-cut and are clouded by many questions. In the end, every woman will make her own decision based on what she thinks are her needs, her belief that a particular therapy might be useful to her, and what therapy (or combination of therapies) fits her lifestyle.

The NCI maintains its position that practitioners of unconventional methods of cancer treatment be held to the same standards as conventional practitioners and scientists—that proof of benefit to patients in a specific disease situation be reported in a timely and thorough way in scientific journals so that others can learn about, assess, and critique the research results. According to the NCI, the "nature of the discovery should be completely and accurately described so that other researchers can verify and expand upon these results."

Robin Marantz Henig is a freelance journalist and author of several books and articles about conventional medicine. Writing for the Library of Congress magazine *Civilization,* she was amazed at the complexity of so-called New Age medicine. Still, she concludes, "Until alternative medicine comes up with its own assessment standards, though, the future status of these treatments will remain unsettled. Without the proper proof, neither critics nor advocates will be able to demonstrate whether these approaches, based largely on whatever inexplicable magic happens between the healer and the healed, actually work."

Ultimately, every woman—each person with cancer (or without cancer, for that matter) needs to make a personal and individual decision about using complementary and alternative therapies. Ideally, she makes these decisions only after a thorough search for information and will base these decisions on information from reliable sources—not hearsay. She utilizes partnerships with the doctors and nurses providing her care; they may not have all the answers, but they may be able to offer some guidance toward useful information-seeking practices. Some excellent books are available that offer a good starting place. My recommendations are as follows:

Bognar, D. *Cancer: Increasing Your Odds for Survival.* Alameda, CA: Hunter House, 1998.

Decker, G. M. (ed). *An Introduction to Complementary and Alternative Therapies.* Pittsburgh: Oncology Nursing Press, 1999.

Gordon, J. S., and Curtin, S. *Comprehensive Cancer Care: Integrating Alternative, Complementary, and Conventional Therapies.* Cambridge, MA: Perseus Publishing, 2000.

Hammerschlag, C. A., and Silverman, H. D. *Healing Ceremonies: Creating Personal Rituals for Spiritual, Emotional, Physical and Mental Health.* New York: Berkley Publishing Group, 1997.

Khalsa, D. S., and Stauth, C. *Medication as Medicine: Activate the Power of Your Natural Healing Force.* New York: Pocket Books, 2001.

Labriola, D. *Complementary Cancer Therapies: Combining Traditional and Alternative Approaches for the Best Possible Outcome.* Roseville, CA: Prima Health, 2000.

Moore, K., and Schmais, L. *Living Well with Cancer: A Nurse Tells You Everything You Need to Know About Managing the Side Effects of Your Treatment.* New York: G.P. Putnam's Sons, 2001.

Sagar, S. M. *Restored Harmony: An Evidence Based Approach for Integrating Traditional Chinese Medicine into Complementary Cancer Care.* Hamilton, Ontario: Dreaming DragonFly Communications, 2001.

— *Pamela Haylock*

CHAPTER **10**

FEELINGS

When they hear the words "You have cancer," some women begin to cry—
and do not stop for days.

I could not cry at first. I wanted to, and the big lump of unshed tears in
my throat and chest was nearly choking me. Even watching sad movies and
peeling onions (I tried both) would not start the tears flowing. I had to
make the immediate decisions before I could relax into tears.

That was simply my individual emotional timetable. It is common for
the woman diagnosed with cancer to experience fear, sadness, anger, and
perhaps guilt. She may agonize over who she is, how she looks, and what
will happen to her. But she will do it on her own timetable.

This is partly because she is who she is, with a background and set of
circumstances that are hers alone. But it is also because the timetables for
cancer therapies are so different. One woman may finish diagnosis and
treatment within a week, and another may still be undergoing therapy
months or even years later.

Thus, one woman may feel an emotion much earlier or later than
another—and both of them are quite normal. That is why this chapter and
Chapter 24, "Feelings after Treatment Ends," work together. What is not in
one chapter is discussed in the other.

NUMBNESS AND DENIAL

The doctor says, "You have cancer." The woman may hear the first few
words and then little else. This normal protective mechanism saves the
woman from the full initial shock of what is happening. She talks, and
moves, and drives home—and may even say, "Oh, I'm just fine, thank
you"—but inside she is numb. None of it feels *real*.

Sometimes that cushioning sense of unreality persists during treatment: "This is not happening." "This is happening, but it won't make any
real difference in my life." Some women continue in this state for years,
and never confront the cancer. In fact, if the treatment is minimal and the

prognosis excellent, the cancer may never make any real difference in their lives. But some women may be truly expert deniers who never notice the elephant in the living room or may be totally distracted by other events in their lives.

Others may bargain unconsciously during therapy: "I'm doing what I'm supposed to do, as hard as it is. Such good behavior means that I deserve not to have this in my life anymore." Then, when treatment is over, these women reward themselves by putting cancer out of their minds forever.

Indeed, it is possible for a woman to choose to live as if the cancer makes no real difference in her life (although she may be ambushed by painful feelings years later). On the other hand, this means she loses the *opportunity* for it to make a real difference in her life. She misses the cloud—but also the silver lining.

The silver lining is that cancer is a chance to change and grow. Because "business as usual" so often does not work after a cancer diagnosis, many a woman must try business as *unusual*. Cancer has a way of shaking up the status quo.

A woman may discover that she likes the new ways better. She may have ignored her own needs for years as she cared for others, but now she must listen to herself more. She may discover, as many women do, that in daring to face the possibility of her own death, she learns to spread her wings. She can see what is important, set new priorities, have more fun, and be less afraid of what other people think. I love the sweatshirt that proclaims on the front, "Rule #1: Don't sweat the small stuff" and on the back, "Rule #2: It's *all* small stuff."

At the same time, life has a sweeter edge. Many a woman experiences a "honeymoon" with life: Never has she felt so in love with the world around her. Holding on to this fresh delight is one of the challenges of long-term cancer survivorship. Of course, there may be easier ways to learn these lessons!

REGAINING CONTROL

When the numbness wears off, the woman may feel more helpless than she ever has in her entire life. Everything is spinning out of control; her once somewhat-predictable life is orderly no more. What goals? What personal calendar? What sense of independence and autonomy? She may feel utterly dependent on people she did not meet until last week who now say she must do such and such if she wants to save her life.

This is the perfect time to remember the famous Serenity Prayer:

God grant me the serenity
to accept the things I cannot change,
the courage to change the things I can,
and the wisdom to know the difference.

Indeed, there are some factors about a woman's experience with cancer that are out of anybody's hands. All she can do is accept that and not waste her energy fighting what cannot be changed. Just doing something—anything—does not help, because her feeling of control is soon revealed as an illusion.

But there are sensible steps a woman can take to establish some real control. She can get information from her doctors, books, and other sources. She can assemble a cancer care team she trusts and think of herself as a key and contributing team member rather than as a victim. She can gather as much support from family, friends, and others as she needs. She can stay as healthy as possible, eat well, and get some exercise so that she feels stronger, more able to do what she must do. She may choose to research and use complementary therapies to help herself feel better.

And she can start looking at herself as a cancer survivor or a cancer victor—or even a cancer "thriver." The National Coalition for Cancer Survivorship contends that survivorship has several "seasons," but that being a cancer survivor begins at the moment of diagnosis. So, right from the beginning, the woman can start saying, as cancer survivor Melinda Sheinkopf does in *Coping* magazine (Summer 1992), "Listen, Cancer, maybe it is your job to take years from my life. I really don't know. But I know it's my job to see you don't take life from my years."

EXPERIENCING FEELINGS

Some people believe that to be cancer survivors they must "think positive" all the time and squelch any negative thoughts. Not true. Susan Diamond, LCSW, a social worker and psychotherapist who leads a support group for women with breast cancer, hates that "positive attitude bullshit. It makes women think they can't admit to their very scariest feelings, even to themselves. Then, if they harbor fears, concerns, and anxieties—and have no way to put them out on the table and deal with them—the women become immobilized and wonder why."

Feelings are energy, power. If we repress painful, difficult feelings, eventually we spend our lives guarding an emotional volcano, terrified lest it erupt and overwhelm us and everyone around us. But released and expressed, in a safe manner, those same emotions become energy for us to use.

How do we let emotions free in a safe manner? Acknowledging and naming feelings, at least to ourselves, is the first step, though often not an easy one. Trying to sort out strong emotions may be quite new for us. Susan Diamond advises: "Make the unspoken spoken. This has the effect of making it smaller and more manageable."

There are many ways to do this, and not all of them require words spoken aloud. We can consciously think—or perhaps write in a journal—about what is happening and what we are feeling: "What's going on here? This feels like the way I felt when...." Our unconscious minds will do much of the work for us.

There are two big myths about feelings and cancer. First, people with cancer may not get the psychological care they desperately need for severe anxiety or depression because they or their health-care professionals wrongly believe, "However much distress he or she is having, it's normal with a cancer diagnosis." On the other hand, people may receive costly services they neither need nor want if their health professionals are convinced that "All patients are so distressed that they need intensive psychiatric help."

The truth is that although most cancer patients undergo some periods of crisis without suffering persistent, severe psychological problems, a sizable minority would benefit from intensive psychological help. If emotional distress is disabling, especially if extreme anxiety or deep depression lasts longer than two weeks, it is urgent that a woman see a therapist.

The chief signs of depression are continuous empty, very sad feelings (sometimes with suicidal thoughts) combined with major changes in eating or sleeping habits. Depression may show itself in severe restlessness or agitation.

Many women do not need or want intensive psychotherapy but still want to gain something positive from their experience with cancer and want support and guidance. A competent, caring therapist or counselor (preferably one familiar with cancer patients) can help a woman sort through painful feelings safely, begin integrating her cancer experience into her life, and perhaps make her life more satisfying than it ever was before. Seeking counseling in no way means a woman is crazy or weak; rather, it means she has the sense to make use of available help.

At some point in their cancer journey, many women draw on spiritual resources to cope with painful feelings. Whether it is against the background of a lifetime of organized religion or a new search for meaning in the wake of crisis, women often find comfort and hope in personal prayer, talks with clergy, spiritual reading, or membership in a church. Feeling the presence of a higher power makes them feel less alone and vulnerable.

On the other hand, some women lose faith after the cancer diagnosis, questioning or blaming God. Harold S. Kushner's book *When Bad Things Happen to Good People* is a thoughtful guide for a woman asking spiritual questions.

Brisk physical exercise and deep relaxation are two strategies for coping with distressing emotions. Reading about feelings may help, as can talking them over with a partner, friends, or family.

And, since most women do not want (or need) to spend every minute dwelling on feelings, distractions of any kind can be a godsend. Hobbies, a movie, a trashy novel, a visit with a friend during which cancer is never mentioned—all these keep a woman aware that life exists apart from cancer. I found that spending a few hours a week working intensely on "cancer stuff" in my support group freed me to focus on everything else most of the rest of the time.

The woman with a sense of humor will find it comes to her rescue now. Laughter cheers her, broadens her perspective, makes her more attractive to be with, and may actually stimulate her body's defenses. Cancer is serious, but her experience with it does not have to be perpetually grim.

Dealing with Fear and Anxiety

Psychology books often define *fear* as the emotional response to a clear external threat and *anxiety* as the response when it is harder to pin down what the actual threat is: those nameless things that go bump in the night. In fact, many people mix the two words or know that the feelings can occur together. Thus I, as a cancer patient, may fear cancer's clear external threats to my health, but I may also feel panicky inside because of "fuzzier" threats to my well-being that I cannot even identify. This anxiety might arise because of how society looks at cancer, because of past experiences with cancer in someone I loved, or even because of something that has nothing at all to do with cancer. But if I can put a name and shape to what terrifies me, it becomes more manageable.

It is fairly common for a woman to feel an intense blast of fear or anxiety soon after diagnosis. She may find that this feeling lessens while she undergoes treatment: She is "doing something powerful," which gives her a sense of control. Thus, it is typical for fear to grow more severe again as the woman finishes treatment and no longer feels "protected."

What do we fear? Death, of course. Indeed, some people with cancer will eventually die of the disease. What is absolutely certain is that every person with cancer will eventually die of *something,* someday—as will every person who never gets cancer. Death is a fact of life. None of us gets out of here alive.

Given the choice, however, most of us try not to think about dying. We cram our feelings about death into an emotional closet deep within. A cancer diagnosis wrenches open that closet door. We can try to ignore feelings and fears that tumble out, or try to cram them back into the closet, but avoiding something so obvious takes a huge emotional toll.

It is far easier to look at death, to put a name and a shape to it. Becoming more familiar with what happens when we die lets us put death in its proper place. So, we can talk about death, read about it, consider it at our own pace, and express our feelings about it. This is not morbid and does not make us die any sooner.

However we come by it, that fundamental awareness of death gives a context to our life. Cancer lets us look at death squarely while we still have time to change the way we live, to make our lives what we want them to be.

Most of us fear protracted, painful dying. Most patients and even many health professionals do not realize that cancer-related pain can be treated effectively now for almost everyone, especially if health professionals use all the information and techniques available to them. Every day, as a nurse practitioner, I see advances in treating pain and, especially, erosion of the belief that cancer must mean pain. As a nurse I cheer; as a cancer patient I am comforted. An excellent resource on pain management is *Cancer Doesn't Have to Hurt* (Hunter House, 1997).

Many of us fear treatment: either what we are going through now or our ability to muster the will and energy to go through it again if necessary. We may have such specific fears as, "What will become of my young children if the cancer returns?" All of these fears are real, normal, and legitimate.

Taking back control over them involves acknowledging that they exist, shedding some tears, talking about them, and taking action when appropriate: drafting a will or making a backup plan for the care of children. It seems to be human nature to postpone this kind of practical "housekeeping," perhaps because of unspoken fears that if we plan for trouble, trouble will come. In fact, however, having our affairs in order allows us to relax and get on with life.

With normal fear or anxiety, a woman *temporarily* feels severe distress. She may not be able to sit still and may notice that her heart is beating fast and her breathing is rapid. She may not be able to fall asleep, or she may wake up in the middle of the night with her mind racing and her stomach churning. She may have no appetite or be starving all the time, or she may have diarrhea. Some women recall feeling paralyzed—"like a deer in the headlights, unable to move." These symptoms happen because the woman's autonomic nervous system, the part of the nervous system that regulates heart rate, digestion, and other "automatic" body functions, is in high gear for a time. If she starts to feel better after a week or two, she probably will do well with basic support from her family, friends, and health professionals. (She may still benefit from a session or two with a psychologist or counselor or from a support group.)

If severe anxiety does not begin to improve or if the woman has little support from family or friends, she needs more help. Anxiety usually comes from an overreaction to the cancer crisis: reactive or situational anxiety. A few sessions with a psychologist or psychiatrist and perhaps short-term use of an antianxiety medicine can ease her through the crisis so she can get on with her life. Learning specific guided-relaxation skills may be part of the program.

Some women suffer anxiety directly related to medical factors (such as from certain drugs, like prednisone, that may be part of their chemotherapy), and their medical doctors may be able to adjust treatment to relieve the anxiety. A few women—often those who have had past problems with phobias, panic attacks, or other serious anxiety—will experience a full-fledged anxiety disorder with little connection to the cancer, and may need more intensive psychological support or medications tailored to the condition. The woman with panic attacks, for instance, may thrive with occasional use of beta blockers, drugs that slow down the heart rate and other symptoms of anxiety. A small daily dose of certain antidepression drugs can work wonders with severe anxiety, although it may take two weeks or more for the woman to notice the difference.

Dealing with Anger

Many women have been brought up afraid to feel intense anger. Our feelings are supposed to be positive, moderate, gentle—in a word, "ladylike." It is okay for us to be peeved, but God forbid that we connect with any deep rage within. Our culture and political systems, too, tend to gloss over female anger. As a result, many women spend their lives performing emotional contortions to "prove" that black is really white.

We may be so accustomed to doing this that we cannot tell what we are feeling anymore. We cannot separate anger from sadness, for instance. Sometimes, when we cannot tolerate one emotion in ourselves, we substitute another less painful one. "Will I die?" might become "I can't believe that the doctor didn't call back." Or if we cannot face our fears about someone perceived as powerful in our lives (Will the doctor stop caring for me? Will the person I love stop loving me?), we may turn our fear to anger and direct it at those perceived as less powerful—such as ourselves or our children—and feel sad or guilty.

Anger is one of the most energetic emotions: It screams for action. Once a woman knows what she is dealing with, she needs to find something to do with this force other than turning it against herself in the form of depression. Even if she cannot resolve the situation, she may be able to channel the energy elsewhere—through physical exercise or joining a cancer political action group, for example.

Dealing with Grief and Depression

Only a leaden lump could go through a cancer diagnosis without feeling deep sadness. Our normal response to any loss is to grieve for it, and cancer brings about inevitable losses—physical losses, of course, and perhaps financial losses. We lose the way things were, and our "innocence" of disease and our own mortality. Often we must change our dreams to fit a new reality.

We cannot sweep our losses under the bed and ignore them, or they will turn into monsters, lying in wait to bite us. So the woman before a mastectomy, for instance, needs to look at her breast and cherish it fully, appreciating what she is losing; afterward, she can mourn what is gone. Even years later she may feel an occasional pang of sorrow—and this does not mean she appreciates any less the fact that she is alive and healthy.

As with anxiety, some temporary severe sadness is considered a normal reaction to these losses. It is an expected step in the process of coping with a cancer crisis, a kind of tunnel we need to get through before we can see anything positive in the experience.

But when does sadness become abnormal? Cancer and its treatments can cause several of the common physical symptoms of a deep depression, such as fatigue and change in appetite. Although that makes it trickier to diagnose depression in the person with cancer, the key symptoms to look out for are more than two weeks of intense and constant tearfulness, withdrawal from family and friends, brooding, self-pity, and pessimism, with nary a break in the storm clouds. (Obviously, it takes most people much longer than two weeks to fully mourn all the profound losses a cancer diagnosis brings.) The person may feel as if it is impossible to climb out of an abyss. In most people with these symptoms, the depression is still a direct reaction—or overreaction—to the cancer.

The woman with this kind of reactive or situational depression usually benefits greatly from short-term psychological support and perhaps antidepressant medication. With depression, women tend to view the world through dismally dark glasses, and psychological support might include not only counseling but also cognitive therapies in which the woman can learn more realistic and hopeful ways of looking at the situation.

Medical factors related to cancer disease or treatment cause or increase depression for many women. Common factors include poorly controlled symptoms (such as pain), tumors that affect hormone balance, abnormal metabolic states (such as infection or too much calcium), and the woman's individual reaction to particular chemotherapy and hormone therapy drugs. Relieving this kind of depression takes good symptom control and other medical changes when possible. When the doctor cannot change the medical situation—such as when a chemotherapy drug causing depression is the best drug available for the cancer—antidepressants may be useful.

Women with serious past depressions are at greater risk for the kind of clinical depression that is not related to the cancer. Many psychiatrists now believe that some glitch in the brain's chemical and hormonal connections—more than deep psychological issues—causes this kind of depression, and they successfully treat many patients with a combination of antidepressants and psychiatric therapy.

One more issue: Many women, at some time during their cancer journey, find themselves wondering about suicide. This may be a brief thought that occasionally flutters through the mind, a fleeting moment of despair, or even a normal way of feeling more in control: "If things get too bad, this is a possibility." However, if a woman finds herself dwelling on suicide and seriously considering how to kill herself, she needs immediate and effective help. In many cases, she is not thinking straight but is feeling overwhelmed by a situation that could get better—a depression that could be treated and cancer or therapy symptoms that could be resolved, often with simple measures.

Suicide that could have been avoided is a tragedy that engulfs not only the woman but everyone around her. She fully deserves every chance to change her mind.

For most women, however, sadness is a distressing feeling that happens now and then during the cancer experience. Good things begin happening to crowd out the sorrow. Time—and seeking out the good things—are often the best cures for the grief of cancer.

Feeling Responsible for Cancer

Human nature wants a universe that makes sense. We feel safer if life is ordered in a way we can control, so that we can avoid things that cause problems. That means we want a cause for every effect, including cancer. When the effect is cancer and when no obvious cause is known (such as smoking for many cases of lung cancer), we keep looking anyway.

Lacking a clear villain outside, many people become convinced that cancer comes from within us, that we are responsible for it. (As the old

Woody Allen line puts it, "I don't get angry, I grow tumors instead.") A common perception is that only "nice" people—"nice" because they have repressed strong feelings—get cancer, despite the fact that most nice people do not get cancer, and plenty of decidedly un-nice people do. The New Age extension of this thinking is that if we get cancer, it is because we somehow *need* it—that cancer fills some kind of emptiness within.

This kind of thinking may comfort the onlookers and help them deal with their own terror of developing cancer. They may believe that if they deal with stress better or express their emotions more effectively, they have "cancer-proofed" themselves.

But this all backfires if we get cancer. We may feel blamed and shamed and responsible for the disease. What did we do wrong? How did we fail? The woman with a cancer diagnosis may not only berate herself for emotional "failings," but may also have to cope with "friends" who try to get her to see the error of her psychological ways.

Cancer patient Treya Killam Weber did the same kind of smug theorizing when her mother was diagnosed with cancer. After her own diagnosis, she acknowledged in a speech entitled "What Kind of Help Really Helps": "When my mother was sick, I was motivated by fear and a desire for self-protection. When I got cancer myself, my theorizing was initially fueled by the 'you create your own reality' philosophy, which generated guilt about my past and a feeling that others must think I had failed in some way by getting cancer. This philosophy also bred the magical hope that if I could find 'the cause,' I could correct it, root out the mistake, cleanse my past, change my future and, hopefully, thus cure myself. This philosophy also implied that the only proof of success at creating my own reality would be if I got well physically."

This touches on the negative side of the theories about feisty "exceptional patients" in such popular books as Bernie Siegel's *Love, Medicine, and Miracles*. These books offer hope because they say that patients who fight the disease psychologically can get well despite enormous odds. But the other side of this viewpoint is that a patient can feel undeserved guilt if the cancer gets worse. ("I just didn't try hard enough; I wasn't exceptional enough.")

What will people looking back from the twenty-fifth century think about some of our current psychological theories about cancer? Will they consider them pioneering work, or laugh at them as we do now at earlier "sensible" theories that a child's blindness was caused by the sins of the parents, epilepsy by demonic possession, TB by an "artistic temperament"?

We do not know what causes many cancers or makes some people live and others die after developing them. Our emotional states and coping styles may indeed influence our immune system responses somewhat, but there seems to be much more involved in a normal cell's turning cancerous and growing into a tumor than a person's mental attitude.

When it comes to cancer, I see "responsibility" as the *ability to respond as best I can*. But I also believe that there is much about cancer that we do not know and much that is totally beyond human control.

If a woman finds it personally helpful to consider that her cancer arose from her own inner need or was a lesson she needed to learn, that is fine—for her. And it is always helpful, of course, to care for our emotional health. We can use a cancer diagnosis to see where we can make good changes. But it makes no sense at all to blame ourselves.

Feeling Guilty

Many a woman strives to get an "A" in the "cancer experience"—whatever that means to her. She sets up expectations for herself that may or may not be realistic and helpful, and then feels guilty if she fails to "perform." If she expects to work throughout treatment, for instance, she may blame herself if she has to take time off. Ironically, if she feels fine during chemotherapy and continues working, she may feel guilty because she is not being "kind enough" to herself! Why do so many of us torture ourselves like this? Are we the products of our upbringing as females? Is this a religious legacy? Do we feel that if we suffer enough and pay our "suffering dues" (and guilt can be very effective suffering), we will get well?

It helps to step back and look at what is happening—and then to laugh gently at ourselves for getting caught up in such tangles. We are doing the very best we can under trying circumstances. We deserve to *appreciate* and *love* and *cherish* ourselves.

HOW WE SEE OURSELVES

How we think of ourselves is our self-image or self-concept, our sense of who we are. We continuously (but usually unconsciously) monitor how well our behavior, feelings, and appearance match this internal picture. Our self-image includes, but is not limited to, our body image: how we "see" our physical selves. For better or worse, cancer almost always changes this image.

In our society, few women have learned to love and value themselves simply because they are who they are. Most of us attach conditions to our sense of self-worth, many of them holdovers from growing up ("Oh, I just love you because you're such a giving person" or "Can't you do anything right?" or "A truly feminine woman always . . . "). We internalize these messages—some of them useful, others quite harmful—from our families and friends, religion, culture, and the media, and they become our self-image.

Given the choice, many of us prefer not to examine this image of ourselves too closely. To do so is scary and unsettling. Although the image may not "fit" perfectly and although it may pinch or even hobble us, we hold on to it.

When cancer comes along, we may suddenly see ourselves as unhealthy, not in control, unfeminine, asexual. A woman who viewed and valued herself because she was a hard-working, productive, and efficient attorney, now can barely move from the couch. Or she may have seen herself as sweet, loving, and giving, and now is so filled with anger that she could explode.

While we may never have fit our old self-image, now the mismatch is so obvious that it is impossible to ignore. Although some of the changes are temporary and treatment related, others are permanent. Being so at odds with that old familiar self makes us feel uncertain and lost.

Some women cling desperately to the old image. No matter how exhausted, a woman may drag herself to work every day during treatment to prove to everyone else—but mostly to herself—that she is perfectly healthy and in control, and that nothing has changed. To her, preserving a sense of normalcy is worth any price. (Unfortunately, many women have no choice but to work throughout treatment no matter how they feel.)

Other women, instead of changing themselves to fit the precancer self-image, prefer to put their emotional energies into crafting a self-image that fits them better. Many cancer survivors echo Chris's sentiment: "I wish to God there were an easier way, but it took cancer shaking me by the scruff of the neck to get me to look at myself. I was trying to live up to something that wasn't me at all. I realized that my self-image was just going to have to learn to live with me, rather than the other way around."

The idea is to save what is "us," to broaden and enrich our definitions of what is acceptable and lovable, and to discard the constricting limits of the old image. Like a truly comfortable walking shoe, an authentic self-image does not bind or distort—it allows us to move forward without pain.

We don't have to start from scratch, and we can take all the time we want. In fact, we may discover the pleasures of an evolving self-image, one that grows with us. Some aspects of the old self-image do not need to change at all. If I have always viewed and valued myself as a fine seamstress, for example, cancer does not alter that at all.

A woman may preserve certain parts of her image but express them differently. Perhaps she continues to feel that having a sense of control is healthy for her and necessary to her vision of herself. Instead of managing a tight time schedule, however, she maintains that sense of control during treatment by obtaining information, participating as a decision-making member of her health-care team, and persisting in a healing package of therapies for herself. After treatment, she may choose an entirely new way of expressing this part of herself.

On the other hand, after a cancer diagnosis she may recognize that, for her, the need to be in control goes far beyond being a healthy, normal coping technique. As she learns to acknowledge the "uncontrolled" parts of herself, a woman may replace some of that need for control with more self-acceptance and spontaneity.

Our concepts of what a "real woman" is need to be expanded and deepened. Culturally, women tend to see themselves as caretakers and to define their self-worth in terms of what they do for other people. Nurse-psychotherapist Diane W. Scott, Ph.D., who specializes in therapy for women with cancer, claims that men with cancer tend to relax and let the women in their lives cosset them, make them special foods, and make the process easier for them. Women with cancer, on the other hand, keep "protecting" others: keeping painful news from them, continuing "business as usual" (career, being a wife and mother, or whatever), making it as easy as possible for everyone else, despite the cost to themselves. Even if women allow themselves to let down a little during treatment, they may expect themselves to be up and running the moment treatment ends.

But, somewhere along the way, a woman may begin to question this picture. At some point, out of necessity, she puts her needs first and discovers that the world does not fall apart. Perhaps she becomes aware of some simmering resentment in herself. She talks with other women with cancer and finds a broader definition of acceptable "womanly" behavior.

How assertive can a "feminine" woman be? During cancer treatment women often discover that they must make their needs known, directly and forcefully. Their very lives depend on it, and there is neither time nor energy to shilly-shally. Support groups may model techniques for clear communication with doctors (and others) and offer opportunities for women to rehearse these approaches in a safe environment. When they see how effective this kind of communication is, some women will not settle for less after cancer treatment ends.

The way society tells it, a woman with breast or gynecologic cancer is less of a woman. She has scars or missing organs and no longer fits the narrow definition of "femininity." But many women with cancer know differently—and they come to realize that it is society's definition that is lacking.

Womanliness is a concept that should include rather than exclude. To fill its own needs, society has given women a limited picture of what "real" women "should" be. Cancer offers us the opportunity to experience some energizing anger, and then come up with a better definition.

Coping with Body Changes

All the philosophizing aside, how does a woman cope with losing a breast, her hair, and a svelte figure, all within a few months? Some losses may be temporary, but that is small comfort to the woman with handfuls of hair on the floor of the shower.

First, she can acknowledge the loss. Even if she is an ardent feminist and convinced intellectually that what our bodies look like has nothing to do with our inner value, it is normal and human to mourn the changes.

It is very hard not to feel alone when we look different. This does not bother some women at all, but others feel much happier if they can either disguise the differences or join other women in the same situation.

To disguise the difference—and even make it a plus—a woman who has lost her hair might use bright scarves, experiment with a frivolous wig, or attend a "Look Good, Feel Better" session. She may feel less invested in appearance than usual, and this can translate into a sense of freedom and daring in her fashion statements. Some women develop a whole new look for themselves after a cancer diagnosis. Or, a woman may just relax with other "baldies" in a support group, take courage from their shared strength, and learn from their experiences.

— Kerry McGinn

PART TWO

BREAST CANCER

Breasts.

Two mounds, mostly fat and glandular tissue, that perch on the large chest muscle. They can nourish babies, bring pleasure to a woman and her lover, fill out clothes—and cause many a woman endless worry.

When a healthy woman is asked what disease she fears most, chances are she will answer, "Breast cancer." It is not the deadliest cancer women get (lung cancer is) and it is not the most common life-threatening illness (heart disease is), but breast cancer has a hold on women's fears that no other disease can match.

However, most women *never* develop breast cancer. Even with family histories of cancer and several personal risk factors, most women do not get the disease.

On the other hand, most of the women who *do* develop breast cancer do not have any particular known risk factors beyond the fact that they are women growing older. The woman who says, "No one in my family has breast cancer, so I don't need to worry," is fooling herself. There is no cause for women to panic about breast cancer—but there is ample reason for every woman to take care of herself.

When it comes to their breasts, many women feel panicky, helpless, hopeless. Every time there is another scary newspaper story about breast cancer statistics, they *know* they will get breast cancer; it is simply a matter of when. They feel so much at the mercy of forces beyond their control that they cannot begin to take action—even if they had some idea what to do.

Some of this sense of vulnerability may have little to do with medical facts. Physically, the breasts are soft, yielding, exposed, and "out there" on the chest—but it may be that we feel more defenseless because of messages society sends us about breasts.

Traditionally, a young girl grows up defining much of her self-image and body image in terms of external cues rather than from the inside out. Do her breasts look like the breasts in vogue during her adolescence? How do other people (family, friends, lovers) react to her breasts? And these external cues keep shifting. Depending on what year it is, the woman's breasts should be bigger or smaller, pointier or higher or droopier. Is this the year of Ms. Super-skinny Model or Ms. Buxom?

The breast has several functions—and there is plenty of misinformation available about each of them, which means more possibilities for a woman to question her self-worth. Did she stop breastfeeding because she "didn't have enough milk"? Does she fail to reach orgasm from breast stimulation? Do her blouses bunch over her breasts?

Add the breast cancer statistics to the equation, and it is small wonder that many a woman with perfectly healthy breasts feels off balance. It doesn't help that some doctors insist that only the things doctors can do, like professional breast exams and mammography, make a real difference in breast health, and that the woman should just "trust the doctor" to take care of her.

But there is plenty we can do. Whether or not there is a breast cancer diagnosis, it is possible to establish our own standards for what our breasts should be, learn to live comfortably with our own breasts (or lack of them), and make a genuine difference in protecting our own breast health.

First, we can ask who is telling us about how our breasts should look and function, and by what right? Often there is a profit motive, as with fashion changes. Sometimes there is a social agenda. For instance, society may extol bigger—and supposedly more "feminine"—breasts when economic factors push women to stay home and nurture a family. And, were it not for society's confusion about women, would the same slang word— "boob"—mean both breast and . . . dunce?

Once we recognize what is happening, we may feel an energizing anger, or we may laugh at ourselves for listening to such silly messages. We are so much more than a pair of mammary glands.

Caring for our breasts means getting accurate information. What is going on in there? What can we do to protect ourselves? What can we safely ignore? And when do we need to take prompt action? A doctor, nurse practitioner, breast health center staff member, or other health professional can teach a woman how to examine her breasts effectively. Books, pamphlets, magazine articles, and videotapes can give her general information.

Finally, we can gather the best possible breast health team. The team includes the woman herself, knowledgeable about what she can do to protect herself. It includes the doctor or nurse who examines the woman's breasts thoroughly and regularly. At the appropriate time, the team adds routine mammography to the program.

Most breast changes are not cancer. But because breast cancer is by far the most common women's cancer and because breast health issues cover so much territory, these issues have received one section in this book. The following four chapters run the gamut: from what is inside the normal breast to the different kinds of breast cancer, from how a woman can examine her breasts effectively to what it feels like to undergo—and complete— breast cancer therapy.

— *Kerry McGinn*

CHAPTER 11

QUESTIONS ABOUT BREASTS

Why should a woman learn about her breasts? Because if she knows something about how they are constructed and how they function, she can understand better what goes wrong with them—and how much goes right. She can examine her breasts more effectively if she knows what she is feeling. Also, a working knowledge of breast terms gives her a language to communicate with health professionals.

The breasts include more than what fits into a bra. Breast tissue extends from the collarbone to the "bra line," from the breast bone to the middle of the armpit (**axilla**), and from the skin to the chest muscle. Except for a tiny bit of muscle around the nipples, breasts contain no muscle of their own. They vary in shape, size, coloring, and skin texture from woman to woman, and in the same woman at different times in her life.

In the middle of each breast is a nipple—which may protrude a little or a lot, be flat against the skin, or even be inverted ("tucked in") and still be functional and normal, as long as that is the way it has always been. Nipples contain spongy tissue that fills with blood and becomes taut in response to touch, cold, a baby's suckling, or even a baby's cry. The pigmented area around the base of the nipple is called the **areola**, which means "ring of color." **Montgomery's tubercles** are the visible pores or tiny lumps on the areola, which are openings for the oil glands that lubricate the nipple and areola during breastfeeding.

Each breast is divided into fifteen to twenty sections, rather like the sections of a halved grapefruit, called **lobes**. **Cooper's ligaments** are bands of strong, flexible, fibrous tissue that separate the sections, passing from the chest muscles, between the lobes, to the skin. They give the breast its support; as they stretch with age, the breast droops. A lacy filigree of tiny fibers forms a network throughout each breast. Doctors interpreting mammograms look for any place where this architecture of fibers has been disturbed.

Fat cells, found between and around the lobes, cushion and shape the breast. The fat cells, fibrous tissue, and other parts of the breast that are not involved in producing, transporting, and storing milk are called the **stroma**. The working part of the breast is called the **parenchyma,** which is where most serious breast problems occur.

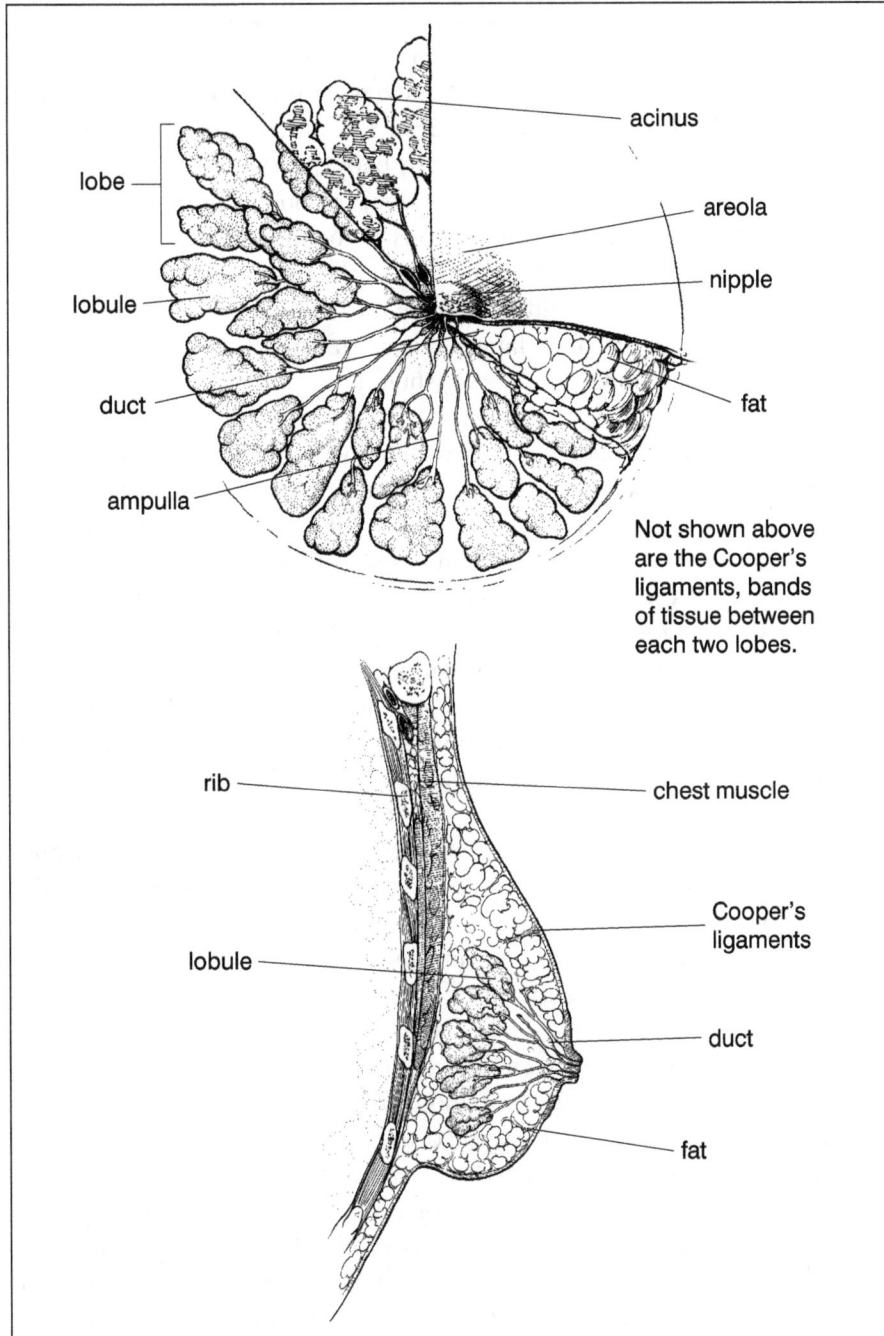

acinus

areola

nipple

fat

lobe

lobule

duct

ampulla

Not shown above are the Cooper's ligaments, bands of tissue between each two lobes.

rib

chest muscle

lobule

Cooper's ligaments

duct

fat

Anatomy of a healthy breast

(courtesy of Breast Cancer Digest, National Cancer Institute)

How does the breast work? Within each lobe are **lobules** (little lobes) that look rather like tiny bunches of grapes. When a mother breastfeeds her baby, the tiny gland cells lining the **acinus** (sac) at the end of each "grape" follow the body's recipe to extract from nearby blood vessels the ingredients they need to make milk. For a few days after birth, the gland cells extract the right amounts of water, sugar, fat, protein, and salts to make **colostrum,** the best fluid for a newborn baby. As the baby grows a little older and needs a different kind of nutrition, the body's hormones instruct the gland cells to use different proportions of the same materials.

After the gland cells extract and combine the right ingredients, the milk is squeezed into the acinus and from there into a small duct, or passageway. Small ducts join to become larger ducts, transporting the milk to an **ampulla** (reservoir) under the areola where it stays until it is time for the baby to nurse.

The breasts are supplied with many blood vessels that bring the ingredients for milk, hormonal messages from the rest of the body (brain and ovaries especially), and the chemical energy for the breast to do its work. The lymph system, the body's second circulatory system, removes wastes from the breast, recycling when possible; thus fluids and tissues that can be reused by the body are swept into the lymph system and eventually back into the blood supply. Lymph vessels connect the two breasts and also drain each breast by way of channels through the axilla, along the breastbone, and up past the collarbone. Along the lymph channels are **lymph nodes,** filter stations that trap cells that cannot pass through; an occasional one is a cancer cell.

The nerves in the breast, concentrated around the nipple, send only one-way messages—that the breast is being touched, perhaps—to the brain. Any reply from the brain comes as a hormone message through the bloodstream. If a baby starts suckling, for instance, the breast nerves send a message to the brain, which then releases a hormone through the bloodstream to "let down" the milk.

Each month, from adolescence to menopause, a woman's breasts prepare for a possible pregnancy. Throughout the menstrual cycle the hormone **estrogen** flows to the breasts from the ovaries and the adrenal glands, but it reaches its peak during the middle two weeks of the cycle, counting from the first day of the menstrual period. Estrogen, the "buildup" hormone, pushes the breast cells to prepare for possible milk production and transport.

When the ovary releases its ripe egg at midcycle, it begins releasing the "secretory" hormone **progesterone** as well. The breast cells begin rehearsing their functions of secreting (producing) and transporting milk. The blood supply increases to the breast to meet the additional needs of the working breast, and some extra fluid—basically blood minus the blood cells—seeps from the tiny blood vessels into the breast tissue. A woman may feel this extra fluid as a sense of fullness, tenderness, and sometimes discomfort.

If no pregnancy occurs, the breasts begin their monthly cleanup during and right after the menstrual period. The extra fluid returns into the body's general circulation via the lymph system. The body reabsorbs unused extra cells and secretions so the whole process can start again. This relatively quiet phase after the period is the best time to examine the breasts.

If pregnancy does occur, preparations for producing milk accelerate. The gland cells multiply, lobules enlarge, ducts lengthen, and blood and lymph vessels become larger. By the end of pregnancy, under the influence of the hormones, the glandular tissue in the breast has crowded out almost all the fat tissue.

After pregnancy (and lactation if the woman breastfeeds), a massive cleanup begins as the cells and structures revert to their prepregnancy state. The lymph system recycles what can be recycled and gets rid of any debris.

A woman's breasts change throughout life. The basic structures are present from before birth, but need the hormonal stimulation of adolescence to begin growing and developing. With pregnancy or lactation, the working tissue crowds out the stroma. After pregnancy and lactation, however, the parenchyma decreases dramatically. The woman may feel as if she has no breasts until the stroma builds up again.

As a woman grows older and especially after menopause, the proportions of parenchyma and stroma inside the breasts keep changing until there is almost no working tissue left. Since fatty tissue shows up clearly on mammograms and working, glandular tissue often does not, mammograms tend to become easier to read as women age. If a woman takes hormone therapy after menopause, however, her breasts will still be influenced by hormonal cycles and will appear on a mammogram and act more like premenopausal breasts.

WHO GETS BREAST CANCER?

Being a woman and growing older are the two biggest breast cancer risk factors for most women. Although men occasionally develop breast cancer, as do a few women under twenty-five, this is very rare. While we know some other risk factors, 75 percent of women who develop breast cancer have no known risk factor except for gender and age. This means that *every woman is at risk and needs to protect herself.*

Like every cancer, breast cancer develops from a series of mutations in the genes, so that the cell "scanning" these genetic "bar codes" gets the wrong information about when to divide (see Chapter 1, "How Cancer

Comes About"). Every day we are learning more about these genetic players in breast cancer. Researchers have the most information about Breast Cancer 1 (BRCA1) and Breast Cancer 2 (BRCA2), two kinds of mutated anti-oncogenes that can be passed down from generation to generation in a few families. These were identified in 1994 and 1995; BRCA3 is known and the CHEK-2 (or CHK2) gene mutation was named in 2002—and there are doubtless more to find. People born with these mutated genes may never develop breast cancer, but they have taken a dramatic first step toward cancer even before birth (see the next section, "Family and Personal Cancer History"). These and other anti-oncogenes and proto-oncogenes can also mutate at any time later in life, beginning a process that could lead to breast cancer.

Discovering these mutant genes helps us learn more about what happens to turn a normal cell into an invading cancer cell. But the big question remains: What causes these genes to mutate in the first place?

Family and Personal Cancer History

Many women worry about breast cancer because they have a relative with the disease. In fact, women are often at much less risk because of family history than they think. The questions to ask are these: How close is the relationship—sister, mother, aunt, or grandmother? (The relationship need not be through the mother's side to increase risk.) How old was the relative when breast cancer was diagnosed—before or after menopause? Did cancer develop in one breast or both? What type of breast cancer was it? In how many relatives and generations has it occurred? Have people in the family developed colon or ovarian cancers? These are two other kinds of cancers that tend to cluster with breast cancer in family patterns.

The woman whose only cancer history is a grandmother who developed breast cancer at age seventy-five may be at minimally increased risk for cancer. This tends to be the garden-variety type of cancer to which all women become vulnerable as they grow older. However, researchers have discovered that about 10 percent of breast cancers occur in true "breast cancer families," in which mutated copies of the tumor suppressor genes BRCA1, BRCA2, or other genes are passed from generation to generation. With its genetic message scrambled, the mutated gene no longer does its normal job of stopping damaged cells from dividing. If a woman inherits this gene, her genes must still undergo other mutations over a period of many years before cancer occurs—and these mutations may never happen—but she has taken a step—even before birth—toward breast cancer and/or ovarian cancer.

Mutated BRCA1 is a severely defective gene on the long arm of chromosome 17q21. The early research indicated that a woman born with a copy of this mutated gene faces an estimated 50–80 percent chance of developing breast cancer by age seventy and a similar risk of ovarian cancer (Later studies have suggested a somewhat lower risk, perhaps 45–60 percent for breast cancer; some researchers speculate that the initial research focused on women with "extreme" family histories of cancer and an especially severe type of gene mutation.) Ashkenazi Jews are one group with a high incidence of BRCA1, with perhaps 2 percent of the women inheriting the gene. Mutated BRCA2, which appears on chromosome 13q, may be present in up to 50 percent of "breast cancer families" and may pose a similar risk of breast cancer but a considerably lower risk of ovarian cancer. Not every female in an affected family will inherit this legacy, since we have two parents and receive genetic information from both. But women who come from families with a pattern of aggressive breast cancers in several close relatives before menopause have difficult questions to answer.

The first question: Although the tests for BRCA1 and BRCA2 are simple blood tests and are quite readily available, does she want to take them to find out whether she carries one of these mutated genes? She may have gone through years of being convinced that breast cancer is inevitable for her—and get good news. Also, while *having* mutated BRCA1 or BRCA2 increases her cancer risk, *knowing* does not increase it at all and gives her the chance to take action that may decrease her risk. On the other hand, the test has come to the marketplace before major ethical issues have been resolved, and there is a possibility of insurance coverage or employment being affected, although some legislators are working on legal protection from insurance discrimination. Test results could influence her if she is planning pregnancy or is concerned about children (daughters especially) she already has. Every woman must decide for herself whether it is better to know, one way or the other, or to suspect but not know for sure.

The second question: If she has a negative BRCA1 and BRCA2 test, what does that mean? Is she home free, without a genetic mutation? Unfortunately, while BRCA1 and BRCA2 are the genetic flaws in a large number of "family breast cancer" cases, they are only part of the picture. Researchers are working on a test for BRCA3 and know about CHEK-2, and there are doubtless other mutations to discover.

Thus, if Mary Jones has a positive BRCA1 or BRCA2 test in a "breast cancer family," and then her sister Jane's test comes back negative, it means that Jane has escaped the family history of gene mutation. On the other hand, a negative result for Rita Smith—with a strong family history of breast cancer but no one who has ever had a positive BRCA1 or BRCA2 test—means much less. While Rita does not have a BRCA1 or BRCA2 mutation, she may still have a not-yet-discovered family genetic mutation that leaves her vulnerable to breast cancer.

The third question: If a woman does carry BRCA1 or BRCA2, what does she plan to do? There is plenty of advice available, but no consensus yet. Some women report high levels of anxiety or depression and feelings of helplessness, lack of control, anger, and paralysis. Others find that this new information energizes them to act on choices they had been thinking about for years and reduces their chronic anxiety.

Deciding whether to take the blood test is not something to do lightly. Many health-care plans that offer the test also offer a coordinated educational and counseling program before, during, and after the test. That is how it should be, because there is much for a woman thinking about the test to consider, learn, and do. At any point in the process, she can decide against the test.

Any woman who knows she carries mutated BRCA1 or BRCA2 or is otherwise at high risk does well to seek out large doses of both accurate information and emotional support. A breast center, a cancer risk counselor associated with a hospital, or a specific program for high-risk women are some options. A clear pamphlet on BRCA1 and BRCA2 is available from the Cancer Information Service (see Resources) or can be read online at http://cis.nci.nih.gov. Other website resources include http://bcresources.-med.unc.edu/genetic.htm and FORCE: Facing Our Risk of Cancer Empowered, at www.facingourrisk.org.

Once she understands her real risk, the woman may decide to work on preventing further mutations by living the healthiest life she can live in order to reduce avoidable risk factors: for example, optimal diet, correct weight, regular exercise, relaxation, stress reduction, and no smoking or alcohol. Becoming politically active in breast cancer organizations that push for answers and learning positive ways of thinking about, and responding to, their risk status helps many women.

Another major strategy is increased surveillance so that any change can be detected as early as possible. This might mean expert training in breast self-examination (and performing it effectively every month), careful clinical examinations every few months, mammography at an earlier age and/or more often than usual, and use of other imaging tools such as MRI.

The woman at high risk may consider using **tamoxifen** or **raloxifene** pills daily in her strategy to prevent or delay breast cancer (see the section "Preventing Breast Cancer" later in this chapter).

The most radical choice for the high-risk woman is **prophylactic mastectomy,** preventive removal of the breasts, usually during early adulthood, to greatly reduce the chances of breast cancer. Because it cannot be reversed and may remove perfectly healthy breasts, this remains a very controversial treatment—and the woman and her doctors need to take time to weigh her risks and options carefully. Several studies are underway to see how much of a difference it makes in a woman's risk and her quality of life. If she decides on mastectomy, it is not enough to perform a subcutaneous mastectomy, which removes the breast tissue but leaves the nipple, areola, and skin intact, because there is still too much tissue where breast cancer can grow. In fact, even a simple mastectomy, the preferred surgery, which removes as much breast tissue as the surgeon can reach plus the nipple, areola, and some of the skin, still leaves some tissue. Simple mastectomy reduces the breast cancer risk to a tiny percentage, but does not eliminate it. The woman who wants reconstructive breast surgery may be able to have it done at the same time as the mastectomy. Insurance companies vary in their coverage for prophylactic mastectomy and reconstructive surgery for women at high risk.

What about breast cancer risks for women with a history of breast cancer or other breast changes? If she has a personal history of breast cancer, a woman faces a higher-than-average risk of developing a second, unrelated breast cancer—although the great majority of women never do. Women with cancers of the ovary also run an increased risk of breast cancer.

Women treated for breast carcinoma in situ who keep their breasts have an average risk of about 1 percent a year of developing invasive breast cancer, although the actual risk depends on the particular condition and her other risk factors. If a woman is diagnosed with a benign breast condition in which the individual cells are atypical but not abnormal enough to be cancer, her risk of later cancer significantly increases.

Do breast biopsies themselves increase risk? No. Women who have biopsies that do not show a specific higher risk condition face the same risk they did before the biopsy. Biopsies themselves have no connection with risk.

Hormonal Events and Taking Hormones

The more menstrual cycles a woman undergoes during her life, the more risk of breast cancer she faces, although the risk increase is rather small. Thus, if she began menstruating at age ten and went through menopause at fifty-five and was never pregnant, she would face about twice the risk of the woman who began menstruating at fifteen, went through early menopause, and had children. Women who have their ovaries removed before age forty-five decrease their risk to some extent.

Childbearing patterns are a factor. Having a first baby before age twenty protects a woman somewhat from breast cancer. Women who do not have children at all are at a higher-than-average risk; women who have a first child after age thirty-five are at still greater risk. One reason for this may be that with normal body wear and tear, abnormal cells become more common as a woman grows older; the hormonal "storm" of pregnancy could nourish these cells so that they outgrow the body's defenses. However, the overwhelming majority of women who get pregnant after thirty-five never develop breast cancer.

What about breastfeeding? Some studies suggest that breastfeeding for a total of two years or more may decrease the risk for breast cancer before menopause, but does not change the risk for breast cancer after menopause.

Miscarriage and abortion, since they are pregnancies that do not continue to term, do not protect a woman from breast cancer but probably do not increase her risk either. Some studies appeared to show that therapeutic abortion increases risk, but later studies that looked at medical records (rather than gathering data by asking women to admit to having an abortion, a less accurate technique) did not find a significant difference between groups with and without abortions.

Because hormones play such a major role in breast cancer, many studies have explored what happens to cancer risk when women change their internal hormone balance by adding either **hormonal birth control** or **hormone replacement therapy** (also called HRT, hormone therapy, HT, estrogen therapy, and/or progesterone therapy) after menopause. Researchers are not concerned that hormone medications might actually *cause* cancer by damaging cell DNA, but they want to be sure that these hormones are not nourishing any stray cancer cells that might be present in the breast.

However, most large studies of birth-control pills before menopause have shown little or no increased risk for most women. Studies have looked especially at certain groups: women using birth-control pills before a first full-term pregnancy or right before menopause, women using birth-control pills for more than ten years, and women with other significant risk factors in their histories.

Huge numbers of women have been using birth-control pills in a variety of combinations since the early 1960s. The current hormone dosages are about one-fifth as high as the dosages in 1960. The Centers for Disease Control's Cancer and Steroid Hormone study did not find any increase in risk even when women with a family history of breast cancer used birth-control pills for several years. A few studies have shown increased risk, and a few have shown decreased risk for certain groups—which means that the final answer is not in yet. (Birth-control pills definitely decrease the risk of ovarian cancer.)

For better or worse, menopausal hormone therapy has become very popular, partly because of aggressive marketing by drug companies who coined the term *hormone "replacement" therapy* and consider menopause a hormone deficiency state rather than a natural process. (Although I have some philosophical arguments with the term, I will use it here to avoid confusion with the other types of hormonal therapy used as treatment for cancer.) Often, HRT has been prescribed for the long term, not only for specific menopausal symptoms such as hot flashes and vaginal dryness, but also because it offers some protection against bone loss (osteoporosis) and seemed to protect against heart disease. Because estrogen-only therapy leads to an increased risk of cancer of the uterus, most HRT for women who still have a uterus now contains progesterone as well.

However, a less-rosy view of HRT began emerging in 2001 and 2002. The biggest bombshell: In July 2002, the large Women's Health Initiative (WHI) study announced it was closing the estrogen and progesterone HRT arm of the research several years early because researchers found the treatment riskier than expected. This study followed 16,608 postmenopausal women, divided into groups, with one group taking progesterone and estrogen HRT pills as a preventive strategy for bone and heart health and the other group taking placebo pills. The study was intended to last for eight years, until 2005. However, unexpected increases in the rates of several diseases in the HRT group, especially of breast cancer but also of heart attack, stroke, and blood clots in the lungs led to the dramatic announcement—and to a deluge of calls from worried women to their gynecologists.

Although the increased risks are modest, study results appear to show that risks of long-term therapy (more than about three years) with estrogen and progesterone outweigh the benefits in this group of women. Meanwhile, in 2001, results of the Heart and Estrogen/Progestin Replacement Study (HERS) in about 2,700 women who already had heart disease failed to show a heart benefit for HRT in this group and, in fact, showed a mildly increased risk of heart problems during the first year.

All these findings need to be confirmed or disproved by more research, and for now, many doctors and women are backing away from estrogen/progesterone HRT as long-term preventive medicine for the bones and heart, at least until we know more. The situation is different for HRT when used as a short-term treatment for severe menopausal symptoms, where the potential benefits are greater and the risks are less. Also, the current studies have not looked at estrogen alone or at the hormones in different forms, such as creams or patches. Finally, while the research predicts risk for groups of women only, it says very little about the risk an individual woman faces. If a woman is taking or considering HRT, it makes sense for her to discuss her specific situation and family history with her gynecologist or other health professional.

As fertility drugs become more common, women and doctors are beginning to ask whether the major hormonal upheaval they cause could increase breast cancer risk. So far, the information comes from anecdotal evidence only—a case of breast cancer here, a case there—rather than from any large studies, so we know very little.

One hormone medication, **diethylstilbestrol** (DES), given to many women years ago to prevent miscarriages, has been linked for years with unusual gynecologic cancers in the daughters of the women who took the hormone. A small increase in breast cancer risk is beginning to appear in these daughters. For decades, DES has not been prescribed for women who might bear children, although it is still used to treat men who have prostate cancer as well as older women with certain medical conditions.

Diet

Many researchers are convinced that a woman's diet could trigger some of the genetic mutations necessary for breast cancer and believe that low fiber and high fat—most kinds of fat, animal or plant—may be the culprits. Worldwide, the higher the average amount of fat in the diet, the higher the breast cancer rate. When women immigrate from a low-risk country to a higher-risk area, their daughters' breast cancer rates tend to approach those of the new country. Animal studies also seem to show increased incidence of breast cancer with high-fat diets, and one theory is that high-fat diets increase the kinds of estrogens related to cancer. Obesity is definitely a risk: After menopause, at least, the more overweight a woman is, the greater her risk of breast cancer. Beyond these connections, however, the relationships between high-fat diets and breast cancer remain unclear, with many conflicting findings.

Findings from the ongoing Harvard study of almost ninety thousand nurses seem to question the connection between a high-fat diet and breast cancer, although some researchers have complained that even the 30 percent and 25 percent "low fat" (a 30 percent fat diet means that 30 percent of the calories in the diet come from fats) diets in the study were not low enough to make a real difference. Other researchers wonder whether a low-fat diet might make more of a difference if it starts in childhood or adolescence or whether some types of fats, such as olive oil and fish oils, might reduce risk.

Another arm of the Women's Health Initiative Study, the same study with the HRT research, has enrolled almost forty-nine thousand women in a diet modification program trial. The goals are reducing total dietary fat to 15–20 percent of daily calories and consuming five servings of vegetables and fruits and six servings of grain each day—and maintaining these changes for over eight years. About 60 percent of the group will continue their normal diets, with the other 40 percent of the group participating in an intensive program of classes and counseling. The big questions: Can and will women make and maintain these diet changes? If they can, will it make a difference in breast cancer or colon cancer risk?

Meanwhile, researchers are looking at many other dietary elements. The theory behind the interest in high-fiber diets is that fiber from fruits, vegetables, and grains helps move food waste products, including some suspected of causing cancerous changes, quickly and easily through the digestive tract before they have a chance to cause problems. Studies are examining vitamin A and the related beta-carotene and retinoids, vitamins C and E, and other vitamin and mineral micronutrients, substances the body needs in tiny amounts. Some of these act as **antioxidants,** combining with free radicals to make these incomplete chemicals in the body unavailable to damage the cells' DNA and begin the breast cancer process. Other studies are exploring whether soy and other specific foods have a potential protective role.

We need to learn much more about dietary factors that either increase risk or protect us, including what happens to our foods before they reach our tables. But for now, the American Cancer Society's guidelines for a commonsense approach to general dietary cancer prevention (see the partial list on page 21) are the best we have for breast cancer prevention.

Lifestyle

There are tantalizing clues that regular physical activity and exercise may lower breast cancer risk. This might happen because exercise decreases obesity, a known risk factor, or because it decreases certain forms of estrogen in the body and reduces stress, or something else entirely. With very high-intensity workouts, women may stop menstruating entirely, reducing their number of hormonal cycles; the negative sides to this are that their bone density may suffer from the hormone lack and that they may even be thrown into premature menopause and become unable to conceive a child. Reports are still preliminary. Among the questions we need answered are these: How vigorous and frequent does exercise need to be to be protective? Are there certain ages at which exercise is especially beneficial?

Alcohol use seems to be related to increased breast cancer risk, particularly in women who drink two ounces or more of alcohol a day most days. An ounce is the amount of alcohol in a glass of wine, a bottle of beer, or a shot of hard liquor. Among the theories of why alcohol increases risk is that liver changes from alcohol alter the body's hormone balance or make the liver less able to detoxify some substance that contributes to breast cancer. However, it is also possible that later studies will show that something else common to women who happen to drink alcohol may be the factor that increases risk.

Some new studies suggest that smoking may raise breast cancer risk somewhat. These reports are preliminary, and more research is essential—

although the wisdom of stopping smoking or never starting has never been in doubt!

Many women with silicone breast implants have questions about their breast cancer risk. To date, implants have not been connected to an increased breast cancer risk, even if there is some leakage from the implants. However, implants do make it more difficult to detect a cancer because mammography does not work as well and any lumps under the implant will be difficult to feel with the fingers.

Environment

It is not only people living near obvious toxic dump areas, downstream from industrial pollution, or in locations with major air pollution who wonder what these environmental poisons are doing to their cancer risk. Breast cancer activists have joined several researchers to question whether substances we as a society have chosen to add to our environment have increased breast cancer risk. Here again, the jury is still out.

One of the big questions is about certain hormone-mimicking chemicals (called **xenoestrogens** or foreign estrogens) found in several pesticides and related chlorinated organic compounds, some plastics, and gasoline. Many researchers argue that these play no role in breast cancer, but others are clearly worried. One theory is that the body's natural estrogen, **estradiol**, can be converted into two distinct products that are very similar in structure but act quite differently. One product is thought to protect against breast cancer while the other is a "bad" form, which some researchers believe is overproduced in women exposed to high levels of xenoestrogens.

Somewhat similar questions arise about hormones and antibiotics fed to livestock and poultry that come to our tables as food, and about fertilizers and other chemicals used to feed and preserve vegetables, fruit, and grains. "Organic" foods have become popular partly because of such consumer concerns. On the other hand, some agricultural specialists point out that organic foods, often from plain, old-fashioned seed varieties, are bred to be naturally pest-resistant, and plants that are more pest-resistant are that way because they contain higher levels of natural toxins, which can be just as harmful as some pesticides.

Low doses of ionizing radiation are a fact of life for every human being, since ionizing radiation comes from natural minerals near the earth's surface, cosmic rays, and other sources. Some people live close to concentrations of radon in the soil, which may increase their risk for some types of cancer but do not seem related to breast cancer.

The breast cells in women under thirty-five are relatively sensitive to high doses of ionizing radiation given to the chest, neck, or head. Thus women who, during their teens or twenties, received radiation therapy to the chest area for Hodgkin's disease need close follow-up years later because they face a somewhat increased risk for breast cancer. This sensitivity to radiation is also a major reason women under thirty-five do not undergo routine mammography, although the mammography radiation dose is very low, and most (although not all) scientists believe that occasional mammograms in women over forty are quite safe.

PREVENTING BREAST CANCER

What does this all mean for the individual woman? She cannot change her family history and she probably will not change her childbearing plans. She can change her diet to lower fat and higher fiber, and she can keep her weight reasonable through diet and exercise. She might use risk data as an additional reason to breastfeed her babies. She can seek current information before taking hormone medications. And she can stay as healthy and happy as possible—it may help and certainly cannot hurt.

Over the last several years, thousands of women without breast cancer but at relatively high risk because of age or family/personal history have participated in breast cancer "chemoprevention" trials to see if certain drugs could postpone or prevent breast cancer in healthy women. The first big study, the Breast Cancer Prevention Trial (or BCPT), began in 1992 and enrolled about thirteen thousand women to take either the drug **tamoxifen citrate** (Nolvadex) or a placebo every day. Tamoxifen (not to be confused with Taxol and Taxotere, which are chemotherapy drugs) is officially known as a selective estrogen receptor modulator (SERM), a weakened estrogen. Tamoxifen probably competes with "real" estrogen, binding to hormone receptor sites on many breast cancer cells and depriving the cells of the estrogen they need.

The study ended before the scheduled five years because preliminary data appeared to show a stunning 45 percent reduction in breast cancer rates in the women taking tamoxifen. In fact, 2.3 percent of the women in the placebo group and 1.27 percent of the women in the tamoxifen group were diagnosed with breast cancer during the study period. Meanwhile, women in the tamoxifen group developed uterine cancer and blood clots, known risks of tamoxifen, at a higher rate than their sisters in the placebo group. Many women receiving tamoxifen dropped out of the study early because of side effects of the drug.

Skeptics point out that the study continued less than five years for a disease that probably takes at least eight years to develop enough to be detected. They ask whether tamoxifen was in fact treating very early cancers rather than actually preventing them. It will take more years to find out whether tamoxifen prevents cancers, postpones them, or treats very early cancers, any of which could be a worthwhile benefit—depending on the risks of treatment in otherwise healthy women.

Two somewhat similar studies in Europe, the Royal Marsden study of 2,500 healthy women in England with strong family breast cancer history, and the Italian study of 5,500 women with a lower initial risk did not show any significant benefit but many more side effects and "adverse events" for tamoxifen. Critics of these studies suggest that these were not large enough or long enough studies to show an effect in women at low to moderate risk.

Hard on the heels of the BCPT closing came the opening of the current big prevention clinical trial, the Study of Tamoxifen and Raloxifene (or STAR). This trial, conducted by the National Surgical Adjuvant Breast and Bowel Project, opened at 193 cancer institutions in 1999. It seeks to enroll twenty-two thousand women past menopause and at high breast cancer risk to take either tamoxifen or another SERM, raloxifene (Evista) every day for several years. Raloxifene has been FDA approved as an osteoporosis treatment since 1997 but has not been approved yet as a breast-cancer treatment.

The goals of this trial are to get further information about using SERMs for healthy women and to discover if one of them works better or with fewer side effects than the other. Critics point to the lack of a placebo group and also voice concern that, as with BCPT, this trial exposes healthy women to somewhat risky drugs. Information on STAR, including enrollment information, is available from health professionals or on the Internet. (One site is www.pinnacleimaging.com/breasthealth/star.)

Women well past menopause who have not been on recent hormone therapy usually tolerate tamoxifen or raloxifene with few side effects. For younger women or those just stopping hormone therapy, hot flashes and other menopausal symptoms are common, with fluid retention and temporary depression occurring fairly often. The major serious medical risks, although rare, are blood clots, eye or liver changes, and uterine cancer, problems that can occur with any estrogen therapy. Uterine cancer, usually found early and cured with treatment, appears to be less of a risk with raloxifene than with tamoxifen, one reason for comparing the two drugs in the STAR trial.

Since the STAR trial enrolls only women after menopause, birth defects are not a concern. However, if tamoxifen or raloxifen are prescribed for a younger woman outside a clinical trial, she must use reliable contraception; although the drugs cause menopausal symptoms, they do not prevent pregnancy (in fact, tamoxifen was originally studied as a fertility drug), but they do cause severe birth defects.

Currently, the American Cancer Society estimates that one in nine women in the United States will develop breast cancer by age eighty-five and that one in eight will develop the disease during her lifetime, up from one in fifteen not many years ago. Breast cancer is diagnosed in about 2 percent of all women under the age of fifty and becomes considerably more common after that age. About 205,000 women and 1,500 men are expected to be diagnosed with the disease in 2002; about 39,600 women and 400 men are expected to die from it. The good news is that the number of breast cancer deaths per year has actually dropped since 1990.

The 11 percent (one in nine) risk figure says that, under present conditions of risk, a white baby girl born today faces an 11-percent chance of being diagnosed with breast cancer at some time up to age eighty-five. White, non-Hispanic women, especially those with higher social and economic status, have the highest rates of diagnosis, with African-American women slightly behind. (However, African-American women are more likely to die of the disease, at least partly because they tend to be diagnosed later and to have less access to treatment. There is also a possibility that breast cancer behaves differently in African-American women than in white, non-Hispanic women. Their death rate has increased while the rate in white women has declined.) Women with Asian roots face a lower risk, but this statistical advantage wanes the more generations the family has been in the United States and the more acculturated it has become. The situation appears to be similar for Hispanic women, but statistics are lacking.

This risk percentage is a cumulative figure obtained by adding a woman's risk of developing breast cancer from age twenty to thirty, plus that from thirty to forty, and so on. *At no one time does the average woman face an 11-percent risk of developing breast cancer.* She faces a small risk during each segment of time. If she does not develop breast cancer during that segment of time, that portion of risk is behind her forever—it is not added on to future segments. During the next segment of time, she faces another small risk. A similar situation: If a woman has to cross eight streets, and she avoids being hit by a car when she crosses the first four streets, the fact that she has remained safe so far does not in any way make it more dangerous for her to cross the fifth street. This is not a case of "luck running out." Because breast cancer is often related to body wear and tear, however, each segment is a little riskier than the one before.

The 11-percent figure is outrageous and scarcely reassuring, but it is not quite as scary as it sounds. The figure partly reflects the rapid increase in longevity for women, who can now expect to live into their eighties and beyond—into the decades at very high risk for breast cancer. For instance,

*Questions
about
Breasts*

203

women face a 1 in 2,500 risk of developing breast cancer by age thirty, and a 1 in 24 risk by age sixty. Ironically, if large numbers of women died young—in childbirth, for instance—the breast cancer statistics would look better.

The fact that the rate is higher now than it was twenty years ago also reflects an increase in detecting breast cancer earlier. However, many people believe that the increasing rate of breast cancer does indicate that something more is going on. They question whether something in the environment, dietary patterns, changes in childbearing patterns—or something else entirely—may be making women more vulnerable.

Statisticians warn against a "The sky is falling, the sky is falling!" approach, either for groups of women or for the individual. Statistics often rise for a few years and then decrease just as unpredictably. And, since a cancer large enough to diagnose has been growing for many years and since the genetic mutations may have begun decades before, statisticians and epidemiologists try to keep a long-term perspective.

For the woman with a family history of breast cancer or another factor that increases her risk significantly, it is especially valuable to think of breast cancer risk as a series of time segments, each with its own small portion of risk. For instance, a condition that "triples" a woman's risk means that, in a decade where she would normally face a 1-percent risk, she might now face a 3-percent chance of developing the disease. When she finishes that decade without the disease, that portion of risk is behind her forever. Also, if the risk condition is discovered when she is forty-five (for example, if a family member develops breast cancer or the woman is diagnosed with a benign condition that increases her risk), she already has several decades of risk behind her. A medical geneticist can use statistical life tables to be much more precise than "triples" or "significantly increases." It also makes sense to remember that statistics tell about groups of women, but say nothing about what will happen to the individual.

BREAST CHANGES THAT ARE NOT CANCER

At least half of all women at some time in their lives experience something about a breast that worries them: discomfort, a lump, or some other change. Probably almost all of these women wonder whether this change could be cancer.

In fact, most of these changes are not cancer and do not in any way increase a woman's risk of cancer.

Many doctors call any noncancerous breast change by the same generic label: **fibrocystic breast disease**. But "breast" is about the only accurate part of the term, since many of the changes have nothing to do with either fibrous or cystic tissue and most of them are not a disease at all. **Benign**

breast change is a better term, along with the name of the actual condition, if possible.

Lumping the lumps together is the problem. Dr. Susan Love, breast surgeon and author of *Dr. Susan Love's Breast Book,* divides benign breast conditions into six categories:

1. Normal physiological changes, like minor tenderness, swelling, and lumpiness

2. Mastalgia, or severe breast pain

3. Infections and inflammations

4. Discharge and other nipple problems

5. Lumpiness or nodularity beyond what most women have

6. "Dominant" benign lumps, ones that "stick out" from the normal lumpiness

Once a woman learns that her breast condition is not cancer, she still wants to know if it could increase her chances of developing cancer later. Prodded by the American Cancer Society's National Task Force on Breast Cancer Control, the College of American Pathologists held a consensus conference in 1985 entitled, "Is 'Fibrocystic' Disease of the Breast Precancerous?" The Board of Governors of the College of American Pathologists later adopted the conclusions as policy.

The pathologists divided the common benign breast changes into three categories, depending on whether they might possibly increase a woman's risk of developing breast cancer later:

1. Nonproliferative changes

2. Proliferative changes without atypical cells

3. Proliferative changes with atypical cells

Nonproliferative breast changes are the most common kinds of changes and do not in any way add to a woman's risk. Except when the breast is developing during adolescence and during pregnancy and lactation, normal breast cells divide at set times to replace old cells and maintain the breast status quo. In nonproliferative changes, the breast cells stick to their normal schedule of division but the total number of cells may pile up somewhat, perhaps because the old cells are not being disposed of quickly enough.

The glandular tissue of the breast normally feels lumpy as it does its work; the breast *normally* gathers in extra fluid every month, which may stretch nerve fibers and send discomfort messages to the brain. These are not considered breast changes at all.

But what happens to many women over the years is that the cell cleanup does not keep up with the cell buildup. The breasts may receive a faulty hormonal message, or overreact to a normal message and overprepare. Or the lymph system and other cleanup agencies may fall down on the job a bit. Instead of being efficiently recycled, the extra fluid and secretions may gather into a **cyst,** large or small, which may pop and drain or may persist from month to month. Cysts are the most common kind of breast lump in women before menopause. Some women are prone to form large numbers of them. A cyst can also press on nerve fibers and cause considerable discomfort.

At other times, breast debris builds up in a benign solid lump called a **fibroadenoma**. This is usually rather round, moves easily in the breast, and may feel rubbery. Part or all of this is usually removed with either a core biopsy or an open biopsy, and the tissue is examined under a microscope, because that is the only way to be absolutely sure of what the lump is. There are several other kinds of nonproliferative breast changes, but as long as they fall into this category they do not increase a woman's risk of cancer.

Proliferative changes without atypical cells occur when, for some reason, the cells divide more often than they should but the individual cells appear quite normal. **Duct hyperplasia,** for instance, means that the walls of the breast ducts and lobules, ordinarily lined with a layer two cells deep, have become thicker. The layer can overgrow slightly, up to four cells in depth, and not affect a woman's risk for developing breast cancer later. If the layer grows to more than four cells deep, however, the hyperplasia is considered to increase a woman's risk slightly, to about 1½ to 2 times the average. Hyperplasia often reverses itself. In another common benign condition called **sclerosing adenosis,** tiny chunks of benign breast debris can take up calcium salts from the body and "calcify." While these are too small to be felt with the fingers as a lump, they can show up on mammograms as microcalcifications; if these look a certain way and appear in clusters, they need to be evaluated, since cancer sometimes shows itself the same way.

Proliferative changes with atypical cells happen when the cells divide more often than they should and the individual cells appear abnormal. Possibly the quality control slips when the breast works overtime to make too many cells. These atypical cells can disappear, stay where they are without causing any trouble, or, once in a while, lead to the ultimate atypical cells: cancer. The more atypical a cell is, the more vulnerable it is to further mutations. Proliferative changes with atypical cells do increase a woman's risk of cancer moderately, two to five times the average, depending on how atypical the individual cells are and how many of them there are.

How are benign breast changes treated? General lumpiness is considered normal and requires no treatment. If a diagnostic procedure is necessary—for a persistent solid lump, some kinds of nipple drainage, or certain changes on a mammogram—and benign changes are found, the doctor needs to describe to the woman what those changes are, especially whether there are any proliferative changes with atypia. With nonproliferative changes, she does not need to do anything except continue a routine breast care program of monthly breast self-exam, regular professional breast exam, and mammography. If there are proliferative changes, particularly with atypia, she can discuss with her doctor whether more frequent professional exams or mammograms are advisable.

Insurance companies have been known to deny a woman coverage for any future breast problem because of a benign breast change that is not a disease and in no way increases her risk of cancer. This is not right or reasonable, but it is legal and it happens. While she has to answer direct questions honestly, and her doctor must too, there is no reason to volunteer anything or to mention a nonproliferative nondisease on an insurance form.

BREAST PAIN

It is the rare woman who does not experience at least a little breast pain (**mastalgia** or **mastodynia**) at some time in her life. If the woman still ovulates or if she takes menopausal hormone replacement therapy, breast pain usually arises because normal cyclic changes bring fluid into the breast which then stretches and irritates the pain nerve fibers. This pain often begins when a woman is in her thirties or forties, after several years of ovulatory cycles, and it is a normal variation that has nothing to do with breast cancer. The balance of hormones may be slightly askew, or the body may be extra sensitive to hormonal stimulation at some time. Another common cause of breast pain is a breast cyst, which irritates nerve fibers but does not increase cancer risk. Very seldom is breast pain the first sign of breast cancer, especially in a young woman.

However, "seldom" does not mean "never." Once in a while, a doctor misses a cancer by assuming breast pain is related to the menstrual cycle and not assessing it fully. Definitely, any pain that is distressing and continues for more than a month or two deserves a thorough evaluation. Some of the questions to ask are these: Is the pain in one breast or both? Pain in both breasts is almost never cancer. Does the pain get worse before the period and better after the period—a typical pattern for normal cyclic pain? Is the pain in one location, perhaps because of a cyst, or throughout the breast? Are there other breast signs or symptoms, like a lump, discharge from the nipple, or any change in how the breast looks?

Sometimes the pain goes away when the woman is reassured that careful examination and appropriate imaging studies do not detect any sign of cancer. Sometimes the doctor finds a cyst, aspirates (withdraws) the fluid, and the pain disappears. The doctor can check also for other causes of breast pain, such as muscle or rib problems or thyroid gland disorders. Often breast pain leaves as mysteriously as it came.

For continuing benign pain, one or a combination of therapies usually relieves discomfort, but every woman is an individual and will respond to a different treatment. The simplest remedy is probably an occasional over-the-counter pain pill. Mechanical treatments include wearing a carefully fitted support bra twenty-four hours a day (although some women feel more comfortable with no bra or with silk or lambswool or another material against the breast), heat and/or cold, and massaging the breast with gentle circular movements to keep fluid moving out of the breast. Regular exercise, too, may adjust hormone balance to relieve pain, and yoga or such Chinese techniques as t'ai chi, ch'i kung, acupuncture, and acupressure can be both useful and enjoyable.

Many women recommend dietary strategies. The basic American Cancer Society diet for cancer prevention (see "Diet" on pages 20 and 21 in Chapter 2), which recommends low fat and high fiber foods as well as many vegetables and fruits, may affect hormone balance positively. Reducing or eliminating salt helps some women. Others swear by eliminating caffeine from the diet, including coffee, tea, chocolate, and cola drinks. Still others add 400 IU of vitamin E or evening primrose oil daily to their diet.

Psychological remedies can often reduce pain or increase a woman's ability to cope with it. They may also enrich other parts of a woman's life. Typical techniques include progressive muscle relaxation, distraction (for instance, a good conversation, a walk in the park, or a novel), guided imagery tapes, and individual counseling.

Pharmacologic treatments might require starting or stopping birth-control pills or hormone replacement therapy, or changing to a different type of pill; adjusting the amounts of estrogen or progesterone may decrease breast tenderness. Research continues on local therapy hormones, such as a progesterone gel that is applied directly to the breast. The drug danazol is effective for severe continuing breast pain, but often has masculinizing side effects like deepening the voice and increasing facial hair; bromocriptine is another possibility. A few women improve with diuretics ("water pills"). Two books that contain more information are *The Informed Woman's Guide to Breast Health* and *Dr. Susan Love's Breast Book* (see Resources).

— *Kerry McGinn*

CHAPTER 12

Detecting and Diagnosing Breast Changes

Until medical science learns how to prevent breast cancer, the best strategy for dealing with it is to find it as early as possible. In truth, even with the "early" detection techniques we have available now, a breast cancer has usually been growing for years before we find it. However, these techniques still give women a very good chance to live longer and perhaps keep their breasts as well.

Early detection means being alert to changes in how a breast looks, feels, and functions. Most of these changes are not cancer, but they need to be evaluated.

A breast lump is the most common change, felt with the fingers or seen on a mammogram. The cancerous breast lump is ordinarily hard ("rock-like"), but it can be as minimal as a soft thickening. Besides a lump, there are other possible signs:

✦ changes in how the breast appears, such as swelling, dimpling, number of visible blood vessels, skin redness, enlarged pores, and nipple alterations

✦ nipple discharges

✦ microcalcifications or other findings on mammograms

What needs to be evaluated by a health professional? Any breast change that lasts longer than a month in a premenopausal woman. In the postmenopausal woman, who is at greater risk for breast cancer, *any* breast change needs to be checked as soon as possible, even if she is on hormone replacement therapy and still experiences monthly breast changes. Pain, especially pain that comes and goes with the menstrual cycle, is usually not the earliest symptom of a breast cancer, but persistent pain definitely needs to be checked.

DETECTING BREAST CHANGES

The "big three" in detecting breast changes, benign or cancerous, are mammography, monthly breast self-examination, and regular examinations by a health professional. No one method of detection is perfect, but the three work together as a team. Each method has advantages and weaknesses. Each finds certain breast changes that the others can miss.

Mammography remains the workhorse of breast imaging techniques, both for screening the woman who does not have any breast symptoms and for giving information when she does. It may save many lives by finding some very small invasive cancers and breast changes with a high risk of becoming invasive breast cancers, even before there is a lump to feel (see Chapter 3).

In specific cases, doctors may order another technique. Ultrasound, for example, is commonly used if the woman with a breast lump that can be felt is under thirty-five or is pregnant or nursing. It can also help when there is a suspicious finding in breasts that shows up poorly on mammograms or when the doctor suspects that a lump is a cyst. Less often, doctors turn to magnetic resonance imaging or one of the other alternative imaging techniques described in Chapter 3.

Women—not health professionals or mammograms—still find more than 80 percent of the breast lumps that can be felt. Unfortunately, too often these lumps are found by chance when they are relatively large. A common scenario is a woman soaping her breasts in the shower and suddenly feeling this...thing.

The idea behind regular **breast self-examination** (BSE) is that after a woman learns what to look and feel for, she becomes so well-acquainted with her own breasts that she can spot very early changes. BSE is not an anxious monthly cancer search. Instead, it means "checking for normal."

What advantages does BSE offer? It involves the person most concerned with her own breasts and most motivated to take care of them. It offers continuing surveillance. If the doctor or other health professional examines the breasts annually in September and a cancerous lump finally becomes big enough to feel in October, the woman who does not perform BSE has lost eleven crucial months before the cancer is detected by her doctor the following September.

When a woman examines her own breasts, her fingers feel from "the outside in." At the same time, her chest wall and other internal structures feel from "the inside out" against her fingers. This gives her an extra sense of her own breasts that no health professional can share.

BSE does not cost anything, and a woman does not have to leave home for it. It is absolutely safe and does not cause discomfort. Plus, many women like the fact that this is a real contribution they can make to their own health.

BSE is available to every woman who has eyes and fingers. That includes women who cannot get routine mammography because they are pregnant, nursing a baby, or too young for mammograms. The American Cancer Society recommends that women begin practicing BSE at age twenty. Depending on their doctor's (and their insurance company's) philosophy, most women do not start routine mammograms until they are forty or even fifty (see "Standard X rays" and "Mammograms" in Chapter 3).

For the woman with "dense" glandular breasts that do not show up well on mammograms, BSE may be the best chance of finding an early cancer. And while the woman with lumpy, difficult-to-examine breasts may find it hard to learn BSE initially, it still may be easier for her to detect changes if she examines her breasts every month than it is for the doctor who checks them once a year.

Some doctors minimize the importance of BSE, usually because they think of it as occasional, halfhearted poking and prodding by a woman who does not know what she is doing. But self-examination, used consistently and effectively by women who are well-trained and motivated, is something else entirely. Doctors and women who put all their trust in mammography may miss many breast cancers completely, especially in premenopausal women.

Obviously, I'm a believer. When I found a tiny breast lump with BSE, it did not show up with mammography. My careful and competent surgeon could not even feel it. I finally convinced the doctor to aspirate a few cells through a needle—and promptly learned the lump was cancer. Of the four doctors I saw during the next few days—two surgeons, one medical oncologist, and one radiation oncologist—*every single one* volunteered that he or she would not have found the lump: "How in the world did you ever find that?" I think it was because my body could feel from "the inside out" and because I was more familiar with my breasts than any doctor could be.

My experience is not unique. Roughly a third of the women in my breast cancer support group, mostly premenopausal, discovered their own tumors, which did not appear on mammograms and which our doctors had difficulty feeling. Of course, that means that the other two-thirds had their cancers detected either by mammography or by a health professional's examination.

Women often avoid BSE because they do not feel competent to perform it. Everything feels lumpy to them and they do not know "what's what." Even with the best training, no woman is competent at first; it takes months to "learn" the breasts. Early on, every woman wonders whether what she is feeling now was there last month or not. But each month brings increasing expertise and confidence, *if* the woman does not get discouraged and give up.

No woman has to interpret or diagnose what she feels. The only conclusion she needs to draw is whether her breasts have changed or not since the previous exam.

Many women do not practice BSE because they are scared of what they will find. It is natural and normal to be scared, but most of the time there will not be any changes, and a woman will feel reassured. If there is a change, it is most likely benign. Should there ever be a cancerous change, the scary thing is *not* finding it. With life and breasts at stake, many women discover that learning BSE—taking concrete action to protect their health—soon crowds out fear and brings peace of mind instead.

PERFORMING BSE

BSE takes about fifteen unhurried minutes once a month. If done less often, it is harder to "remember" the breast; if done more often, it is too soon to recognize a change. Women who still menstruate schedule it about a week or so after their period starts, when their breasts are most at rest hormonally. Women past menopause or who are pregnant or lactating can choose any day of the month that they will remember easily. Those who have undergone hysterectomies but still have functioning ovaries have to listen to other bodily cues; it makes sense to avoid times when symptoms such as bloating or breast tenderness indicate more hormonal activity.

It is very helpful for a woman to have BSE training, especially with a doctor or nurse who will take the time to "map" a woman's breasts for her. A woman's personal doctor or nurse practitioner, a breast health center, American Cancer Society BSE trainers, or a women's health group can teach her what she is feeling and what is normal for her. Some women get a breast model with simulated lumps to use each month to "reeducate" their fingers before feeling their own breasts.

Each month, a woman can jog her memory with the "seven Ps" of BSE:

+ *positions* to assume while inspecting and palpating (feeling) the breasts

+ *perimeter* (boundaries) of breast tissue to be examined

+ *palpation* using *pads* of the fingers

+ *pressures* of the fingers

+ *pattern* of the search

- ✦ *practice* with feedback

- ✦ *plan of action* for breast health

What initially seems awkward soon becomes second nature. There is nothing difficult about the BSE eye and hand movements.

Inspecting the Breasts

To examine her breasts visually, the woman first stands with her arms relaxed at her sides in front of a large mirror in a good light. As she faces the mirror, she carefully inspects her breasts: their symmetry, shape, color, skin texture, pattern of blood vessels, and so on (see the illustrations on pages 214–218).

Skin over a tumor can appear stretched, shiny, and large-pored; in fact, this condition is called *peau d'orange,* skin of the orange. A cancer's need for nutrition can lead to increased numbers of blood vessels in the vicinity, and these may show through the skin. Nipples and areolas get special attention: any rashes or discharges? an "outie" nipple that has become an "innie"?

The woman turns slowly, bringing first one breast forward to examine and then the other, so that light and shadow help disclose any changes in breast contour. Then, since other positions do a better job of accentuating any breast swellings or puckerings, the woman raises her arms above her head, with her elbows back, or clasps her hands behind her head. This tightens the chest muscles, elevates the breasts, and stretches the skin. She pivots slowly, first in this position and then with her hands pressing firmly on her hips. Puckerings, "dimples," or changes in the shape or direction of the nipples can result from a tumor pulling on one of the Cooper's ligaments that attach from the chest wall to the skin.

A woman can also bend forward at the hips and check the symmetry of the breasts as they hang. Most women normally have one breast a little larger than the other, but the two should look relatively similar. Only if the size *and* symmetry have changed is it significant. The woman with large or pendulous breasts can lift each one with the opposite hand so that she can see the underside.

Feeling the Breasts

POSITIONS After she has looked carefully at her breasts, the woman lies down in the best position for palpating her breasts effectively. Many women accidentally discover a breast lump while they are showering—but when a woman is standing up, gravity pulls the breast tissue down so that it

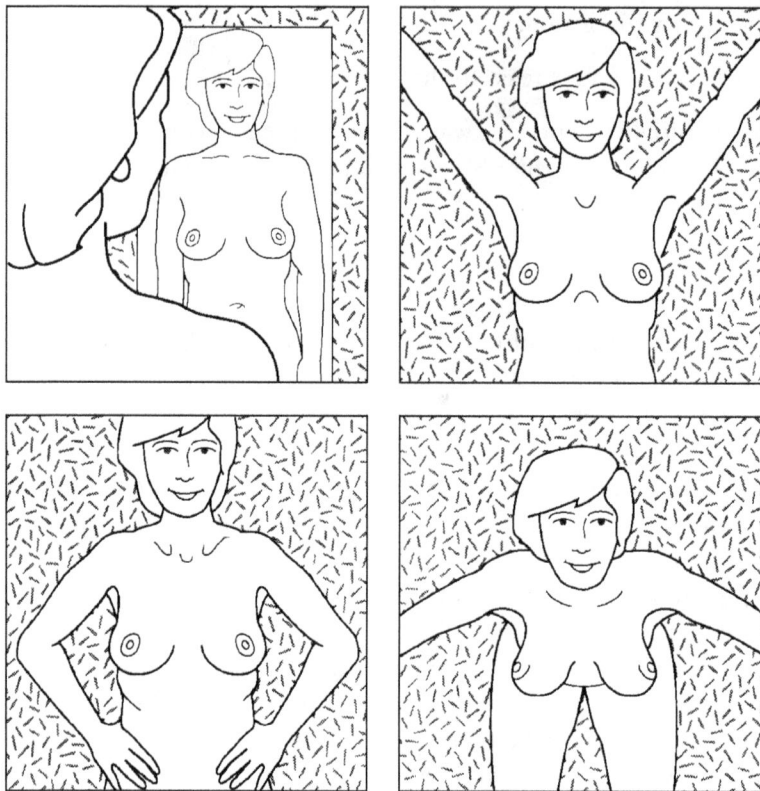

Breast Inspection Process

(this series of illustrations—continued on pages 215, 216, 217, and 218—
courtesy of The Informed Woman's Guide to Breast Health)

bulges at the bases and is difficult to examine. The idea with BSE is to support and spread the breast evenly so that all the tissue can be felt against the firm background of the chest wall.

A small-breasted woman may be able to do this just by lying flat on her back. If breast tissue bulges to the side when she does this, she can place a small pillow behind the shoulder of the breast she plans to examine.

The MammaCare Method, one popular program of BSE training, refines this further. A woman always palpates her breast with the opposite hand. Thus, when it is time to examine the outer half of her right breast, she turns onto her left side, bends her knees, and lets her right shoulder fall back slightly until the nipple "floats" at the top of the mound of breast. (A pillow behind her back makes the position comfortable.) She rests the back of her right hand on her forehead.

When she is ready to check the inner half of the breast, from nipple line to breastbone, the woman keeps the examining fingers in place on the

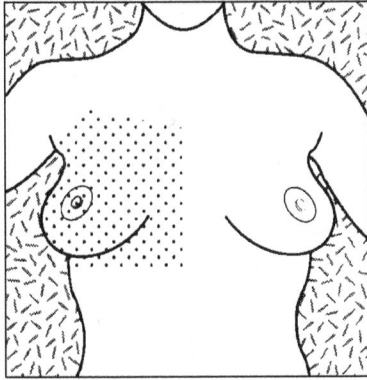

Shaded area is perimeter for BSE

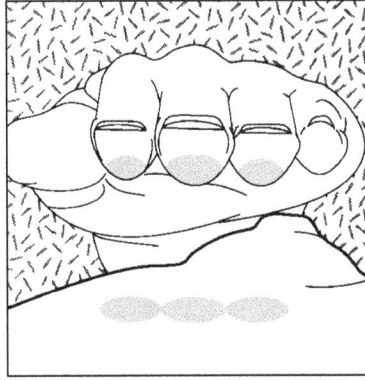

Palpation with pads of fingers

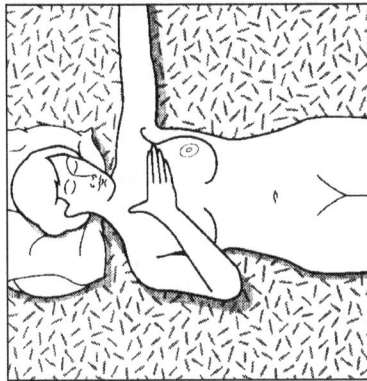

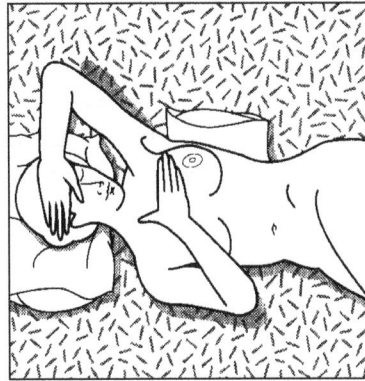

Breast Self-Examination

breast so that she does not miss any area, while she pushes the pillow away and rolls onto her back. She holds the other arm out to the side.

PERIMETER The area to check on each breast is bounded by an imaginary line down from the middle of the armpit to the bra line just below the breast, along the bra line to the middle of the breastbone, up the breastbone to the collarbone, along the collarbone, and back to the middle of the armpit. The upper, outer **quadrant** (quarter) of the breast is the most common site for breast cancers, but cancer can occur anywhere in the breast area.

PALPATION (WITH PADS OF THE FINGERS) If a woman applies corn-starch, powder, oil, or lotion to the breast, it is easier for the fingers to glide over the breast and feel any changes. That is why so many women discover lumps when they are soaping their breasts in the shower. If she loses that slippery feel during the examination, she can relubricate the breasts.

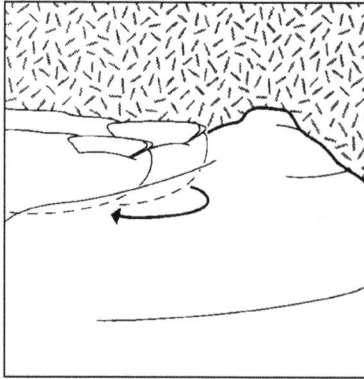

Light-pressure circles

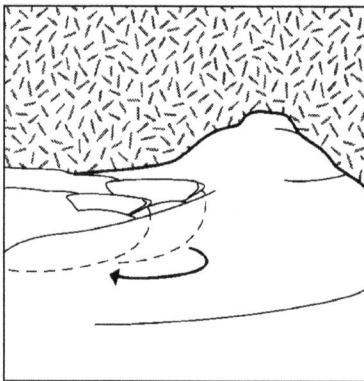

Medium-pressure circles

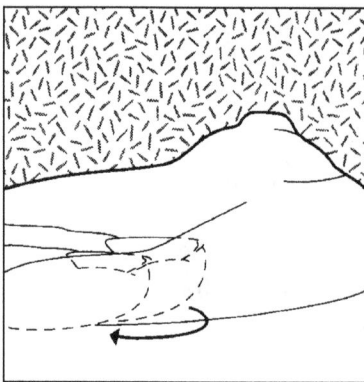

Deep-pressure circles

After she lies down, the woman places the flat areas of three or four fingers (not the thumb), from the last joint to the end of the finger, on the tissue to be examined. She uses the hand opposite the breast to be examined and lays the fingers flat and parallel to the chest wall. She moves the soft pads of her fingers in small, dime-size circles over all the breast tissue and does not lift them from the breast between circles. The pads of the fingers are more sensitive than the fingertips, and using more than two fingers stabilizes the tissue so that a lump cannot skitter away from probing fingers.

PRESSURES At each spot, the woman makes circles using three different pressures. The light-pressure circle just moves the skin without jostling the breast tissue underneath. The medium-pressure circle presses midway into the tissue. The deep-pressure circle probes deeply and firmly into the breast, down to the ribs or to the point just short of discomfort. Changes can appear at any depth, and this thoroughness gives a woman the best chance of finding anything that is there.

PATTERN OF SEARCH There are three common patterns of search. Most women find that they become more familiar with their breasts if they use the same pattern each month, but any one of the three, used carefully and consistently, can be effective.

The MammaCare pattern searches the breast in parallel vertical lines, like "mowing the lawn." Lying on her side, the woman moves her fingers in their small circles and different pressures along an imaginary line from the middle of the armpit down to the bra line. At the end of that strip, the fingers move inward one fingerbreadth and start up from the bra line to the collarbone. The fingers repeat vertical strips up and down until they reach the nipple. They are held in place over the nipple as the woman rolls onto her back, and then continue their parallel strips until they reach the breastbone.

The second pattern involves examining the breasts along imaginary concentric circles. The fingers begin their journey at the top of the breast, far from the nipple, and move a fingerbreadth clockwise or counterclockwise to continue. When that entire circle has been examined, the fingers move inward a fingerbreadth to begin the next, slightly smaller ring, and so on until the nipple is reached. It is very important to feel carefully under the nipple, in the armpit, and along the collarbone for any lumps or changes.

The third pattern divides the breast into twelve sections like a clock, and draws imaginary lines from the nipple to each of the "numerals." The fingers move along each imaginary line making their dime-size circles: from "12" to the nipple, back from the nipple to "1," over to "2," and down the line to the nipple again. Again, it is crucial to check under the nipple, in the armpit, and along the collarbone.

Whichever pattern she uses, a woman also checks for any nipple discharges. Most doctors are more concerned about spontaneous discharges—stains on the bra or nightclothes—than with those that are "milked" from the breast, so trying to "express" a drop or two of fluid from each breast is no longer a routine part of BSE.

Many discharges in women who are not pregnant or breastfeeding still come from benign changes. Nonmilky discharge from both breasts or from several ducts of one breast typically means little and will cease by itself. Milky fluid that begins more than a year or so after the end of pregnancy or breastfeeding usually calls for tests of a woman's hormonal system, all the way up to the pituitary gland in the brain. Greenish-gray drainage from both breasts almost always comes from a benign condition called **duct ectasia**.

Doctors tend to worry more about cancer when a persistent, spontaneous discharge comes from one duct of one breast, especially if it looks watery or bloody (pink, red, or black). Like any other breast change, any discharge should be investigated.

PRACTICE WITH FEEDBACK The woman with very easy-to-examine breasts may have her skills checked once by a health professional and then feel quite confident performing BSE. On the other hand, the woman who normally has very lumpy breasts usually finds it takes her much longer to become reasonably familiar with her

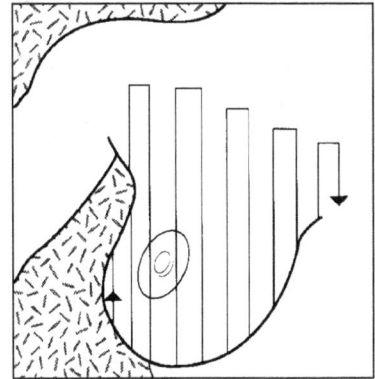

Vertical pattern

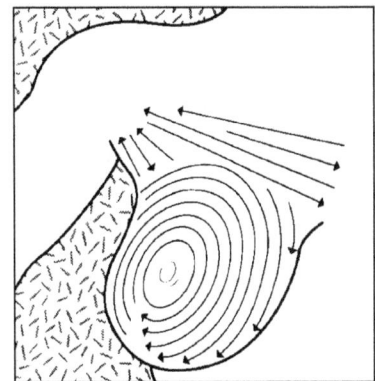

Concentric rings

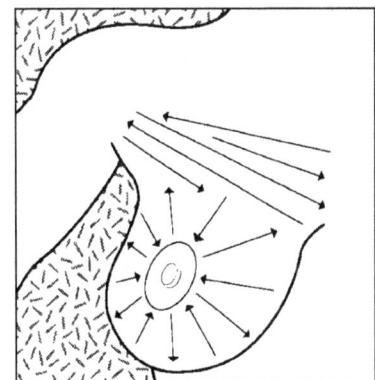

"Clock" pattern

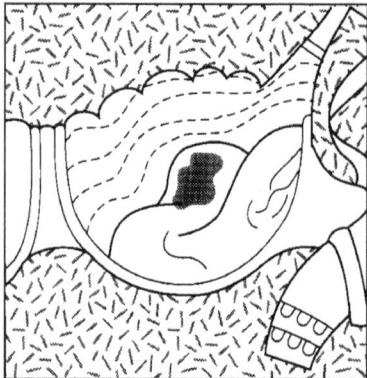

Nipple discharge around bra

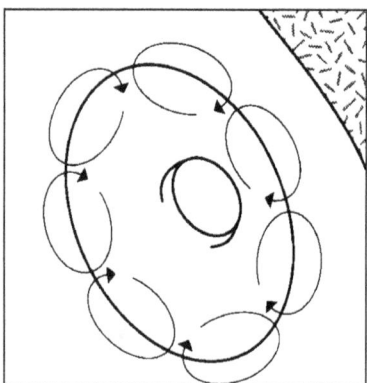

BSE around areola

breasts and comfortable with her skills. Her doctor will probably have similar difficulty: Some breasts are just much harder to examine than others.

It often helps if the woman with harder-to-examine breasts draws a simple "map" of her breasts. This might be just two large circles with smaller circles for nipples and areolas. She can mark on it, perhaps with an X, any area that feels different from her average breast tissue: firmer, lumpier, or a specific lump. That way she does not have to remember everything until the next month, but has a guide to help her check whether there is any change. The good news is that many breasts become much easier to examine after menopause, as the tissue becomes less glandular.

PLAN OF ACTION BSE is not just an exercise for eyes and fingers, of course. Unless there is also concentrating and questioning going on, it is a waste of time. A woman looks and feels for anything that has changed since the previous month and for any obvious differences between right and left sides. She feels for the normal breast tissue, which is often some combination of soft fatty tissue, ridgy ("corrugated") fibrous tissue, and lumpy glandular tissue (rather like partially cooked rice). She checks for any dominant, three-dimensional lump or new thickening and looks for any kind of visible change. Many women normally have a thickened natural "underwire" under both breasts and perhaps some thickening at the upper, outer portion of each breast.

What if she finds something? First she checks the same area of the opposite breast to see whether there is something similar, and thus presumably normal, there. If she discovers something new in one breast, she reports it to a health professional right away. In most cases, it will be a benign change. In the case of cancer, however, this prompt action could save her life.

Knowing ahead of time what she will do if she ever discovers a breast change is part of a woman's breast health plan of action. The other part is setting up with her health professional a reasonable schedule for the rest of her breast care. How often she should have mammograms and routine professional breast examinations depends on her age and individual risk factors.

Having a plan gives a woman some sense of control over her breast health. This plan of action can truly make a difference.

PROFESSIONAL BREAST EXAMINATION

When it comes to detecting breast changes, a woman contributes her intimate knowledge of her own breasts. What the health professional offers, in contrast, is experience with a wide variety of breasts.

The gynecologist, internist, family doctor, or nurse practitioner usually carries out the professional exam along with a regular physical. A sensible plan for the woman under forty with no special risk factors or breast complaints is to have her breasts examined at least every three years, then at least annually after age forty. A breast surgeon or general surgeon is an option for the woman with special needs, such as frequent benign lumps.

A professional breast examination need not be lengthy, but must contain at least the following elements: a breast history of risk factors and past problems, taken during the first visit; questioning about any current breast concerns; visual inspection under good light, with the woman standing or sitting with arms both down and raised; careful palpation of all the breast tissue, including in the armpits, beneath the nipples, and along the collarbone, while the woman lies down with arms behind her head.

Some health professionals use additional positions or spend time teaching the woman. A few try to extract nipple discharge with a suction device, either to look at or to send to the cytology lab for an experimental Pap smear–type analysis.

The examination must be carried out with respect for the woman's dignity and modesty. If the exam does not meet the minimum standards of thoroughness and concern for the patient, the woman needs to speak up or change doctors. I once had a surgeon whose idea of an adequate annual breast exam was placing the palms of the hands flat against the breast for ten seconds. I did not agree, told the surgeon so—and took my business elsewhere.

DIAGNOSING BREAST CHANGES

If a breast change is detected, what then?

In the case of a lump that can be palpated but feels as if it could be fluid-filled, a needle can be inserted into the lump and any fluid withdrawn into the syringe (fine needle aspiration, or FNA). This makes a cyst collapse, and sometimes gets rid of breast pain. This FNA, modified so that the needle reaches several areas in the lump, can also obtain some cells from a solid lump. To get more tissue without an open biopsy, the doctor may be able to do a core biopsy, using a needle wide enough to extract one or more small cylinders of tissue (see "Fine Needle Aspirations, Core Biopsies, and Guided Needle Biopsies" in Chapter 4).

A persistent, dominant lump that can be felt needs to be either removed entirely in an open surgical biopsy or followed very carefully by the doctor for several months. This includes the lump that does not collapse after an aspiration and the needle-biopsied lump in which the pathologist cannot find cancer cells. A positive-for-cancer result is considered trustworthy, but with such a small tissue specimen, a negative result needs to be followed up.

For the breast change that can be detected only by mammography, the radiologist and the surgeon can collaborate on a needle localization biopsy or a stereotactic guided needle biopsy.

Nipple discharges can be checked for cancer cells; if these are present or if the doctor is otherwise concerned, an open biopsy can be performed at the area under the nipple.

After any diagnostic procedure (except sometimes an FNA that clearly shows cyst fluid and in which the cyst collapses), the biopsied tissue is sent to a pathologist for examination and diagnosis.

IF BREAST CANCER IS DIAGNOSED

If the pathologist finds very abnormal cells that have not broken through into neighboring tissue—that are confined within a duct, for instance—the diagnosis is carcinoma in situ. But if the highly abnormal cells have invaded neighboring tissue, there is a possibility they have strayed into the lymph nodes or even beyond.

Thus, with any diagnosis of invasive cancer, both the woman and the tumor go through a thorough workup. For the woman, it is the beginning of the staging process, in which her doctor discovers how extensive the cancer is. To stage the cancer using the TNM information, the doctor needs to know the size of the tumor (T), whether any lymph nodes have cancer in them (N), and whether there is any known metastasis to a distant organ (M) (see the section "Staging a Cancer" in Chapter 4).

If the whole lump has been removed, the size of the tumor is known. The doctor may be able to feel lymph nodes in the axilla or along the collarbone that are either hard and swollen or fixed (attached) to the skin. If not, the lymph-node information must wait until the pathologist has some axillary lymph nodes to examine under the microscope.

When there are "positive" lymph nodes but no known distant metastasis, many doctors divide this group further when looking at prognosis and deciding on treatment. They first consider the number of positive lymph nodes, and often treat women with four or more positive nodes more aggressively than those with one to three positive nodes. Doctors tend to target women with ten or more positive nodes with the very strongest therapy. Second, doctors look at how many tumor cells are in each positive node, from a tiny number (micrometastasis, an amount filling less than about one-tenth of an inch) to enough to block the entire lymph node or break out of the node—a more serious sign. Finally, they consider how close to the breast the positive lymph nodes are, and their concern is greater when they are in Level III, at the point in the armpit farthest from the breast, than when they are in Level I, right next to the breast.

Occasionally, there is an obvious clue that the cancer has metastasized to one of its common target organs: bones, lungs, liver, or brain. Even if there are no symptoms, like bone pain or shortness of breath, many cancer doctors routinely order baseline tests: a chest X ray to rule out lung metastasis, a bone scan to check the bones, and perhaps a computerized tomography study of the liver. Many women also undergo baseline blood tests for such tumor markers as CA 27-29 or CA 15-3.

Meanwhile, if the whole tumor has been removed, the pathologist grades the cancer according to what the cells look like and also examines both individual cells and the entire tumor to get as much information as possible about how the tumor is likely to behave.

One common way of classifying breast tumors, the Scarff-Richardson-Bloom classification, assigns one to three points to each of three tumor characteristics: how many cancer cells are dividing at one time (a measure of how fast the tumor is growing), how different the cells are from normal cells, and how much the cancer forms "*tubules*." The lower the score for each characteristic, the better. The pathologist totals the three scores, with a score from three to five considered Grade I, the least different from normal cells; from six to seven, Grade II, the middle grade; and from eight to nine, Grade III, the least like normal cells.

The tumor may be sent to an outside laboratory for additional tests (see the table on page 223). All this information from the woman and the tumor is used in making treatment decisions.

CARCINOMA IN SITU: THE IN-BETWEEN DIAGNOSIS

When a pathologist looks at a breast biopsy slide and sees a place where highly abnormal cells have broken through the duct wall, the diagnosis is obvious: invasive cancer. However, if the abnormal cells are confined inside the duct with no evidence of a breakthrough, the pathologist calls it **carcinoma in situ** ("at the site"). The two common types, depending on how

Types of Invasive Breast Cancer

Invasive ductal carcinoma, NOS: The most common kind of invasive breast cancer (70% of all breast cancer cases). NOS, or "not otherwise specified," simply means the tumor has no unusual cellular characteristics and does not fall into one of the categories below. Usually appears as a hard breast lump.

Medullary carcinoma: An invasive ductal carcinoma (6% of all breast cancers). It appears to be confined (encapsulated) and often contains many small white blood cells. May grow large, but has a better-than-average prognosis.

Comedocarcinoma: An invasive ductal carcinoma (5% of all breast cancers) that fills the ducts with tumor plugs before invading the duct wall. Prognosis is better than average.

Mucinous carcinoma: An invasive ductal carcinoma (3% of all breast cancers) that contains mucus-producing cells that make the tumor look glistening. Very good prognosis.

Tubular carcinoma: An invasive ductal carcinoma (2% of all breast cancers) that contains characteristic tubular structures ringed with a single layer of cells. Better-than-average prognosis.

Invasive lobular carcinoma: Arises at the ends of the ducts or in the lobules (5 to 10% of all breast cancers). Otherwise looks and acts like invasive ductal carcinoma, NOS. Better-than-average prognosis.

Invasive Paget's disease: Rare cancer in ducts beneath nipple that originally appears as itching and is characterized by an eczema-like rash around the nipple (fewer than 1% of all breast cancers). Prognosis dependent on the individual case.

Inflammatory carcinoma: Most serious breast cancer (1 to 4% of all breast cancers), with skin over breast appearing acutely inflamed and swollen because skin lymph vessels are blocked by cancer. Least favorable prognosis.

---

the cells look and their pattern of growth, are **duct carcinoma in situ** (DCIS, also called noninvasive or noninfiltrating ductal carcinoma or intraductal carcinoma) and **lobular carcinoma in situ** (LCIS or lobular neoplasia). If Paget's disease of the nipple is very localized, some doctors consider it an in situ disease.

Pathologists often discover carcinoma in situ near an area of invasive breast cancer or find tiny areas of invasion when they are carefully examining slides that show mostly carcinoma in situ. When any invasive cancer at all is found, the disease is treated as invasive cancer.

Carcinoma in situ is one of the most controversial areas in breast health today. The first big question is whether these changes represent an early but "real" cancer that has not shown its hand yet, or whether they are cancer "markers" that say the tissue is not cancerous now but is at risk for cancer later. *Carcinoma* means cancer, of course, but the condition got its name

Prognostic Tests for Breast Cancer Tumors

Aside from the visual examination of the breast cancer tumor, which the pathologist does to see how large the tumor is, what the cells look like, what the blood supply to the tumor is, and so on, the tumor is often subjected to several tests, including the following:

Estrogen and progesterone receptor measurements tell whether and to what degree the cancer cells have "receptors" to the female hormones estrogen and progesterone on the outside of the cell. Each hormone "status" is measured as a number, and scores above a certain point are considered "positive." Positive receptor status for one or both hormones correlates with a better prognosis and a better response to hormonal therapy.

Flow cytometry analyzes the DNA content of the tumor. Tumors that have the normal amount of DNA (diploid) tend to be less aggressive and have a better prognosis than those with abnormal amounts of DNA (aneuploid).

Cell cycle analysis measures the percentage of cancer cells in the "S-phase" of the normal cell cycle, which is when the cell is preparing to divide. The more cells in this phase, the faster the tumor is dividing, so the prognosis is less good.

Abnormal tumor protein analysis looks for tumor proteins, including the enzyme cathepsin-D (low levels are associated with better prognosis).

Oncogene levels, growth factors, and so on measure such factors as HER-2/neu oncogene, with high levels of "expression" associated with faster tumor growth and poorer prognosis.

Each day brings word of new prognostic tests to detect or measure a factor that could be related to prognosis so that doctors will know how aggressively to treat an individual woman's breast cancer.

---

years ago, before pathologists saw it very often. The cells are certainly very abnormal—but they have not yet shown that they can behave like full-fledged cancer cells, with the ability to invade neighboring tissue and spread beyond the breast. There is even the possibility that changes like this can reverse themselves. So what does that make carcinoma in situ?

The good news is that, by itself, carcinoma in situ does not threaten a woman's life; by definition, it has not left its own neighborhood. However, breasts that have produced cells this abnormal are at high risk of producing other highly abnormal cells. So the second big question is how much of a risk, either of more carcinoma in situ or of later invasive cancer, this poses for the woman.

Probably the biggest question of all now, especially in the case of duct carcinoma in situ, is this: How do we treat it? Because it takes several years for an invasive cancer to develop and because we do not know yet just how in situ changes fit into the picture, it may take many years to get clear answers.

Duct Carcinoma in Situ

With the use of screening mammograms, doctors diagnose duct carcinoma in situ (DCIS or intraductal carcinoma) much more often now than they used to. While DCIS may sometimes show itself as a lump or even a nipple discharge, it is often found because of a suspicious cluster of microcalcifications on a mammogram. Like a breast lump, these microcalcifications must be biopsied, and they can mean anything from the most benign of changes to invasive breast cancer.

To reach a diagnosis of DCIS, the pathologist looks through the microscope and sees slides with one or more "thickened" ducts, rough circles with obviously abnormal cells built up around the edge but all clearly inside the duct. Sometimes DCIS slides also show a dark clump of dead cells occupying the center of the ring of abnormal cells, a **comedo** (or blackhead) **DCIS**.

Doctors used to consider DCIS a single condition, but just about everyone now agrees that it covers a broad range of diseases, from relatively mild abnormalities to much more dangerous disease. Pathologists look at several factors, including the **nuclear grade** of the DCIS, or how different the cells are from normal cells. A DCIS that is made up of cells that look especially abnormal, and that perhaps have the wrong number of chromosomes, is more likely to return after treatment or to be associated with invasive breast cancer.

Because **necrosis,** or a clump of dead cells, means that the cells are dividing fast enough to outgrow their blood supply and die, comedo DCIS is a sign of more aggressive disease. Larger areas of DCIS, more than an inch in greatest diameter, also tend to be somewhat more dangerous. DCIS typically occurs in only one breast but it is often multifocal, appearing in more than one duct but in the same general area; less often, it is multicentric, appearing in widely separated ducts.

Surgeons at one time always treated DCIS with a mastectomy, which gives almost a 100 percent cure rate. But many women really wanted to keep their breasts and wondered why the breast-conserving treatment of lumpectomy was an option for invasive cancer but not for the less serious condition of DCIS. In the late 1970s, a few surgeons began offering selected women the possibility of removing only the area and a margin of normal tissue around it. To be considered for this therapy, the woman needed to have a small area of DCIS (an inch or preferably less in greatest diameter) that had shown up clearly on a mammogram. She could not have other major breast cancer risk factors, such as a family history, and she had to be truly committed to keeping her breast, willing to comply with close follow-up, and fully aware that she faced more future risk of DCIS and invasive cancer than she would with a mastectomy.

Then, in the mid-1980s, the National Surgical Adjuvant Breast Project Protocol began a large clinical trial called B-17 to compare the results of two different breast-conserving treatments for DCIS. One treatment was surgical removal of the area only. The other treatment included the same surgery with several weeks of follow-up daily radiation therapy to the whole breast, in the hope of destroying any stray abnormal cells left and "sterilizing" the remaining breast tissue. First results, published in 1993, seemed to show much less recurrence when radiation was added. In fact, the study was ended early because the results seemed to favor radiation so strongly, although longer follow-up has shown some problems with the study, as evidenced by some less rosy outcomes.

The major question is whether this is the right treatment for every woman—or even most women—with DCIS. One alternative is to subdivide women with DCIS into groups based on how aggressive their disease appears to be, and to use this as a guide for recommending treatment. For instance, the Van Nuys Prognostic Index (VNPI) rates each case of DCIS from one (best) to three (worst) on three factors related to the likelihood the disease will return: tumor size, the size of the margin of disease-free tissue around the DCIS in the surgical specimen, and a combination of tumor grade factors. The three numbers are added up for a total score, or prognostic index, with three the lowest possible score and nine the highest.

VNPI proponents argue that the woman with a score of three or four should do well with just a lumpectomy. This score would mean a small area of DCIS, a generous disease-free margin all around the surgical specimen (to avoid leaving nearby clusters of DCIS in the breast), and "good" tumor grade. With this group of women, the chances of recurrence are very low once the actual area of DCIS is gone, and radiation does not seem to make a difference. If she foregoes radiation, the woman also misses its side effects and cost, and she still has radiation as an option if she ever develops invasive cancer in that breast. Some doctors question how effective radiation—which targets cells as they divide—is with these less-aggressive cells, which do not divide that often.

The middle group seems to do better with the combination of surgery and radiation, but then should have a fairly low recurrence rate of about 1 percent each year.

Finally, the doctors contend, women with a score of eight or nine tend to have a high recurrence rate, even with lumpectomy and radiation. Despite the combined therapy, more than half of these women have a recurrence within five years. With a DCIS area over an inch and a half, abnormal cells right at the edge of the surgical specimen, and "bad" tumor grade, the woman may want to think seriously about a mastectomy, which would offer her an almost-certain cure.

Many recurrences are more DCIS, but close to half are invasive cancer. If DCIS or invasive cancer is diagnosed in a breast that has already been treated with radiation therapy, mastectomy is the likely treatment because the breast has already received all the radiation it can safely get. (Even if women who have been treated for DCIS develop invasive breast cancer later on, it usually is detected relatively early and the woman is likely to survive long-term.)

Should tamoxifen be a part of DCIS treatment? Several clinical trials going on now look at treatment options with and without tamoxifen in women with more and less agressive DCIS, with and without radiation. Results of one early trial seem to show some decrease in "breast cancer events" with tamoxifen at five years: invasive breast cancer in the same breast 2.1 percent with tamoxifen, 4.2 percent without it, and some drop in invasive breast cancer in the other breast. However, the group of women studied had such a variation in the sizes of their tumors, the surgical margins (known now to be crucial), and the tumor grades that it is difficult to tell what the statistics really mean. Newer trials attempt to compare more similar groups, but it will take time to get meaningful results. Every woman is different, and, where one woman may happily face relatively high risk of recurrence if it means she can keep her breasts, another with "good" DCIS may strongly prefer a mastectomy, perhaps with breast reconstruction later. Second opinions are crucial, and pathology slides can be mailed safely and quickly to another medical institution if necessary.

Although DCIS is not life threatening in itself, it means that the woman faces increased risk for both more DCIS and invasive breast cancer—and all the anxieties this risk brings. The treatments, surgery, and radiation can be emotionally traumatic. Unfortunately, while she may go through many of the emotions familiar to the woman diagnosed with invasive breast cancer, she may have less emotional support. Some women find it helpful to ask their doctors about a possible "buddy" who is either going through treatment or has "been there, done that."

Lobular Carcinoma in Situ

Like DCIS, lobular carcinoma in situ often occurs at the ends of the breast ducts. While it does not itself invade neighboring tissues or spread beyond the breast, LCIS puts a woman at increased risk for developing invasive breast cancer later on. It is often diagnosed in premenopausal women.

There the similarity to DCIS ends. LCIS frequently does *not* show up on mammograms (or as a lump) and is often discovered when the pathologist looks at slides after a breast biopsy for something else. Typically, the condition occurs in both breasts. If it is not in both breasts yet, both breasts are at equal risk for developing new areas of the neoplasia. However, the size and number of areas of LCIS do not appear to affect the woman's prognosis in any way: Widespread LCIS in both breasts is no more likely to be associated with invasive cancer than a tiny area.

Traditionally, the treatment for LCIS has been a double mastectomy. The other conventional option has been removal of one breast and a biopsy of the "mirror image" location on the second breast to see whether there is more neoplasia there.

But about forty years ago, a group of doctors at New York's Columbia University noticed that, of the women who for some reason did not have any breast surgery beyond the biopsy, very few ever developed invasive cancer. Since then, "treating" LCIS with close follow-up only—professional breast examination every few months—has become common. The woman performs BSE every month and gets her routine mammograms (LCIS does not show up on mammograms, but a lump or other breast problem could). The invasive lobular carcinomas tend to be relatively slow-growing, and the idea is to find any as early as possible.

Paget's Disease of the Nipple

Paget's disease of the nipple is a rare condition that shows itself with an eczema-like rash around the nipple. Until recently, doctors considered the nipple condition a "beachhead" established by an underlying breast cancer. Now many view it as a condition that can sometimes be an in situ change, sometimes an invasive cancer. If it is in situ, it does significantly increase a woman's chance of developing invasive cancer later.

Breast-conserving treatment includes removing the Paget's area with a clear margin of disease-free tissue around it. Sometimes a portion of the nipple can be saved, but usually the entire nipple is removed. After she finds out how extensive the breast surgery will be, the woman may want to check with a plastic surgeon to see what options are available for her and whether it is worth it to her to conserve the breast.

— *Kerry McGinn*

CHAPTER 13

TREATING INVASIVE
BREAST CANCER

*"You have breast cancer. You have three options. You can do
nothing—but that is not a good option—or. . ."*

Later, I suggested to my surgeon that a cup of tea might have helped. Or at
least a brief pause after the words "breast cancer." But in no way could I
quarrel with his immediate emphasis on options. The woman diagnosed
with breast cancer must choose (and fairly soon) between mastectomy and
breast-conserving surgery (popularly called lumpectomy), with or without
radiation. If she opts for mastectomy, she decides whether or not to
undergo reconstructive surgery at the same time and, if so, what kind. And
that's just for starters.

But "fairly soon" does not mean the choices have to be made the day or
even the week of diagnosis—and they should not be made then. Many
women, on hearing they have breast cancer, feel an urgent need to take
action, to "do something." But this is one time when it is much better to
think about it for a few days.

Some women may immediately react with "Get rid of it—take off my
breast tomorrow." For others, it's "You can do anything else, but you can't
take my breast." Whatever that first desperate urge, it makes sense for a
woman to resist it, to take the time to find out about all the options, and to
think about what each would mean in her life. She may eventually choose
to follow her original impulse, but then it will be a real decision with which
she can live comfortably and confidently. Waiting two weeks or so after
diagnosis before further surgery usually makes no difference in a woman's
prognosis.

Many women rely on their surgeons to offer some guidance, perhaps a
strong recommendation one way or the other—and that is as it should be.
As oncologic surgeon Peter Richards, M.D., of California Pacific Medical
Center in San Francisco, puts it: "I tell a woman about all her options, but if
I believe strongly that she should follow one of them, it would be remiss of

me not to tell her what I think and why. She's paying for my experience and knowledge. She has to make the final decision, but my recommendations serve as a reference point for her and are part of the data she should have."

However, if both mastectomy and breast-conserving surgery are possible options, it makes sense to consult a radiation oncologist before making a decision. While surgeons are beginning to recommend limited surgery much more often than they used to, radiation oncologists are those most likely to speak up for lumpectomy with radiation. It is worth hearing what each of them has to say. (Note: Because *lumpectomy* is a shorter, simpler term that rolls off the tongue more easily than the preferred *breast-conserving surgery,* we use the two terms interchangeably in this book.)

LOCAL TREATMENTS: MASTECTOMY OR LUMPECTOMY/RADIATION

As with any cancer, treating invasive breast cancer may involve either or both local treatment (getting rid of any cancer cells in the breast area itself) and systemic treatment (destroying any cancer cells that have strayed outside the breast area). The local therapies for breast cancer are primarily surgery and radiation, with chemotherapy sometimes used as a local therapy to shrink a breast tumor before surgery or radiation. The systemic possibilities are chemotherapy, hormone therapy, and biological therapy.

During the last several years, doctors have learned that either one of two possible strategies can work equally well to eliminate cancer cells in the breast itself. One strategy involves removing the whole breast (**mastectomy**). The second conserves the breast, cutting out only the obvious area of cancer with a wide margin of clear tissue around it (**lumpectomy**) and then giving several weeks of radiation treatments to the breast to destroy any residual cancer cells. Sometimes, radiation is given even after a mastectomy if, for instance, the breast tumor was deep in the breast near the chest wall, or in certain other situations.

Mastectomy

Until a few decades ago, the standard treatment for breast cancer was the **Halsted radical mastectomy**. This surgery, named after the surgeon who developed it in the late nineteenth century, removes the breast itself, the lymph nodes in the armpit, the chest wall muscles, and other lymph nodes. The theory was that breast cancer started in the breast, moved out to all the lymph nodes, and only after conquering the last lymph node did it spread out to the rest of the body. Surgeons followed the dictum, "The

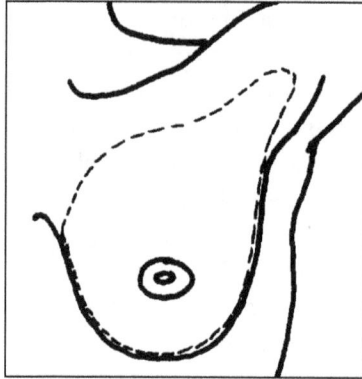

Modified radical mastectomy,
area of breast tissue to be removed

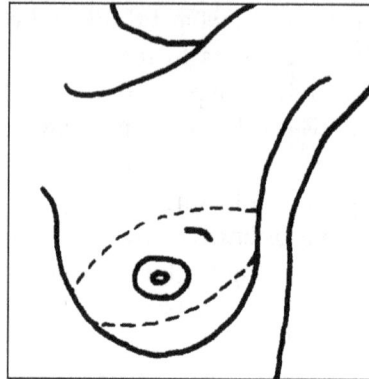

Skin incisions (modified radical)

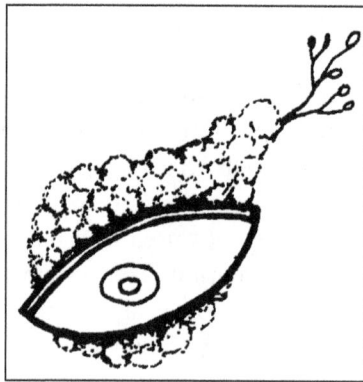

Breast and axillary tissue removed
(modified radical)

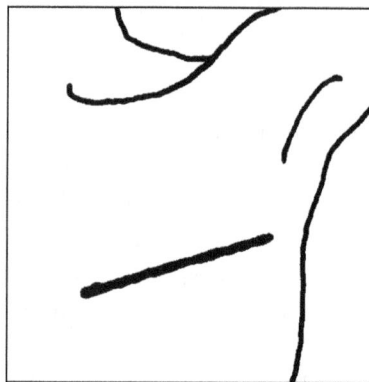

Mastectomy scar
(modified radical)

(this series of illustrations—continued on page 231—courtesy of Susan Schoen)

more you take, the better off she will be," and tried ever more extensive surgeries. Eventually, even the Halsted radical looked almost conservative. The Halsted procedure left a woman with a long scar down one side of her chest, a "caved-in" appearance, and, often, lingering disability from the missing muscle.

In time, doctors learned that this kind of mutilating surgery did not increase women's survival rate and began pushing for less drastic operations. If there is a mastectomy now for invasive cancer, it is almost always a **modified radical mastectomy,** which removes an island of skin over the breast (including the nipple and areola), as much of the actual breast tissue as possible, and one or more of the lymph nodes from the axillary area. The chest muscle is left intact. If reconstructive surgery is not done at this time, the area where the breast used to be will be flat, but not caved-in; some surgeons may leave some extra skin for possible reconstructive surgery later. The scar typically runs horizontally or diagonally from near the breastbone into the armpit.

A prophylactic (preventive) mastectomy or a mastectomy for a small carcinoma in situ removes the same tissues except for the lymph nodes and is called a **simple** or a **total mastectomy**. Sometimes, for a prophylactic mastectomy, the surgeon leaves the nipple and areola intact; but cancer can grow there later. Occasionally, if a large invasive cancer has also spread to the chest wall muscle, the surgeon will remove part of that along with the breast and lymph tissue in a **radical mastectomy**.

Breast-Conserving Surgery

A breast-conserving surgery spares most of the breast and cuts out only the cancer and a piece of tissue around it. Ordinarily, when a biopsy, which removes minimal tissue, is followed by a cancer diagnosis, the surgeon wants to cut out a somewhat wider swath of breast tissue (**wide excision**).

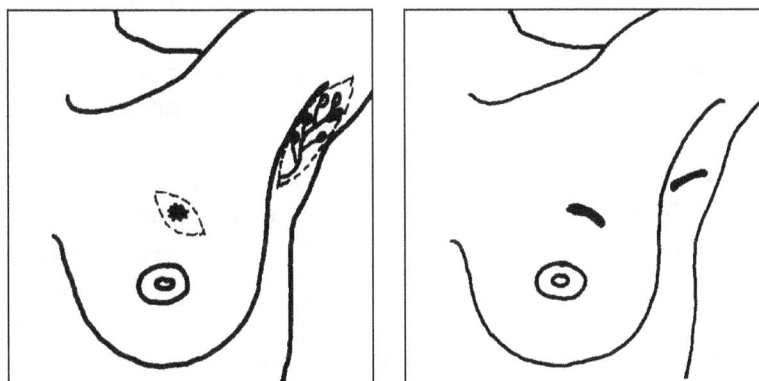

Lumpectomy, breast and lymph
node tissue to be removed

Lumpectomy/axillary
surgery scars

Depending somewhat on how much tissue is removed (but mostly on the surgeon labeling it), this can be called a lumpectomy, **tylectomy, segmental resection, quandrantectomy,** or **partial mastectomy**; there are no precise definitions for what's what. Usually the rest of the breast tissue moves over to fill in the empty spot, and the surgery leaves a minimal scar.

Years ago, doctors discovered that when they performed a lumpectomy and then simply sent a woman on her way, the cancer recurred in the breast in about 40 percent of patients. This prompted doctors to add several weeks of daily breast radiation treatments to the regimen. With lumpectomy/radiation, the local recurrence rate is about 10 percent. With mastectomy, it is about 8 percent, but the recurrences may be harder to treat.

Treating
Invasive
Breast
Cancer

Many invasive cancers have large areas of duct carcinoma in situ around them. For a time, some surgeons thought they could remove just the cancer itself with a small margin of surrounding tissue and that the radiation would eliminate the rest of the abnormal cells. But cancer showed up again at the same location in over a quarter of these women. The theory is that radiation, which neatly dispatches stray cancer cells and tiny clusters, does not deal adequately with large clumps of abnormal cells. What this means for surgeons is that they must be careful to remove any DCIS around the cancer so that the margins are truly "clean."

If the lumpectomy is performed because of invasive cancer, the surgeon usually also removes from one or two to all of the lymph nodes in the axilla. This involves a separate incision, one or more inches long and just below the hollow of the armpit, so that the surgeon has good access to the axilla.

Axillary Surgery

Most of the immediate discomfort and long-term side effects of either a modified radical or a lumpectomy come from this lymph-node surgery. The surgeon often cannot reach the axillary area without injuring and occasionally severing one or more of the nerves that transmit sensation. Because of the stretching and pulling the surgeon has to do, many women have numbness in the armpit and along the back of the upper arm for at least several weeks; if the numbness remains after several months, it is probably permanent (and feels peculiar when a woman shaves under her arm).

Of more medical concern is the possibility that removing lymph nodes from the arm may affect the drainage of lymph fluid from that arm, so that the arm swells with **lymphedema** (see Chapter 25). Once in a great while, the axillary surgery permanently damages a nerve that regulates movement.

If removing the lymph nodes causes these problems, why do surgeons do it—especially now, when well over half of the women with a new diagnosis of breast cancer do not have any cancer in their lymph nodes?

A common path for breast cancer cells leaving the breast takes them through the axillary lymph channels where they can get trapped in the lymph nodes. These axillary lymph nodes are more common escape routes than the lymph channels along the breastbone or the collarbone and are much easier to reach surgically.

Until quite recently, most surgeons reasoned that since the lymph nodes could have cancer cells trapped in them, removing them would help cure the cancer—so they removed all the lymph nodes under the arm near the cancer: a **lymph-node dissection**. But, in fact, removing all the lymph nodes proved to have little or no effect on curing the cancer, and the side effects of the full dissection were much greater than when a smaller number were cut out. Not only was the lymph drainage system from the arm seriously injured in most cases, but the woman also lost lymph nodes (most of them cancer-free) that were an important part of her body's defense system.

However, with the coming of systemic therapies for breast cancer, surgeons and oncologists began making treatment decisions based partly on information that currently comes only from lymph nodes. Are cancer cells present in the lymph nodes (node-positive) or not (node-negative)? Unfortunately, while surgeons can make an informed guess before surgery that a node that feels swollen and hard to their examining fingers probably is "positive," they have no way of telling whether the nodes they cannot feel have cancer in them or not. Even when surgeons are "sure" before surgery, the microscope slides often prove them wrong.

How many lymph nodes are positive? Is a node positive because of a small number of cancer cells that can only be found with a microscope (**micrometastasis**), or is it obviously overrun with cancer cells? Have cancer cells made any lymph nodes stick together or become "fixed" to other tissues? Examining the lymph nodes helps stage the breast cancer and gives doctors clues about the woman's prognosis as well as what treatment to give her.

Many surgeons now compromise with **lymph-node sampling,** removing only a few of the lymph nodes. The lymph nodes occur at three clumpy levels in the axilla. The surgeon who takes out node-containing tissue from the lower two levels nearest the breast minimizes damage, but still gets the necessary information. Later the pathologist discovers exactly how many lymph nodes have been removed (often about ten, out of a normal total of thirty to sixty).

Some surgeons still prefer to remove all the axillary lymph nodes, at least partly to prevent the possibility that a lymph node with a hidden nest of breast cancer cells will become severely enlarged and cause problems later. For the same reason, some radiation oncologists believe in giving radiation therapy to the axillary area if the lymph nodes have not all been removed.

Sentinal lymph node sampling or biopsy (SLNS) is the new technique more and more surgeons are using when there is no evidence of "positive" lymph nodes before surgery. The idea behind this technique is that if cancer cells leave the breast via the lymph system, they will travel along a specific drainage path and reach the closest node on that path first. SLNS attempts to identify this closest, or "sentinal," node or two for removal by the surgeon; if there are no cancer cells there, chances are excellent that all the lymph nodes will be clear.

Commonly, a few hours before surgery the surgeon injects a tiny amount of radioactive sulfur into the tumor still in the breast. This drains from the tumor along the lymph path. Then, a few minutes before the lymph-node surgery, the surgeon injects a blue dye around the tumor (or around the localization wire if the cancer showed only on mammography) and the area is massaged for a few minutes so that the dye moves toward the lymph nodes. Meanwhile, the radioactive substance makes the lymph nodes mildly radioactive so that the surgeon, using a hand-held radiation-detecting probe, knows where to cut. The first lymph node, embedded in fat, shows blue and the surgeon removes it and perhaps one or two more. The pathologist checks these immediately for cancer cells; if none are found, no more axillary surgery is done. Of course, the surgeon must remove more tissue if the node tests positive for cancer. Occasionally the node looks negative on the first look but is found to be positive on further testing, which may mean more surgery is necessary later.

As SLNS moves into the surgical mainstream, more surgeons are incorporating it into their practice, but it takes training and experience to learn the technique. A woman interested in SLNS may need to search to find a surgeon competent and comfortable with the procedure. Many surgeons remain concerned that SLNS, even in experienced hands, may miss positive lymph nodes if the cancer cells "skip" the first node(s).

Some doctors reason that since more women now are receiving chemotherapy or hormone treatment regardless of node status, removing nodes that do not feel positive should be unnecessary most of the time. Too, information about the tumor itself from the pathologists and from laboratory tests becomes more helpful all the time. But....

If there is a reasonable chance the node information will make a difference in treatment, it probably makes sense to do some type of axillary surgery. The Kaufman axillary treatment scale (KATS) is one method being investigated to fine-tune "reasonable chance." This scale assigns a number value to tumor size, patient age, and tumor grade for the cancer, all information available before breast-conserving surgery or mastectomy. For instance, a very small, low-grade cancer in a woman over seventy will receive the lowest—or best—score.

Patients are then divided into three groups by their scores. Women with the lowest scores are considered at such low risk of positive axillary nodes that they receive no axillary surgery or radiation. The middle group undergoes SLNS, and more surgery if the sentinal node(s) prove positive. The highest-scoring group faces a high risk of positive nodes and receive a full axillary dissection rather than SLNS.

Axillary surgery remains one of the many controversial topics in breast cancer therapy—and controversy will probably continue for some time.

Deciding on Local Treatment

The National Cancer Institute says in its 1990 Consensus Conference statement: "Breast conservation treatment is an appropriate method of primary therapy for the majority of women with Stage I and Stage II breast cancer and is preferable because it provides survival equivalent to total mastectomy and axillary dissection while preserving the breast." Basically, lumpectomy/radiation is worth considering for most women with Stage I or II disease, but it is not necessarily the best treatment for *every* woman.

On the other hand, neither mastectomy nor lumpectomy/radiation makes sense as the first treatment for the woman with either Stage IIIB or Stage IV breast cancer, since her problem is not the local disease. To handle the spread beyond the breast that is causing her problems, she needs systemic therapy (see the table on page 237 for descriptions of the different stages).

QUESTIONS TO ASK YOUR PHYSICIAN

Aside from any medical factors, a woman and her doctor may want to consider the following aesthetic, practical, and psychological issues:

1. *How large is the tumor in comparison with the breast, and where is it located?* A surgeon can usually remove a one-inch tumor with a margin of surrounding tissue from a medium-size breast and the result will look fine. However, it may be impossible to perform a lumpectomy with a large tumor in a small breast and have any kind of aesthetically pleasing results, although reconstructive surgery may be possible. (Another possibility is shrinking a tumor with chemotherapy before surgery so that it is small enough to be removed with a lumpectomy.) When the tumor is located near the nipple, the surgeon may have to remove not only the nipple and areola but a large area around it.

2. *Is there any evidence that the cancer in the breast is multicentric (has clusters of cancer cells at widely separated places in the breast)?*

3. *Is there any problem with getting radiation therapy?* Are you pregnant or breastfeeding, in which case radiation therapy is definitely not an option? Can you get to treatments reasonably easily? Is there any problem spending the time each weekday for several weeks? Have you ever had radiation to this area before? (If this is a recurrence in a breast already treated with lumpectomy/radiation, you no longer have this option.) Do you have any medical

conditions such as a rheumatologic disorder (lupus erythematosis, rheumatoid arthritis, or scleroderma, for instance), which some radiation oncologists believe get worse with radiation therapy? Are you under thirty-five or so, in which case you need to review with the radiation oncologist any increased risks because your breast tissue is more sensitive to radiation than an older woman's is? Some women initially feel uncomfortable about the thought of radiation—but how do you feel about the therapy once you know more about it?

4. *How easy are your breasts to "follow" over time?* Not everyone agrees that this should be a factor, but the woman with breasts that are unusually difficult to examine mammographically or with the fingers may want to consider this. Do you have risk factors that might make you especially vulnerable to a second primary cancer in the breast? If you keep your breast, you want a reasonable chance that it will remain trouble-free and that any problem will be detected early.

5. *How committed are you to keeping your breast—and why?* How do you feel about yourself in general, and about your breasts in particular? If you undergo mastectomy, you will lose the nipple and areola sensation of that breast—how important is that to you? If you feel strongly that you want to have a breast mound of some sort, would you be comfortable with either a breast prosthesis or the risks and benefits of reconstructive surgery? Does it matter to you that, after a lumpectomy, you can change your mind later and have a mastectomy, but the reverse is not possible?

6. *Is money a factor?* The least expensive treatment is usually a modified radical mastectomy with a day or two of hospitalization and without radiation or reconstructive surgery. Radiation is a big-ticket item and makes the lumpectomy/radiation combination (or, of course, mastectomy/radiation) considerably more costly. Reconstructive surgery ranges widely in price, with the "flap" surgeries almost always more expensive than implant procedures.

Researchers have compared several aspects of how a woman's choice of breast-conserving surgery or mastectomy affects her later. So far, the results are anything but clear-cut. One study "proves" that women with mastectomies have much poorer body image a year after surgery than women with lumpectomies, while another finds little difference. One study shows "definitively" that women with mastectomies feel safer and less anxious than those with lumpectomies, but the next study refutes it.

Staging System for Cancer of the Breast

Stage	TNM	Description
0	Tis N0 M0	Carcinoma in situ (Tis) with no positive axillary lymph nodes (N0) or known distant metastasis (M0)
I	T1 N0 M0	Earliest invasive cancer, with tumor smaller than 2 cm, or ¾ inches (T1) and no positive axillary nodes or known distant metastasis
IIA	T1 N1 M0	Either a tumor smaller than 2 cm with one or more positive axillary lymph nodes (N1) and no known distant metastasis
	T2 N0 M0	*or* a tumor 2–5 cm, or ¾–2 inches (T2), with neither positive nodes nor known distant metastasis
IIB	T2 N1 M0	Either a tumor 2–5 cm with positive axillary node(s) but no known distant metastasis
	T3 N0 M0	*or* a tumor larger than 5 cm or 2 inches (T3), with no positive axillary nodes or known distant metastasis
IIIA	T1-2 N2 M0	Either a tumor 5 cm or under with fixed (stuck to other tissues) axillary lymph nodes on the same side (N2) but no known distant metastasis
	T3 N1-2 M0	*or* a tumor larger than 5 cm (T3) with free or fixed axillary lymph nodes but no known distant metastasis
IIIB	T(any) N3 M0	Either any size tumor with chest lymph node involvement (N3) but no known distant metastasis
	T4 N(any) M0	*or* a tumor that involves the chest wall or breaks through the skin (T4) with any number of positive axillary lymph node(s) but no known distant metastasis; this includes inflammatory carcinoma
IV	T(any) N(any) M1	Known distant metastasis (usually bone, lung, liver, brain) or involves the skin or chest wall beyond the breast area

Before deciding on a course of action, many women consult a second surgeon, a medical oncologist, and/or a "second opinion" service, such as one at a breast health center, to get varying points of view.

Whatever she chooses, it is normal for a woman to wonder occasionally if she made the right choice. But most women, most of the time—if they make a careful, thoughtful decision based on what they have heard from their doctors and what they personally think and feel—will be reasonably happy with whatever they choose.

SURGERY

In some ways, breast cancer surgery is like the other cancer surgeries discussed in Chapter 7, but it has its own peculiarities.

The woman is almost always put to sleep with general anesthesia for any procedure that includes removal of axillary nodes. When she wakes up, she usually has a protective, bulky bandage covering the surgical sutures or tape strips holding the outer layers of skin together. She may have IV access for a day or so for antibiotics and pain medicine. She may have one or more drainage tubes from the breast or underarm area, each connected to a suction bulb, although tubes are becoming somewhat less common.

Some surgeons put a sling on the arm to hold it in place, but most want a woman to start using her arm fairly soon so that it does not stiffen up. As she starts moving and stretching the arm over the next several weeks, the discomfort will become worse at first but then will gradually subside. Many women undergoing either a mastectomy or a lumpectomy will be pleasantly surprised by how little pain there is in the breast area. They may be less happy with the strange sensations in the armpit area and along the back of the arm, if the surgeon has performed any major axillary surgery.

Some of the sensations in the armpit may be less painful than strange: numbness, "pins and needles," or pinching/pulling feelings. Many women continue to have peculiar discomforts in the axilla once in a while for the rest of their lives, although lasting axillary problems have become much rarer with the smaller axillary surgeries common now.

A few women complain of more severe pain—often shooting, sharp, or burning pains—and for longer periods, perhaps as the result of some nerve damage during surgery. Researchers are just beginning to study this **post-mastectomy pain syndrome**, which seems to happen at least as often after lumpectomy/radiation as it does after mastectomy. Therapies that have proven effective in clinical trials include rubbing the area with 0.025 percent capsaicin treatment and taking amitriptyline pills; amitriptyline is an antidepressant, but in this case it is used because it works so well on nerve damage pain. These treatments require a prescription. Some women report a "phantom limb" sensation where the breast was removed, which sometimes responds to regular, gentle massage of the scar and the breast area.

A woman may feel more comfortable lying on her back or on the opposite side for several weeks after a mastectomy. This puts gravity to work, draining fluid away from the area.

Depending on her surgeon, the surgery, and her response, the woman may go home the day of surgery, the next day, or several days later. The final pathology report should be ready within a few days.

If a woman has both breasts removed at the same time (bilateral mastectomy), she needs to have hospital bedside equipment placed where she can reach it easily. Until she is able to raise her arms, she will not be able to wear clothes that have to be pulled over her head; pieces that can be pulled on from below and have loose sleeves and generous armholes (a zippered housecoat perhaps) work best at first.

Many women have heard of research studies suggesting that breast cancer prognosis for the premenopausal woman was rosier when the surgeon performed breast cancer surgery during the second half of her menstrual cycle. One theory: The cancer cells might be "stickier" then and less likely to leave the breast area during surgery. Other studies to prove or disprove this have come up with conflicting results, with some rather large studies showing no difference. A study of 900 women underway now (NSABP Menstrual Timing Study) may answer the question once and for all.

The woman who will likely receive chemotherapy after surgery may be interested in having her tumor tested in a chemosensitivity assay to get more information about the chemotherapy drugs likely to work best against her particular cancer (see "Why Use Chemotherapy?" in Chapter 8). This takes at least a day or two of preplanning, since the pathologist will need the mailing materials before surgery so that a fresh (not frozen) piece of the tumor can be sent. The best scenario: a cancer diagnosis before the surgery from a fine needle aspiration or core biopsy, leaving most of the tumor to be removed in the surgery. If, soon after mailing the specimen, the doctors learn that chemotherapy will not be necessary, a quick call cancels the assay.

RADIATION THERAPY

When radiation therapy is given after a breast-conserving surgery for invasive breast cancer, it is considered the primary local treatment for the disease. It can also be used as secondary—but important—therapy along with mastectomy in certain situations. For example, when the tumor is located at the edge of the breast tissue, the surgeon may want radiation to that area as extra "insurance" (see Chapter 7 for more information about radiation).

The linear accelerator is the usual radiation machine. There should be no discomfort during the actual process. Probably the most difficult part for the woman is raising her arm, which can be uncomfortable if radiation starts soon after surgery.

If a woman is to undergo chemotherapy, breast radiation may be given first, may be postponed until she finishes, or may be given midway through; occasionally the two are given together. Otherwise, radiation begins a few weeks after a lumpectomy, when the surgical site is relatively healed.

The first part of the treatment plan typically includes six weeks or so of radiation to the whole breast area, from collarbone to bra line and from breastbone to axilla. Divided doses deliver a total of about 4,700 rads.

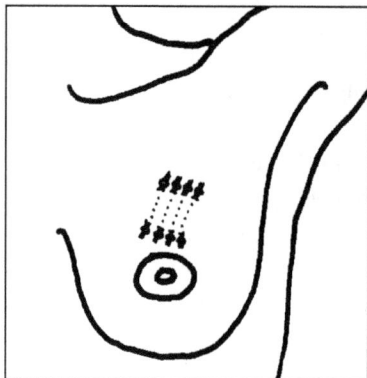

Internal radiation
(courtesy of Susan Schoen)

This period of radiation to the whole breast may be followed by a booster dose concentrated on the immediate area of the tumor. This is usually given in the form of daily "electron beam" sessions for a week or so. The radiation may be delivered by the same linear accelerator, but with the high-energy field adjusted downward so the rays are not moving so fast. The radiation area is smaller, and there may be more skin damage because the electron beam releases its energy at a shallow level closer to the skin. Otherwise, for the woman, it is about the same as the earlier treatments. If the tumor was deep or quite large, the booster dose sometimes involves the placement, for thirty hours or so, of tiny radioactive seeds into minute tubes threaded through the skin into the tumor area (see "Internal Radiation" in Chapter 7).

Radiation to the breast area after a lumpectomy for cancer is considered (ironically) quite "benign"—it does not usually cause serious side effects. Almost everyone feels some fatigue and eventually has temporary skin redness at the radiation site. The breast often is temporarily swollen and sensitive, and it usually becomes permanently firmer and less droopy than it was before treatment. If there is much radiation to the axillary lymph nodes, the woman may be more vulnerable to lymphedema.

Some women develop a few lung symptoms like a mild cough during radiation; a few show radiation pneumonitis or lung inflammation, with a dry cough and slight fever, three to six months after radiation. Rib fractures can occur but are rare and heal by themselves. Several months after radiation, many women develop assorted arthritis-like aching or shooting pains in the breast area, the chest wall, or the connection points between rib and breastbone. The worst part of these symptoms is that they may terrify a woman into believing her cancer has returned. What they often mean is that the body is slowly (and rather clumsily) regenerating after the treatment. A call to her doctor usually brings reassurance.

When radiation is used along with a mastectomy, the treatment field may be smaller, the number of treatments fewer, and ordinarily no booster is necessary.

SYSTEMIC TREATMENT

Many oncologists believe that cancer cells begin escaping from the breast fairly early in the course of the disease, but that the body's defenses can usually demolish the occasional cell and keep the cancer in check. Systemic treatment for breast cancer—either chemotherapy or hormonal therapy—is recommended when the oncologist either knows or suspects that the body "system" outside the breast harbors more cancer cells than it can destroy without outside help.

Breast cancer is often a slow-growing and unpredictable disease, and short-term studies do not give long-term results. This is why the statistical picture can be so muddy. Five-year survival—although it is an excellent sign—is not synonymous with cure. Thus, statisticians do not talk about cures but look at or combine such factors as five-year survival, ten-year survival, death rates, and disease-free interval. It is the best they can do.

Hormonal Therapy

Since the female hormones seem to play such a major role in breast cancer, one plausible strategy for fighting the disease is to shift the body's hormonal balance in such a way as to discourage cancer growth. The first attempts to do this included removing the ovaries of some young women with fast-growing breast cancers so that the estrogen from the ovaries would no longer be available to "feed" the cancer cells. In fact, this kind of surgery is making a small comeback, especially in Europe. It is a much simpler surgery than it used to be because it can often be done through a laparoscope (a lighted tube inserted through a small skin opening). In premenopausal women with estrogen-receptor-positive tumors, at least, some early studies seem to show results similar to those of chemotherapy. Removing the ovaries causes immediate menopause.

More common in the United States is hormone therapy with the drug tamoxifen (Nolvadex). Like other hormonal manipulations, tamoxifen does not kill cancer cells directly, but instead prevents them from growing: It is a siege weapon rather than a gun or a bomb. Initially, researchers thought that the drug worked as an estrogen blocker, simply starving the cancer cells that needed estrogen to grow. Now it appears the mechanism is not so straightforward. Tamoxifen is a **selective estrogen receptor modulator**, or SERM, an estrogen-like hormone that may fool the cancer cells into accepting the "impostor," or it may act in some way researchers have not yet discovered. For instance, it sometimes appears to work on cancers that are classified as estrogen-receptor negative. (One theory is that some of the cells may have mutated to be positive.)

Taking two tamoxifen pills daily appears to give at least postmenopausal women with breast cancer a decided survival edge. In this age group, it is statistically more effective at extending life than chemotherapy, although an individual woman may do better on chemotherapy. Postmenopausal women taking tamoxifen add an average of two years to their lives—which means that many of them add far more than two years, and some may be cured.

Tamoxifen appears to markedly decrease both local recurrences and second unrelated cancers in the remaining breast tissue. It may also have mildly protective effects on bones and possibly the circulatory system. There is some increased risk of cancer of the lining of the uterus, as there is with any estrogen hormone therapy, so the woman needs regular follow-up visits with her gynecologist. Fortunately, uterine cancer is almost always easily detected and treated if it does occur. There may also be a slight risk of liver changes and blood clots.

Most women well past menopause who have not recently been taking hormone therapy seem to tolerate the pills so well that even if a woman is not at especially high risk, doctors feel quite comfortable prescribing the drug. The original recommendation of two years of treatment has stretched to five years; some caution that, after five years, the benefits are reduced and the risks become greater.

Some premenopausal women, women not far past menopause whose hormonal balances may still fluctuate, and women who have recently stopped menopausal hormone therapy do not tolerate the drug so easily. They may complain of hot flashes, night sweats, and similar menopausal symptoms for which hormone replacement therapy is not usually an option. Nausea, bloating, and breast tenderness and swelling for a few weeks is common, although these symptoms eventually subside. Some women report depression for some months, though this is often difficult to distinguish from the emotional upheaval many women go through as they finish primary breast cancer treatment. Tamoxifen can cause birth defects if a woman becomes pregnant while taking it, though it does not bar fertility.

If tamoxifen does indeed increase cures and/or disease-free survival time, many women will gladly put up with the side effects. For premenopausal women, that is the unanswered question. Many thoughtful oncologists have no doubt it works, but others are still waiting for convincing scientific evidence that tamoxifen increases survival in premenopausal women. One of their concerns is that younger women taking the drug over a longer period of time may be more at risk for serious side effects that are as yet unknown.

Another SERM, raloxifene (Evista), has fewer years of testing, but may work similarly to tamoxifen and may pose less risk of uterine cancer. Aromatase inhibitors, a class of hormone drugs that affect the adrenal glands—and through them the ovaries and breasts—often work very well to treat metastatic breast cancers. Now these drugs, such as anastrozole (Arimidex), letrozole (Femara) and exemestane (Aromasin), are being tested against early breast cancers as possible alternatives to the SERMs.

They are showing such good early results that they might someday become the first choice in treatment. Since so many glands profoundly affect our hormone balance, and potentially a breast cancer's environment, there are paths aplenty for researchers and oncologists to follow.

Chemotherapy

Weighing the pros and cons of chemotherapy can be even more difficult than deciding on hormone therapy. It is a less "benign" therapy than hormonal therapy, with more obvious side effects and toxicities; it is not something that an oncologist, in good conscience, prescribes to everyone. On the other hand, **adjuvant chemotherapy** (given when there is no known distant metastasis) adds an average of about three to five years to the premenopausal woman's life; that means some cures and some much-extended lives.

Another way of looking at how much chemotherapy is likely to help reduce the risk of cancer recurrence is to realize that, statistically, it reduces risk by about 20 to 30 percent of whatever the risk is without chemotherapy. This means that the group of women at highest risk of recurrence benefits the most from chemotherapy. That is, the woman with a large, aggressive tumor and enough positive lymph nodes so that she falls into the group with a 70-percent risk of recurrence would see her statistical risk decrease to 50 percent or so. (As always, of course, this refers to groups of women and does not say anything about what will happen to an individual woman.) On the other hand, the woman with a small, slow-growing cancer and no positive lymph nodes might see her risk decrease from 10 percent to 8 percent, still a reduction but not nearly as dramatic.

The woman well past menopause often does better with hormonal therapy and is less likely to receive chemotherapy, although if her tumor is estrogen- and progesterone-receptor negative or especially aggressive, she may be a chemo candidate. Some oncologists contend that the reason for the relatively dismal showing for chemotherapy in this age group is that doctors give gentler and much less potentially effective doses of the drugs.

For the premenopausal women with positive lymph nodes, no matter how few or how minimally positive, most oncologists will recommend a course of chemotherapy. There may be no circulating cancer cells, but few oncologists are willing to take that chance.

It is much harder for both the oncologist and the woman to decide on treatment when the woman is either premenopausal with negative nodes or in her fifties and not far past menopause (when her cancer may have premenopausal "roots"). In these cases especially, the oncologist must consider the type of tumor, its stage, and any other prognostic factors such as hormone receptor status to make an informed recommendation, based on the statistical likelihood that there are cancer cells that need to be killed and that chemotherapy is the weapon of choice.

Many premenopausal women with node-negative tumors, especially those in certain subgroups of women—those whose cancers have a high expression of HER-2/neu oncogene, for instance, or other signs of a more aggressive tumor—face relatively high risk that their cancer will come back. It is also conceivable that a pathologist missed seeing a tiny micrometastasis. The National Cancer Institute currently advises oncologists to consider a course of chemo for any premenopausal woman with invasive breast cancer, regardless of her lymph-node status. But it is up to the woman and her oncologist to decide together.

The traditional chemotherapy regimens for Stage I or II breast cancer combine two or three drugs: cyclophosphamide (Cytoxan), either methotrexate or doxorubicin (Adriamycin), and often 5-fluorouracil (5-FU). A woman may be on CMF or CAF or AC, names created by combining the first letter of each of the chemotherapy drugs she is taking. Adriamycin is somewhat stronger and has more serious side effects than methotrexate, so it is given when the oncologist wants a more powerful drug. Newer chemotherapy agents, given often now for more aggressive breast cancers of any stage, include paclitaxel (Taxol) or docetaxel (Taxotere), members of the taxane family, originally derived from the yew tree. Other agents are coming out of clinical trials and into community use. But, as chemo drugs and dosages go, these breast cancer chemo regimens are considered relatively tame (see Chapter 8 for general information about chemotherapy).

Tame, however, does not mean ineffective, or fun.

Ordinarily, these drugs can be given in the doctor's office or at an outpatient infusion center (typically a room or rooms linked to a hospital where people go to receive chemotherapy, blood, or other fluids through the vein), so the woman does not need to be hospitalized. Cyclophosphamide can be injected into a vein or taken as pills. The other drugs are given into the vein, either "pushed" slowly with a syringe or dripped from an IV bag.

A typical course might be eight repetitions of a three-week cycle, with intravenous injections of all three medications on day one and nothing else for the next twenty days. When Cytoxan is taken as pills, a twenty-eight–day cycle is common, with injections of both methotrexate and 5-FU on days one and eight in the oncologist's office. The Cytoxan pills are taken at home every day from day one through day fourteen, and then no medications are taken as the body recovers from day fifteen to day twenty-eight.

The courses of adjuvant chemotherapy are getting shorter now, and usually last from four to six months (although one year is not uncommon). Chemo usually starts within a month after surgery and often before any radiation, since this seems to be a particular "window of opportunity" for destroying cancer cells. An alternative strategy, especially with a somewhat larger or more aggressive tumor, is to begin treatment with several months of chemotherapy, then perform the surgery, and finish off with more chemo: a kind of treatment "sandwich" called **neo-adjuvant therapy**.

The common temporary side effects of the non-taxane drugs are fatigue, digestive tract complaints, and hair loss (hair thinning with CMF, usually complete loss with Adriamycin, although it may be worth trying the suggestions in Chapter 8 under "Hair Loss"). Chapter 8 gives information on dealing with all these side effects. Loss of menstruation and menopausal symptoms often occur in premenopausal women; these changes are more likely to be permanent if the woman is over forty.

Weight gain (much more often than weight loss) happens so often with breast cancer chemo that it may be a side effect of the drug. Although it is not inevitable, it is common for a woman to gain 20 pounds or more, and the weight may take a long time to come off.

No one is quite sure why weight gain occurs. It may be that these particular chemo regimens bring about some changes in the woman's metabolism that make it easier to gain weight and harder to lose it. Possible contributing factors might be menopausal changes, frequent snacking to keep ahead of queasiness, or lack of exercise. Also, some women take the steroid pill prednisone as part of their chemotherapy, and that causes weight gain.

Besides general side effects, there are some special cautions with the breast chemo drugs. If a woman is taking Adriamycin, her oncologist may order special heart function tests. Ordinarily, however, heart damage occurs only when the cumulative dosage of the drug exceeds a certain amount and oncologists are careful to keep below that amount. In fact, the possibility of heart damage is the "dose-limiting" factor for Adriamycin, although oncologists may be able to protect the heart if they need to go beyond the "safe" dose of Adriamycin, by adding dexrazoxane (Zinecard) to the later doses of chemotherapy. Giving these high doses is usually done only with cancer that has spread to distant organs. Many women taking Adriamycin complain of nightmares and other temporary psychological changes.

The woman taking Cytoxan will be cautioned to drink about three quarts of fluids on the days she receives the drug. The end products of Cytoxan are notoriously rough on the bladder as they pass through and can cause a severe bleeding irritation called **hemorrhagic cystitis**. While the woman may feel "waterlogged," drinking all these fluids dilutes the Cytoxan and washes it out of the body before it can cause problems.

Taxol and Taxotere can cause brief severe muscle aches. More serious are the strange nerve symptoms of burning, tingling, or numbness that sometimes occur, usually in hands or feet or near them. This peripheral neuropathy usually goes away eventually but can be permanent. Certain medicines relieve these symptoms fairly well for many women.

During the last few years, oncologists have added other chemotherapy drugs to their breast cancer arsenal, with new drugs appearing from time to time. Each has a different profile, and the woman's primary source of information about side effects is the oncologist. Oncology nurses can be a rich resource, as can pharmacists, the Cancer Information Service at (800) 4-CANCER, and many breast cancer advocacy groups. A clear and accurate Internet resource for information on many chemotherapy agents (as well as all sorts of other cancer topics) is the British website www.cancerbacup.-org.uk/info.

When the woman has an especially high-risk cancer (such as a very fast-growing tumor or many positive lymph nodes), the oncologist may use special treatment protocols with new drugs or higher doses of standard drugs than usual. The highest doses of chemotherapy are given only when a woman's supply of white blood cells can be "rescued" by stem cells, "baby" blood cells donated by the woman earlier and then stored until the time for a stem-cell transplant (see "Stem-Cell Transplants" in Chapter 14). But the oncologist can give doses that are higher than standard doses by adding granulocyte colony stimulating factor (G-CSF, filgrastim, Neupogen), which stimulates the bone marrow to produce more white blood cells faster to reduce the chance of serious infection (see "Side Effects of Chemotherapy" in Chapter 8). This makes it much safer to give these relatively high doses, although not everyone agrees that these high doses are any more effective than standard doses.

Biological Therapies

Biological therapies appear to be coming into their own in breast cancer therapy. For the woman whose breast cancer cells "overexpress" or have too much of the HER-2/neu receptor protein—usually a young woman with a very aggressive cancer—the monoclonal antibody trastuzumab (Herceptin) binds to these target cells so that the body correctly sees them as "bad" and "not belonging," and attacks them. Trastuzumab (the "mab" at the end shows that it is a monoclonal antibody) is given into the vein for a brief period each week. With the first dose, about 40 percent of women feel as if they are catching the flu, with fever and chills, nausea, body aches and diarrhea, but major symptoms tend to be rare with later doses. Heart problems can occur, sometimes serious ones, especially in women who already have heart disease or if the agent is given with one of the chemotherapy drugs, like Adriamycin, that can damage the heart. At least with metastatic breast cancer, trastuzumab is not considered a cure, but it has given many women extended comfortable time. The hope is that it will work even better earlier, when the foe is less formidable. Trastuzumab is effective only in women who overexpress HER-2/neu, and not in all of them. But its success in this group makes researchers eager to discover, and then clone in the laboratory, antibodies to other breast-cancer proteins.

Theratope cancer vaccine is a more general biologic therapy being tested against several types of cancer, including breast cancer. The theory behind the vaccine: Cancer can grow because the body is not recognizing and mounting a defense against the small amount of certain antigens on the cancer, substances which would normally bring about an immune response. If a large amount of an antigen were let loose in the body, however, the immune system might "get the message" and start attacking the antigen wherever it is, including on the cancer. Theratope is a specific carbohydrate antigen cancer vaccine produced in large quantities in the laboratory and then injected into the patient. A large Phase III clinical trial of Theratope in metastatic breast cancer is underway, with results expected in 2004.

Other biologic therapy agents are in the clinical trial pipeline, including anti-angiogenesis agents to block a cancer's ability to make new blood vessels to nourish itself. Over the last several years, research companies have been accumulating the know-how and the experience to begin making some real contributions to breast cancer therapy.

SPECIAL SITUATIONS

Pregnancy and breastfeeding, Paget's disease of the nipple, and Stage III breast cancer are three situations that deserve special attention.

Pregnancy

Breast cancer diagnosed during pregnancy is fairly rare—unless, of course, it happens to you. In fact, it is becoming more common as women delay pregnancy into years of greater overall risk.

Until recently, most doctors believed that the huge hormonal changes in pregnancy "fed" breast cancers and advised the pregnant woman with breast cancer to have an immediate therapeutic abortion and then undergo cancer treatment. To many people's surprise, later studies showed that, when breast cancers with the same stage (size and lymph-node involvement) were compared, there was little difference in prognosis whether the breast cancer was diagnosed during pregnancy or at some other time.

The big problem is that breast cancers are harder to detect during pregnancy, which leads to delayed diagnosis and more advanced cancers at diagnosis. It is too easy to confuse cancer changes with the normal breast changes of pregnancy, and screening mammography is not an option. Any dominant lump or spontaneous, persistent nonmilky discharge from one breast duct still needs to be checked out carefully. Fortunately, breast biopsy under local anesthesia is safe at any time during pregnancy.

The woman who is near the end of pregnancy when the cancer is diagnosed can deliver her baby and then undergo either mastectomy or breast-conserving surgery/radiation and systemic therapy as needed (although some doctors worry that radiation may be less effective on this actively changing breast tissue). Most doctors advise against breastfeeding.

When the cancer is diagnosed earlier in the pregnancy, the woman who continues her pregnancy is usually limited to mastectomy as local treatment, since radiation therapy is not safe for the developing baby. With special care for the anesthesia given and how the woman is positioned on the operating table, a mastectomy under general anesthesia does not usually seem to cause problems for the baby. Any reconstruction surgery should be delayed both because the longer surgery is risky for the baby and the remaining breast needs to reach its normal size and shape so the surgeon has something to match.

Once in a while, a woman may be able to have lumpectomy surgery, then receive chemotherapy through delivery and, finally, radiation after delivery. Giving chemotherapy during pregnancy is very controversial, and many doctors automatically recommend therapeutic abortion before any chemotherapy. Others point to apparently normal babies born to women who have received chemotherapy during pregnancy.

Most doctors agree that pregnancy, especially early pregnancy, seriously limits the drug choices, and they do not know yet whether there are any long-term effects on the baby. Side effects of chemotherapy on the blood cells could also increase risks of infection or bleeding if the baby is delivered at an unexpected time. Adding chemotherapy fatigue to normal delivery and new baby fatigue is another issue, but so is the fact that chemotherapy may end the woman's chance to have another pregnancy. Hormonal therapy is not an option during pregnancy because it causes both miscarriages and birth defects.

Making treatment decisions about breast cancer is hard enough at any time; being pregnant makes it even more complicated and emotionally challenging. The woman and her partner need all the information and support (and the most knowledgeable, empathetic doctors) they can find.

Breastfeeding

When a woman breastfeeds, her breasts normally change so much that detecting a cancerous change continues to be difficult. In case of a persistent suspicious lump, ultrasound or MRI usually does a better job of imaging the area than mammography does. A biopsy can be done during breast-feeding but is riskier because bacteria introduced by surgery grow very well in breast milk and can cause severe infection. Many surgeons urge the woman to stop breastfeeding at least temporarily before surgery and to receive antibiotics. If cancer is diagnosed, most doctors recommend weaning the baby and then undergoing standard treatment.

Paget's Disease of the Nipple

Paget's disease of the nipple is a rare condition in which a rash on the nipple that looks like eczema signals highly abnormal or cancerous cells within and under the nipple. These may be confined to a duct as carcinoma in situ (see "Carcinoma in Situ: The In-between Diagnosis" in Chapter 12) or may have invaded other tissues as invasive cancer. Other signs and symptoms include itching or redness around the nipple, nipple discharge, and a lump or thickening either under or near the nipple or areola. Mammograms may show microcalcifications or other suspicious changes.

Surgery almost always removes at least the nipple, the areola, and a portion of tissue underneath. Because this leaves a crater in the breast and because of fear of more disease elsewhere in the breast, surgeons have traditionally performed a mastectomy, especially if there is a lump or suspicious change in the woman's mammogram. The surgeon who suspects invasive cancer will probably remove at least some lymph nodes under the arm.

Some surgeons are beginning to use breast-conserving surgeries, including removing the nipple and a wedge of tissue along the specific duct, for small areas of Paget's disease without a lump or mammogram changes. Reconstructive surgery may fill in the nipple/areola area. Because the disease is so rare, we do not have large-scale studies to tell whether or not radiation therapy decreases the risk of later problems.

Stage III Breast Cancer

Stage III breast cancer, also known as **locally advanced breast cancer** (LABC), does not have any known distant metastases but fits one of these categories: (1) the tumor is over two inches in diameter; (2) the tumor can be any size but with one or more lymph nodes "fixed," or attached, to each other or to other tissues; (3) the tumor can be any size but has obviously spread to the lymph nodes along the same side of the breastbone; (4) the tumor is **inflammatory breast cancer,** in which the breast is generally red and swollen because tumor cells block the lymph vessels in the deep skin layers; or (5) after mastectomy the cancer has recurred in the breast area with obvious changes in the skin or chest wall. (For postmastectomy recurrences, see "Local Recurrence or Metastasis" in Chapter 14.)

Stage III breast cancer is divided into IIIA, when the problem is a large tumor or fixed lymph nodes, and IIIB, when the skin, chest wall, or chest lymph nodes are involved. About 10 to 20 percent of women have LABC when their cancer is first diagnosed, often because earlier signs or symptoms were not detected or were ignored. About 1 to 4 percent of women have inflammatory breast cancer, the most aggressive form of breast cancer, which grows so quickly that it may not produce any signs or symptoms until the sudden swelling and redness appear; the skin may look swollen and shiny, with enlarged pores like the skin of an orange (peau d'orange).

Treatment aims at decreasing the high risks of both recurrence in the breast area and spread to distant organs. Neither surgery nor radiation works well as the first therapy. What seems to work much better is a "sandwich" approach, beginning with several cycles of chemotherapy (called neoadjuvant, primary, or induction chemotherapy when it is the first cancer treatment). This is given before surgery or radiation and is followed by several more cycles of "maintenance" or adjuvant chemotherapy after all the known cancer has been removed or destroyed. Neoadjuvant chemotherapy acts as both systemic therapy to destroy cancer cells that have left the breast and as local treatment to shrink the breast tumor before the regular local therapies of surgery and/or radiation.

Neoadjuvant chemotherapy also lets the doctor measure directly how effective the drugs are in shrinking the tumor or, in the case of inflammatory breast cancer, in decreasing the redness and swelling. This helps in plans for more treatment, sometimes very high dose chemotherapy with stem cell or bone marrow transplant rescue (see "Stem-Cell Transplants" in Chapter 14).

The surgery usually removes the breast and underarm lymph nodes and may take more tissue (such as part of the chest muscle if the tumor is very close to it). Breast-conserving surgeries may be an option if the tumor shrinks dramatically with neoadjuvant chemotherapy, but this is very controversial.

Doctors differ in how they time treatments. With inflammatory breast cancer, for instance, some doctors prefer to "sterilize" the skin and underlying tissue with radiation before cutting into it with surgery. For any LABC, radiation is a common therapy, either along with neoadjuvant chemotherapy or after mastectomy. (For information about Stage IV breast cancer, cancer that has spread to distant organs, see "Local Recurrence or Metastasis" in Chapter 14.)

— *Kerry McGinn*

BEYOND BASIC TREATMENT FOR BREAST CANCER

Most women have all sorts of other questions about living with breast cancer. How do I get my arm moving again after surgery? What about an external breast prosthesis or reconstructive surgery? What kind of follow-up care do I need, and what can I do for myself? What if the cancer returns or I have metastatic cancer? How does a bone marrow transplant work? This chapter discusses these questions and more.

REGAINING ARM MOBILITY AFTER BREAST SURGERY

After either a mastectomy or a lumpectomy with more than one or two lymph nodes removed, it may be hard at first to move the arm on that side freely. It hurts along the upper arm when the woman tries to reach above shoulder height. If the doctor told her to restrict arm movement for a couple of weeks to protect the new surgery (a controversial precaution), she may have a stiff shoulder. The worst scenario occurs when, to avoid pain, she avoids raising the arm for several weeks and the shoulder joint becomes "frozen."

But while avoiding movement actually leads to more pain, carefully stretching those muscles and keeping the shoulder joint mobile slowly gets rid of the discomfort. Ordinarily, a woman can regain a comfortable and full "range of motion" and reasonable strength by six to eight weeks after surgery—or at least be well on her way. She begins exercising her arm and shoulder, sensibly and gradually, as soon as her surgeon gives the go-ahead, and then increases her range a little every day. A book that addresses the physical problems following breast surgery is *Recovering from Breast Surgery*, by Diana Stumm, P.T. (see Resources).

The doctor may give her a set of exercises. In some hospitals, a physical therapist routinely sees patients after breast cancer surgery. The woman can request a Reach to Recovery volunteer through the local American Cancer Society unit to visit her, demonstrate exercises, and leave her literature.

One standard exercise involves standing a few inches from a wall, bending the elbows, and placing the palms of both hands on the wall at about shoulder height. Then the woman "walks" her hands up the wall as far as they will go, and then back down; the crucial element is that the arm has to move from the shoulder and that she does not lean back at all. The idea is to have the arm protest a bit, but not "scream." The woman does this several times a day, moving a little higher each day. (Light pencil marks on a washable wall let her appreciate her accomplishment.)

In pendulum exercises, the woman bends at the waist and swings her arm slowly from the shoulder: front to back, side to side, and/or in increasing circles in front of her. Scratching her back as high as she can reach toward the opposite shoulder blade helps the shoulder regain another kind of mobility.

Heat, such as in a shower, can make it easier to stretch; some women find an ice pack before or afterward also helpful. A bag of frozen peas covered with a piece of cloth makes a good reusable, moldable ice pack.

Should the shoulder show any signs that it is "frozen" with adhesions because it has not been used, prompt physical therapy is essential. Freeing a frozen shoulder is not a do-it-yourself project.

BODY IMAGE AFTER MASTECTOMY

Many women are bothered sometimes by how they see themselves after a mastectomy. For some, body image after mastectomy is persistently, overpoweringly negative. They look in the mirror and see someone ugly, "less a woman," undesirable. The focus narrows to a tiny piece of themselves; they become "the scar." Concentrating on the scar sometimes means they have found a way to ignore the more painful reality of a cancer diagnosis.

Certainly, every woman with a mastectomy needs time to mourn the lost breast. Many begin to accept the changes by touching the scar, massaging it, making it physically part of themselves. Some dream about the lost breast; some find dance or other movement helps make them feel "whole" again. When distress is severe, counseling may be helpful.

The major strategy for positive self-image is broadening the focus. A woman is infinitely more than her breasts. Now is the time to look at all the rest of herself. Broadening the focus also means looking outside herself, at the world, to see what she can contribute. If a narrow scar a few inches long looks pretty small when compared to a whole woman, it looks even smaller when compared to a whole world.

Many women—even those with supremely healthy body images—want to minimize the physical results of a mastectomy, either by wearing an external breast form or undergoing reconstructive surgery. But it is an individual preference.

When my friend Betsy had both breasts removed, for instance, she was quite happy (as was her husband) to "go bare": "My breasts weren't big to begin with. The mastectomy scars look quite nice, I'm not lopsided at all since both breasts are gone, and I just feel 'freer' this way. I don't have to worry about breast prostheses and don't have to undergo more surgery. This is just right for me."

THE BREAST PROSTHESIS

While some women feel quite happy "going bare," many feel lopsided and unattractive and want something to take the place of the missing breast. An **external prosthesis** (breast form), properly fitted, can not only make the woman's clothes fit better, but can also balance the weight of a remaining breast so that she does not get backaches.

That is what Sheila wanted, and got. "I could not face the thought of more surgery, but I had visions of some scenario like a breast form falling out of my swimsuit. With the new technology, though, I have a prosthesis that feels like a normal breast, is the same weight as my natural breast, and stays in place on my chest with special strips. It's a comfortable, easy solution for me."

For at least the first two or three months, until the surgical area is completely healed, a woman needs something lighter than a "real" weighted prosthesis. Women can wear home from the hospital a specially designed comfortable camisole with one or two built-in, detachable, light breast forms in individual pockets; the Softee (Ladies First, Inc.) is available from some surgeons and breast care centers; call (800) 497-8285 for a list of nearby providers. A Reach to Recovery volunteer can bring the woman a temporary breast form, a simple fabric casing into which she can put the appropriate amount of Dacron "fluff." At first, before the woman can wear a bra, she can have this pinned under her nightgown. After a few weeks, when she can wear a bra, a comfortable alternative against the skin is a fluff of lambswool, purchased at a drugstore or more cheaply from a dancers' supply company. A light foam rubber "sleep breast" is another option at that point, or it can be the permanent choice for the woman who does not need to balance a heavy breast.

The permanent prosthesis matches the remaining breast closely in both shape and weight and can look very natural under clothing. It can be an expensive investment, although if the doctor writes a prescription it is often covered by health insurance, at least in part.

The fact that a prosthesis is relatively expensive has lured many entrepreneurs into the market, and that means that a woman can choose from many different models. Some of the newer breast forms stick securely to the breast with Velcro strips and some kind of adhesive. Others are made of tiny beads so that the breast "moves" like a real breast. Often, a simpler, less expensive prosthesis may fit a woman's needs quite nicely.

Many local ACS units have a display of breast forms and a list of local merchants who provide expert and sensitive fitting. Prostheses can also be ordered by mail, although the woman loses the advantage of receiving a personal fitting.

A woman may be able to wear most of her clothes "as is" over her regular bra and prosthesis. Some bras and swimsuits are made with a special pocket for the breast form that does not adhere directly to the skin. Otherwise, clothing can be easily altered. Many women look for or make pretty nightwear, perhaps with Greek draping on one side, for instance, in which they feel attractive without a prosthesis.

If a bra rides up—either because one side is lighter than the other or the woman has a double mastectomy—it can be anchored with a "V" of elastic sewn to the bottom of the bra and attached (with a stitched-on garter, perhaps) to panties or a girdle.

BREAST RECONSTRUCTION

For other women, an external prosthesis is not enough. Either before a mastectomy or at any time afterward, these women turn to the reconstructive (plastic) surgeon for help. They want to look "normal"—"like myself"—again. They find the absence of a breast or a major indentation in the breast after a lumpectomy to be a constant and unwelcome reminder of the cancer, when they want to move on with life. Or they feel "less like a woman" without breast curves, and flinch at changing at a gym or having a sexual partner see them without clothes. Perhaps they find an external prosthesis an intrusive nuisance, or uncomfortable. Or they suffer from backaches or other problems from not having a breast on one side.

Virtually every woman—no matter how old she is, how long ago she had breast surgery, and how much the chest area was damaged—is a candidate for some kind of breast reconstruction if she wants it.

Anne thought that people might laugh at her for wanting breast reconstruction at age sixty-five, "But the people I cared about thought it was a great idea. They knew it was important to me, my gift to myself. Before this, I wore a good prosthesis, but it never felt like 'me.'"

"I didn't expect or want to be a beauty queen after reconstruction, so my expectations were pretty reasonable. I really like the way I look and feel now. Sure, it's not quite the same as my other breast, but I'm mighty happy with it—in clothes and even out of them."

On the other hand, many women do not want reconstructive surgery. They may be quite content without it, or even be strongly opposed on feminist grounds, and see no need for it. They may not want any more surgery, or may be concerned about possible risks. It is strictly an individual choice.

What does reconstruction offer? The first step is to create a breast mound, using one of several possible techniques. The challenge is making a breast that looks like a breast, with some droop and a normal "crease" underneath. If the woman simply wants something that looks normal under clothes, a mound may be enough for her, but many women want a nipple and areola as well. Finally, making the reconstructed breast reasonably symmetrical with the other breast may mean surgery to make the remaining breast smaller or less droopy.

Implants

How does the surgeon make a breast mound? Occasionally, if the woman has enough skin remaining after the breast is removed, the surgeon may be able simply to slip a breast-shaped implant into a pocket in or under the chest muscle. While it is easier initially to put an implant above the muscle, it is more prone to slippage, rupture, and other complications there. If the woman can flex her breast—an unusual talent indeed—the implant has been placed in the chest muscle. An implant can be inserted during the mastectomy surgery or in a separate surgery later. Inserting an implant is a relatively simple procedure but, as with any surgical procedure, carries with it the risks of possible infection, bleeding, and buildup of fluid in the area.

When a woman does not have enough skin remaining after a mastectomy to fit over a standard implant, she may undergo **tissue expansion**. The idea behind a tissue expander is that the body will recruit more skin over a gradually expanding implant—rather like what happens to the skin of the abdomen during pregnancy.

When first inserted in a pocket in the chest muscle, the silicone tissue expander looks like a small, collapsed balloon, connected to a port that rests under the skin. Over the course of several weeks, the expander is filled with sterile saline (salt water) injected by syringe through the skin and into the port, two or more ounces at a time. Each injection, spaced every week or so, stretches the skin a little as the new breast enlarges. (It is rather like

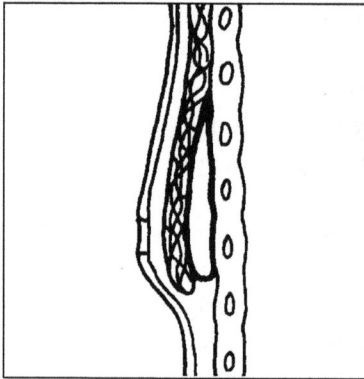

Tissue expander before expansion

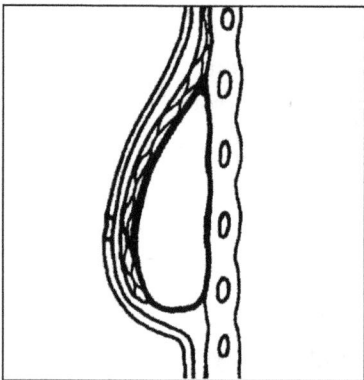

Tissue expander after expansion

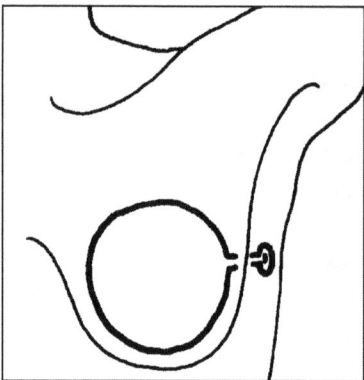

Tissue expander in place
(illustrations courtesy of Susan Schoen)

being thirteen years old again, but the process is certainly faster!)

This tissue expander is often a temporary measure to prepare the chest pocket for a final silicone gel or saline implant, inserted during a second surgery. Some, however, are made so that the expander stays in place permanently while the port is removed. There are many kinds of expanders, including **double-lumen expanders,** ones with an inner empty chamber for saline and an outer chamber filled with a small amount of silicone gel to give the breast a more natural shape.

After the expander has reached the desired size, the surgeon often continues inflating it until it is about one-third overfilled and then leaves it that way for several weeks. The theory is that this helps the breast develop a natural droop when the permanent implant is inserted or the permanent expander is deflated to its final size.

Many women complain of minor discomfort and a "tight skin" sensation for a few hours after each injection. The major complaints come during the overinflation period, when the breast can be quite uncomfortable and can look rather like a large baseball perched on the chest. The same surgical complications can occur as for the regular silicone gel implants.

How do these assorted implants compare with a "natural" breast? It very much depends not only on the surgeon's skill but also on how an individual woman's body responds. The implanted breast rarely matches the other breast perfectly; it is typically firmer and has less of a droop—"perkier" or "more youthful" is how the surgeon might put it—but many look and feel quite natural, both in and out of clothes. It is important to remember, however, that while the "real" breast may change with aging or weight gain or loss, the implanted breast stays the same.

The body normally forms a fibrous scar capsule around any implant. However, in some cases the body is too enthusiastic about "walling off" this "intruder" and, in time, the new breast begins to feel rock-hard. This **capsular contracture** is the most common complication of implant surgery; whether or not it occurs depends on the woman's body and the type of implant.

As the dust raised by the sensational 1990s media and lawsuit publicity begins to settle, it grows easier to learn the real risks of breast implants—and what does and does not need to worry the woman considering breast reconstruction.

A Brief History

Breast implants filled with silicone gel were first marketed in the 1960s and, when the U.S. Food and Drug Administration began requiring premarketing approval for new medical devices in 1976, silicone implants were "grandfathered" in—that is, since the implants were already in use and considered safe, the manufacturers did not need to apply for approval.

In the 1980s, a few anecdotes began appearing about connective tissue disease or related disorders in women who had experienced rupture or slow "bleed" of their silicone-gel implants. The theory was that these problems, often involving muscle or joint pain, fatigue, and other symptoms, occurred because of the body's reaction to silicone gel. The first multimillion-dollar suit against implant manufacturers was filed and the issue snowballed, with more women claiming problems and more lawsuits, public outcry, fear, and distrust.

In 1992, after impassioned public hearings, FDA Commissioner David Kessler temporarily banned silicone-gel implants altogether, except for use in clinical trials of breast reconstruction after breast cancer. Saline breast implants remained available but faced new safety tests. What got lost in the shouting was Kessler's clear statement that the ban was imposed *not* because there was any clear scientific evidence that the implants were unsafe, but because they had not yet been proven safe. Now the manufacturers would have to carry out clinical research under very strict conditions to see whether the implants were indeed safe, something that should have been done years before. Finally, in 1999, the Institute of Medicine (IOM) completed an independent review of all known scientific research of silicone breast implant safety. It found ample evidence of complications in the breast implant area: infection soon after surgery, later capsular contracture with discomfort and disfigurement, implant deflation or rupture, and need for additional surgery. The review found no evidence of increased connective tissue disease or cancer in women with breast implants compared to the general population. Similar studies, carried out in Britain and other countries, found similar results.

As of the year 2000, silicone-gel implants were freely available in the United States for women seeking breast reconstruction or needing replacement of another implant, and Mentor (manufacturer) silicone-gel implants were available on a limited basis for women seeking breast augmentation.

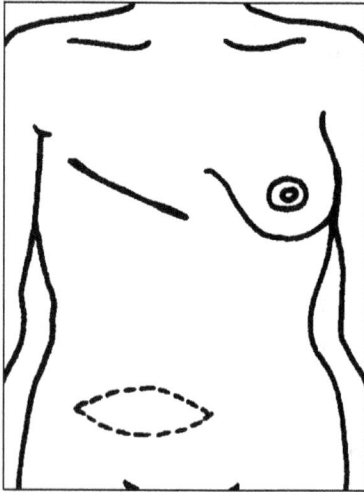

TRAM flap areas of surgery

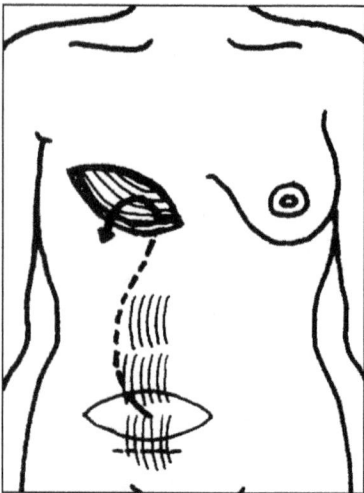

TRAM flap procedure

(these illustrations—continued on page 259—courtesy of Susan Schoen)

Saline implants from either Mentor or McGhan were freely available for anyone. Full information is available on the FDA website: www.fda.gov/cdrh/breast-implants.

One thing that most people agree on is that current implants are not lifetime devices. They must be replaced from time to time, perhaps every ten to fifteen years or so, even if there is no obvious problem, because older implants are more likely to leak. If there is evidence of leakage, the implant is usually removed. However, because the body normally forms a fibrous capsule around the implant, even if there is leakage, the leakage usually stays within the capsule and does not travel elsewhere in the body.

Muscle Flap Reconstructive Procedures

There are various **muscle flap reconstructive procedures** that use a woman's own tissue, moving skin, muscle, and sometimes fat to create a new breast mound. These are lengthier surgeries that require an expert surgeon. They involve considerably more surgical pain than the implant procedures and entail relatively long periods of recuperation.

The TRAM flap (transverse rectus abdominus myocutaneous flap) technique is sometimes called "tummy tuck" surgery because it uses abdominal tissue to make the new breast. To be eligible for the surgery, the woman needs an ample supply of abdominal skin and fat; the surgery not only gives her a new breast (or breasts) but also flattens her abdomen somewhat.

During the operation, the surgeon prepares an island of skin and fat atop a large vertical abdominal muscle. The muscle is cut at one end while the other end remains attached to its original site and blood supply. The whole "flap" is then tunneled under the skin to the mastectomy site where the surgeon shapes it into a breast mound and stitches it in place. The abdominal wound is closed.

The surgery takes several hours. For the first few days, the woman usually requires considerable pain medication for the abdominal pain where the muscle was cut. (Many women report they felt better at first than they expected, but others say they were not at all prepared for how much it hurt.) It may be hard for the woman to stand up straight at first.

The woman will have a large scar on the abdomen, as well as any breast scars. With such major surgery involving the abdomen and the blood supply, possible problems include infection or a flap that dies because it does not get an adequate blood supply, although problems such as these are rare. The woman often wears an abdominal binder for the first weeks and may have trouble performing sit-ups later.

A good TRAM flap looks very natural. It is soft, droops nicely, and often matches the other breast closely. The day after surgery, a woman sometimes feels miserable enough that she wonders why in the world she ever underwent the operation, but a few weeks later, she usually loves the results. The tissue is her own, only one surgery is needed for the breast mound, and she does not have to worry about the possible complications that come with an implant.

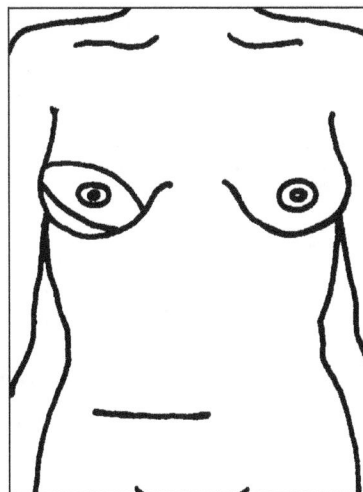

TRAM flap areas of surgery

Muscle flaps can come from other parts of the body besides the abdomen. The **LATS flap** (latissimus dorsi flap) technique, for instance, rotates the fan-shaped latissimus muscle from the mid-back along with an attached island of tissue, tunnels it under the armpit skin, and shapes it into a breast mound. The island of skin from the back fits over the mound. Since the latissimus muscle does not have overlying fat, however, a silicone implant is also usually necessary. There is a back scar and perhaps some decreased muscle power for some activities.

Although they require a surgeon specially trained in microsurgical procedures, the **microsurgical free flap procedures** are becoming more popular. The surgeon cuts completely free the tissue from the abdomen, back, or buttocks, shapes it into a breast mound, and uses microsurgical techniques to attach the blood vessels to blood vessels on the chest wall. Because the free flap does not carry its own blood supply with it, there is an increased risk that it will not "take."

More about Implants and Flaps

However the breast mound is made, the surgeon has a choice of techniques for making the nipple and areola later, when the breast shape has settled. The nipple can be constructed from the nipple of the other breast (one nipple makes two); sometimes it comes from a small flap of breast skin twisted on itself or from the ear lobe or from somewhere else in the body. The areola can come from a doughnut of skin removed from elsewhere, often from the thigh, and/or from medical tattooing of minute dots with a dye to match the areola. Since the new nipple and areola have no nerve supply, they do not have any sensation.

There are two bodies of opinion about whether reconstruction should be done at the time of mastectomy, if possible. One point of view holds that it is safe to do it at the same time and that it saves the woman both an extra surgery and some unnecessary mourning for her lost breast. The other point of view is that, if there is a chance the woman will undergo chemotherapy, she could be at greater risk for infection because of the reconstructive surgery, and that she will appreciate her new breast more if she waits.

In any case, to be happy with the results, a woman needs accurate information and reasonable expectations beforehand. Besides listening to the reconstructive surgeon, who is typically sincerely enthusiastic, she might want to talk to a woman or two who has undergone the same surgery. There is plenty of information readily available, both pro and con. The Food and Drug Administration, (800) 532-4440 or (301) 827-4420, has a hotline and a packet of information available. ACS, the Cancer Information Service, the Y-ME Breast Cancer Support Program, the American Society of Plastic and Reconstructive Surgeons, and the National Women's Health Network (see Resources) are other sources. Among the books available are Bruning's recently updated *Breast Implants: Everything You Need to Know* and Berger and Bostwick's *A Woman's Decision: Breast Care, Treatment, and Reconstruction* (see Resources).

FOLLOW-UP AFTER BREAST CANCER

Even if a woman is presumed cancer free after treatment, she usually sees at least one doctor every three months or so for about two years. Then, unless there is a sign of more cancer, the schedule often stretches out, perhaps to every six months for a few years, and then to every year. Touching base regularly becomes part of her program for life.

During her visits, the woman tells her doctor any concerns she has. In both asking questions and doing the physical examination, the doctor pays special attention to:

+ the area where the cancer occurred, including the incision site, remaining breast tissue, nearby lymph nodes, and chest wall

+ the other breast (if intact)

+ the organs that are especially vulnerable to breast cancer metastasis (bones, lungs, liver, and brain)

- organs at some increased risk for a new cancer, such as the ovaries and uterus (which makes it wise to have a gynecological exam at least every year) and the colon

- her physical and psychological coping with cancer and the changes in her body

Unless the woman has had both breasts removed, almost every doctor will want mammograms of the remaining breast tissue, from every six months to every year or two, at least in women under seventy. Beyond that, however, the thinking about what blood work, X rays, and other imaging studies to order for the woman with no symptoms has changed over the last few years and is still controversial.

One expert doctor may rely on high-intensity surveillance, with periodic complete blood counts, blood chemistry panels, tumor markers such as CA 27-29 and CA 15.3, plus chest X rays, bone scans, and sometimes liver ultrasounds or CT scans and lung CT scans. These are to look for any red flag values that might mean something is wrong with the bone marrow, bones, liver, or lungs. (An abnormal value does not necessarily mean cancer, and it may drift back into normal range as inexplicably as it left or may mean something else entirely, such as an arthritis change on a bone scan.) This doctor believes that the tests make a medical difference for the woman and also make her feel more secure. Meanwhile, another doctor, just as expert, may choose the minimalist approach, continuing physical exams, mammography, and any tests necessary to monitor potential side effects from treatment, but bypassing other blood and imaging tests.

In 1994, a Consensus Conference on Follow-up in Breast Cancer met in Italy to hear doctors, patients, ethics experts, policy makers, and others talk about what kind of follow-up worked best. One major piece of evidence was the large-scale clinical trial carried out by the Interdisciplinary Group for Cancer Care Evaluation in multiple cancer centers that studied care after breast-cancer treatment. This study found that, except for mammograms, careful histories, and physical examinations by doctors, routine follow-up tests accomplished very little—at high cost—for most women. As a group, the women with minimal follow-up, who were not tested unless a symptom appeared, did as well as the women in the intensive follow-up group.

The researchers concluded that most problems occurred between tests and that, if a test happened to show disease spread, it rarely showed it far enough in advance of symptoms to make a difference in either survival or the quality of the woman's life. The Conference did make an exception in considering routine liver ultrasound or CT scans sometimes appropriate for women diagnosed before age thirty-five with aggressive cancers. Obviously,

*Beyond
Basic
Treatment
for Breast
Cancer*

261

if the woman has a specific complaint, appropriate tests are needed to follow it up.

Monthly breast self-examination is even more important after breast cancer than before. The procedure for examining the breasts does not change after lumpectomy/radiation, although the radiated breast is likely to feel firmer than the other (see "Performing BSE" in Chapter 12). The woman needs to pay special attention to the incision and the underarm area, looking for any visible changes and feeling with care. A palpable lump or other changes in the incision area may be from scar tissue, but this is also the prime site for a local recurrence, often easily treated, so the doctor needs to evaluate *any* change.

LOCAL RECURRENCE AND METASTASIS

Some women must face breast cancer more than once. This cancer may be a totally new primary cancer, completely unrelated to the first, and the woman will go through the diagnosis and treatment process again. The other two scenarios are local recurrence and distant metastasis.

Local Recurrence

In a **local recurrence,** surgery or radiation did not destroy some cancer cells in the breast the first time around. These cells seem to have stayed within the breast area, but they continue dividing until they become large enough to detect.

This happens more often after breast-conserving surgery like lumpectomy than after a mastectomy, but is usually less serious and easier to treat after a lumpectomy. After lumpectomy, recurrence typically appears within the breast tissue near the scar, and only rarely in the skin or the lymph nodes, and often is detected from two to six years after the first treatment. Whether the woman had positive underarm lymph nodes before does not seem to matter.

A lump or mammography change signals a local recurrence. The oncologist stages the recurrence, as was done for the original tumor, by the tumor size, the presence or absence of positive lymph nodes, and any known distant metastasis. Unless the recurrence is quite large, involves the skin or chest wall, or has spread to distant organs, it remains a Stage I or II breast cancer, depending on its size and lymph-node status.

Local treatment this time may be different because one or more of the local therapy options have already been exhausted. For example, if the initial treatment was breast conserving therapy with radiation and the new local recurrence is invasive cancer, a mastectomy is the usual treatment, since radiation cannot be used in the same place again. The oncologist may recommend systemic treatment, such as hormonal therapy, depending on such clinical factors as the woman's age and the stage and grade of the tumor, although these recurrences are typically small and often do not need systemic treatment. The systemic treatment and the prognosis are the same as they would be for a primary tumor of the same stage and grade.

It is uncommon for cancer cells to be left in the local area after as much of the breast tissue as possible has been removed in a mastectomy, but it can happen. Then there may not be any place for the cells to grow except on the chest wall, the skin, or the lymph nodes under the arm or along the breast bone, and it can be much harder to get rid of them in those places than in breast tissue. These local recurrences tend to appear in the first two years after the mastectomy and are more common if the woman had positive lymph nodes at the original surgery. They quite often occur at the same time as, or shortly before, distant metastasis arises, although plenty of women never have another sign of cancer once the recurrence is treated. The recurrences show themselves as lumps in the skin or other skin changes, a lump under the skin, or a swollen lymph node. Unless there is distant metastasis as well, these local recurrences are classified as Stage IIIB, locally advanced breast cancer.

If it has not been used before, radiation is the mainstay of local therapy. Often the visible disease is removed surgically and then the remaining tissue receives radiation. Usually, all signs and symptoms of the local recurrence disappear, at least for a time, although they may return in the same place. Sometimes doctors add **hyperthermia,** in which small rods are implanted into the tumor and super-heated, to the radiation treatment. Systemic therapy is controversial and depends on many factors, including the treatment given before. Since there is no one commonly accepted protocol for treatment in this situation, the woman may want to check with a comprehensive cancer center to see what the possibilities are.

Distant Metastasis

What about **distant metastasis,** Stage IV cancer? Stage IV cancer is cancer that has spread to one or more distant organs, most often the bones, the lungs, the liver, or the brain (although any organ is a possible target). Stage IV breast cancer also includes cancer that has obviously spread to the lymph nodes around the collarbone.

Whether the cancer was originally diagnosed as metastatic or its spread was discovered later, it obviously is not good news, but it is not hopeless. For one thing, wherever the cancer spreads, it is still *breast* cancer—and breast cancer that metastasizes to the lung is not as lethal as most primary lung cancers. However, many of these organs are vital to life, which means that the cancer has become directly life-threatening.

Despite this, treatment can often keep women healthy and comfortable for extended periods. Most women with metastatic breast cancer live for many months or years (and some live decades) after diagnosis. While some aggressive breast cancers move quickly, it is quite common that a woman receives therapy for an isolated metastasis, remains symptom-free for months or years until another metastasis appears, receives more treatment, remains symptom-free, and so on.

Local therapy often includes radiation, especially for specific bone metastasis, where two to three weeks of daily treatments may alleviate pain completely. Radiation also decreases symptoms of brain metastasis. Surgery may remove isolated nodules in lung, liver, or brain, and is often a good way to repair a bone weakened or broken because of cancer. Drainage tubes and medication can remove fluid that has collected around the lung or heart and prevent it from collecting again.

Systemic therapy depends on many factors, including whether the tumor is estrogen-receptor positive or negative, how long the woman has gone without obvious disease, what therapies she has received already, where the metastasis is (and whether there is more than one), what symptoms (if any) she is having, what other medical problems she may have, and—especially—what she wants. Treatment ranges from doing nothing except relieving current symptoms to giving extremely high-dose chemotherapy, with rescue from the woman's stored bone marrow or peripheral-stem blood cells in the hope of cure or long-term remission (see the next section, "Stem-Cell Transplants").

Chemotherapy and hormone therapy are the most common systemic treatments. Chemotherapy can involve the same drugs and schedules as in Stage I or II cancer, but—since quality rather than quantity of life becomes more of a factor with metastatic cancer—the protocols may use fewer drugs or may use pills such as capecitabine (Xeloda), which a woman can take at home. If the woman has a hormone-positive tumor and has already taken tamoxifen, one of the aromatase inhibitor drugs might be a first choice, since they work well with few side effects. For the woman with a tumor that overexpresses HER-2/neu, trastuzumab (Herceptin) is commonly used. It seems likely that within a few years, several new biologic therapies will be available and effective to treat the cancer itself.

Other kinds of therapy target specific metastases. For instance, bone metastases cause not only pain and possible fractures, but also can release too much calcium into the bloodstream, a very serious condition called hypercalcemia. Treatment usually includes bisphosphonates, the same class of drugs used to treat the bone thinning of osteoporosis; pamidronate (Aredia) and zoledronic acid (Zometa) are two of many bisphosphonates. For the woman with several areas of bone metastases, injection of the radioactive agent strontium-89 chloride (Metastron) may offer excellent pain relief for months and can be repeated many times if needed.

New clinical trials appear often, and women with metastatic disease may be eligible for studies with bigger curative payoffs. A woman's doctor, breast-cancer advocacy groups, and the Internet information sources can steer her to these options; the National Cancer Institute's www.cancer.gov/clinical_trials is one good source.

And some women, using all sorts of methods, thrive on beating the odds, defying the statistics. As the Wellness Community, a nationwide support network of cancer patients, says, even if a woman has only a 1-percent chance of survival, she may very well be in that 1-percent surviving group.

At some point, however, the woman with metastatic breast disease may have to decide how hard she wants to fight—and the only correct answer is what she wants to do. She needs to know that, should pain become a problem for her, there are almost always good solutions for it, if her health professionals pursue them aggressively. (Cancer-pain management is evolving so quickly and creatively that it is hard for doctors to keep up with it.) Many other symptoms can be treated effectively as well. Symptom relief is a special interest and area of expertise for many oncology nurses, so the smart woman asks the nurses as well as her doctor for help. Even when cure is not possible, comfort always should be. *Cancer Doesn't Have to Hurt*, by Pamela Haylock and Carol Curtiss, covers the subject well (see Resources); www.cancer-pain.org is another fine information source.

STEM-CELL TRANSPLANTS

The idea behind stem-cell transplants for breast cancer is that very high doses of chemotherapy—which can only be given if there is some way to "rescue" the white blood cells in the body from the effects of that chemotherapy—might be enough to cure the cancer or at least let women live longer with it. For a stem-cell transplant, now much more common than bone-marrow transplant, the woman gives blood in a process like a long and complicated blood donation. The "baby" or "stem" white blood cells are drawn off from the collected blood, and the rest of the blood is returned to her. These stem cells are stored until the high-dose chemotherapy is given and the woman's white blood cells diminish dramatically. At that point, the stem cells are given back to her in a blood transfusion and, if all goes well, grow and flourish to renew the body's white blood cell

Beyond Basic Treatment for Breast Cancer

defenses against infection. (A bone-marrow transplant also provides a concentrated supply of white blood cells to "rescue" the bone marrow, but is done less frequently now that stem-cell transplants are available; the bone-marrow "harvest" requires a more painful and complex procedure to draw out the cells from deep in the bone and cleanse them.) The bad news is that, so far, most large-scale clinical trials in the United States, Canada, Italy, and other countries comparing high-dose chemotherapy to standard doses have shown about the same survival in both groups, with no survival edge for the women receiving the higher doses. (Final results from several trials are not due until 2004 or beyond.) A few trials have shown early results that seem to indicate a positive difference for the high-dose chemotherapy in some groups of women, such as those under age forty-five with many positive lymph nodes but no evidence of distant metastasis.

A few years ago, stem-cell transplants appeared to be the coming thing in high-risk breast cancer, expensive but worth every penny. This may happen again, if other clinical trials show a survival advantage, perhaps with refinements in the chemotherapy treatment or a more-focused selection of the women receiving them. However, at the moment, the general recommendation is that a woman desiring high-dose chemotherapy and stem-cell transplant receive it only in the setting of a careful clinical trial.

— *Kerry McGinn*

PART THREE

THE GYNECOLOGIC CANCERS

The word **gynecology** comes from the Greek words *gyne* and *gynaikos,* which mean "woman," and *logia,* meaning "study." In the strict sense of the word, a gynecologist would be one who is deeply involved in the study of women. In reality, gynecology is limited to studying disorders of the female reproductive system. It would be wonderful if gynecologists actually were steeped in the study of women—but that's just not always the case.

SELF-ADVOCACY IN WOMEN'S HEALTH CARE

My earliest memories of learning what it meant to be female were the awkward attempts my mother and I made to talk about having periods—menstruation. The awkwardness was not my mother's fault: No one had ever told her anything. She later told me that when she got her first period, she thought she was bleeding to death.

I remember being introduced to female and male anatomy through a book that used pictures of dogs as the anatomical models. Given my age-group, and that of my mother, I know we were not unique in the hard time we had figuring out how to discuss this subject. How *do* you talk when the parts of your body you need to talk about are called "private parts"? Children learn not to talk about these parts of their bodies, and they learn that they should not touch or think too much about "down there." These are taboos that confuse children *and* adults. Cultures around the world treat sex in different ways: Each cultural and ethnic group is likely to have its own taboos and expectations with regard to talk about genital parts.

My mother had her very first Pap smear at sixty-five and her first mammogram at sixty-seven. I had problems accepting that, regardless of the fact that I am a cancer nurse specialist, as a daughter I could only do so much to influence my mother. When I tried to talk with her about Pap smears and mammograms, she said, "My doctor never told me that I needed it." "But Mom," I said, "there are all kinds of ads and articles about Pap smears, mammograms, and cervical, uterine, and breast cancers in newspapers and magazines. How could you think that these messages don't apply to you?" She had no answer—and I wanted to scream.

My mother was just like millions of women of her generation. In general, women (and men too, to be fair) are not very good advocates for their own health-care rights. In their book *Generations,* Strauss and Howe refer to my mother's generation as the "silent generation." Her generation's silent, go-along attitude is reflected in their attitude toward health: "Whatever happens is meant to be and I have no control." Physicians and other health-care providers are perceived as the experts—they have more education and should be looked to for advice and guidance when it comes to health matters. If something, like a Pap smear, is not advised by the doctor, many women are unlikely to get one on their own. Nor are these issues likely to be brought up by the less-educated person. Not only is this level of trust misplaced and misguided, it also puts most of the responsibility on the doctors and nurses. In today's health-care system in the United States, as in many other countries, the responsibility for a person's health rests mainly with that person. No woman could be forced to get a Pap smear or a mammogram. But a good doctor will certainly help a woman get one if she requests it.

No woman should rely on doctors, nurses, or anyone else to make decisions about her health and health-care needs. Each woman has to be her own advocate—or have a friend, partner, daughter, or son who takes an advocacy role on her behalf if she cannot do it for herself. That is the point of this book: to help you, the reader, get an idea of what is possible and necessary and to help you take an active role in ensuring that you or someone you love gets the best information and the best care possible when questions about cancer arise. You can separate facts from myths. You *can* make decisions. And you can feel you have made the best choice from the available options.

The real question is, how do we convince our mothers, sisters, cousins, and friends that early detection measures are worthwhile? What makes some women willingly have screenings or do breast self-examination? What makes others avoid these self-care measures?

Are they are too busy? Are medical checkups too expensive? Do insurance policies refuse to pay for screening tests? Do women fear that there may actually be something wrong? And, if there is something wrong, can they pay, or afford taking the time off, to have treatment?

Or are women embarrassed to have their "private parts" examined? Do they want to avoid the cold metal speculum used for gynecologic examinations or avoid sitting in a cold, boring exam room with nothing on but a silly-looking paper gown, waiting for a busy and sometimes impersonal doctor? The reasons women fail to get routine checkups are probably combinations of all these things, with different reasons more important to some women than to others. But this is behavior our generation and the generation of our daughters must change.

THE NORMAL FEMALE REPRODUCTIVE SYSTEM

The female reproductive system includes the external genitalia—what we used to call "the private parts." The **vulva** consists of two folds of skin called the **labia,** which cover the openings of the vagina and **urethra** (the

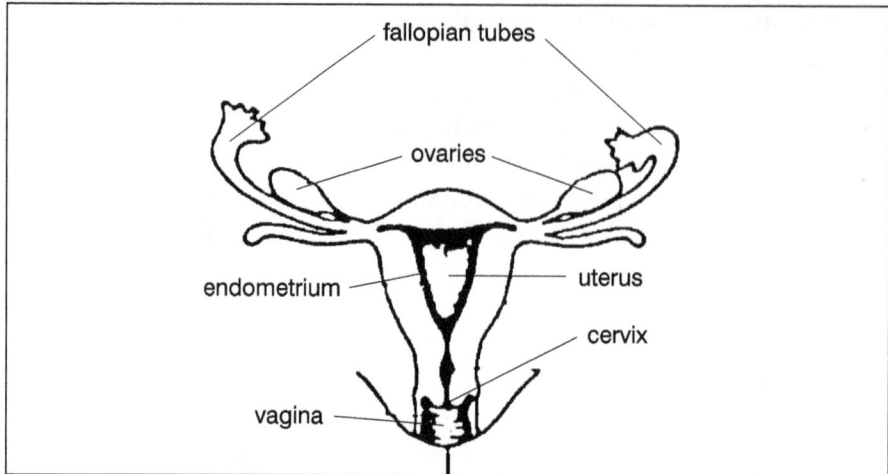

The normal female reproductive system
(reprinted from the NCI booklet What You Need to Know About Cancer of the Cervix*)*

tube leading from the bladder to the outside of the body) and the clitoris. The **vagina** is a stretchy canal that extends from the vulva to the **cervix,** the opening between the vagina and the uterus (womb). The **Bartholin's glands** in the lining of the vagina produce and secrete a lubricating mucous.

The two **fallopian tubes** (sometimes called uterine ducts or oviducts) carry **ova** (eggs) from ovary to uterus. Usually, fertilization takes place in a fallopian tube. The fertilized ovum, or **zygote,** travels on to the uterus and is embedded in the uterine wall (**endometrium**), resulting in pregnancy. If the ovum is not fertilized, the uterus prepares to shed the endometrium through the menstrual cycle and the process of menstruation. This whole process is directed by hormones, some of which are produced by the ovaries.

Estrogen and **progesterone** are hormones produced by the ovaries. (The word *hormone* is derived from the Greek word *hormao,* which means "I stir up" or "I set in motion.") Estrogen is responsible for the development of sex characteristics in teen girls: growth of pubic hair, enlargement of breasts, and the beginning of menstruation. The main function of progesterone is to prepare the uterus to receive a fertilized ovum. Progesterone secretion stops if fertilization does not occur and starts again when a new ovum begins developing in the ovary. This is a regular cycle that happens about every twenty-eight days throughout a woman's childbearing years. After menopause, hormone production in the ovaries slows down, but there is still some estrogen production there as well as in other hormone-producing organs, such as the adrenal glands.

CANCERS OF THE FEMALE REPRODUCTIVE SYSTEM

The gynecologic cancers affect the organs of a woman's reproductive system. They account for about 13 percent of all cancers in women and 6 percent of all cancers (including men, women, and children) diagnosed in the United States. Any of the female reproductive system's organs may be the site of a specific type of cancer.

In the United States, cancers involving the uterus are the most common (about 39,000 new cases per year, or 6 percent of all cancers in women), followed by cancers of the ovary (over 23,000 new cases per year, or about 4 percent of all cancers in women) and cervix (13,000 new cases per year, or 2 percent of all cancers in women). Many gynecologic cancers have high cure rates due to new techniques for detecting precancerous problems early, new methods of treatment, and better understanding of the usual patterns of these cancers. A woman with a gynecologic cancer has a better chance of successful treatment today than ever before.

— *Pamela Haylock*

CHAPTER 15

CANCER OF THE OVARY

"Why did Gilda die?" This is the title of an article in *People Magazine* from June 1991. The article describes the problems American comedienne and actress Gilda Radner had before finding she had ovarian cancer. Her trouble started as "stomach and colon problems." At first, her symptoms were thought to be emotional—she even called herself "the Queen of Neuroses." Then she thought she had Chronic Fatigue Syndrome. After reading about Gilda's death, you might wonder whether her life could have been saved by taking a simple blood test for the tumor marker CA125. Maybe if she had been quizzed about her family history, ovarian cancer might have been considered much sooner. Gilda Radner had symptoms for over a year before she was finally correctly diagnosed.

WHAT IS CANCER OF THE OVARY?

Lifetime statistics indicate that one of every seventy newborn girls will develop ovarian cancer at some time in her life, with half of all cases occurring in women older than sixty-five. Ovarian cancers in children are extremely rare, but do occur. In girls under fifteen, ovarian cancers make up about 1 percent of all cancers. Since they are so uncommon, they will not be covered here. The symptoms of an ovarian mass in young girls often mimic other problems, such as appendicitis. Suffice it to say that girls who have abdominal pain along with other symptoms, such as abdominal tenderness, nausea, and vomiting, should be carefully evaluated by a skilled gynecologic surgeon.

There are over twenty-three thousand new cases of ovarian cancer in the United States each year. Cancer of the ovary is responsible for more deaths than any other gynecologic cancer and the fifth most common cause of death from women's cancers. Just under fourteen thousand women die of this disease each year in the United States alone. The major reason so many women die from cancer of the ovary is that so few have early symptoms of disease. On the other hand, women who are diagnosed with early stages of ovarian cancer have a very good chance of long-term survival.

These numbers might be misleading and cause women undue concern. In reality, ovarian cancer is fairly rare. The gynecologist in a general OB/GYN practice sees, on the average, only one case of ovarian cancer over several years. New discoveries in the biology of cancer cells and information about how this cancer acts promise new approaches to early detection and treatment.

The ovary is a complex organ. The two major functions of ovaries are to release **germ cells** (eggs, ova) regularly and to produce steroid hormones. Each special function of the ovary is performed by certain cell types, and each of these types of cells can turn into a cancer cell. Because of this complexity, tumors arising from the ovary are complex too. Still, 90 percent of ovarian cancers develop from the surface epithelium on the outside of the ovary. These cancers are referred to as **ovarian epithelial cancer.**

Epithelial Cancer of the Ovary

The International Federation of Gynecology and Obstetrics (FIGO) divides ovarian epithelial tumors into three categories: **benign tumors, cancers with low malignant potential** (LMP), and **tumors with very clear malignant characteristics**. The low malignant potential tumors are usually found in younger women. These LMP ovarian cancers make up about 15 percent of all ovarian epithelial cancers, and most—around 75 percent—are found at an early and more curable stage of disease. The average age at diagnosis is about forty years, as compared to fifty-three years for the other forms of epithelial ovarian cancers. Other forms of ovarian cancer include **malignant clear cell tumors,** which are found in about 5 percent of women with ovarian cancer.

Nonepithelial Cancer of the Ovary

Nonepithelial cancer of the ovary usually occurs during childhood and teenage years. These cancers are diagnosed and staged in the same way as epithelial cancers. Most of these are called **germ-cell** and **stromal cancers,** and they account for about 10 percent of ovarian cancers (see chart on page 275).

Germ cells are involved in the development of the sexual organs of a fetus. Some of these cells stop developing during fetal life; they might be dormant for many years and eventually give rise to both benign and malignant tumors inside the ovary.

Stroma refers to structures that provide support for organs. In the ovary, various kinds of tissues form stroma. Stroma called **granulosa cells** and **theca cells** surround the site on the ovary where the ovum is released each month. Granulosa-cell tumors occur most often in women after menopause. The symptoms include an abdominal or pelvic mass, abdominal pain, and bloating. Most women with stromal tumors also have abnormal uterine bleeding. Treatment for women who still want to have children consists of removing the cancerous ovary and fallopian tube. Other women usually have a total hysterectomy, which includes removing both ovaries and fallopian tubes.

Sertoli and **Leydig cells** resemble cells of the male testes. Tumors involving these cells account for a very small number of ovarian cancers. Most occur in women twenty to forty years of age. These tumors produce hormones that cause a woman to take on male sex traits like facial and chest hair. Treatment consists of removing the affected ovary and fallopian tube.

Overall, the long-term outlook or prognosis for women with these ovarian cancers seems to depend on which type of cell is involved—the "histology"—and the size of the primary tumor. Treatment for these cancers discovered at early stages is offered with the intent to cure, and like other ovarian cancers, consists of surgery followed by chemotherapy. Younger women with Stage I and some with Stage II cancers who wish to have children may have the option of surgery that preserves the uterus and the opposite ovary. Women diagnosed at Stage II and beyond will generally undergo total abdominal hysterectomy and removal of both ovaries and fallopian tubes. A chemotherapy protocol will follow, likely lasting for a period of three to six months. Sometimes a course of radiation therapy is one of the treatment options a woman is offered. A disadvantage of radiation therapy directed toward the pelvic area is the loss of fertility. For the most up-to-date treatment information, women should check one of the many Internet sites devoted to providing this information. The National Cancer Institute's CancerNet is always a good place to start: http://cancer-net.nci.nih.gov

THE NATURAL HISTORY OF OVARIAN CANCER

"Natural history" refers to the way a certain form of cancer behaves when it is allowed to go its own way, without any form of treatment. Cancer of the ovary, of course, starts with the ovary. The epithelial cancers, which are the most common, begin on the epithelial (skinlike) surface of an ovary. They commonly spread through direct extension: Tumor cells penetrate the tissue surrounding the ovary and invade structures next to the ovary. These struc-

Germ Cell (Nonepithelial) Tumors of the Ovary

Type	Description
Dysgerminoma	Endodermal sinus tumor; embryonal carcinoma. Less than 5% of ovarian cancers. Usually occurs at 10–30 years of age. 25% have metastases at diagnosis. Both ovaries may be involved. hCG (human chorionic gonadotropin) and AFP (alpha-fetoprotein) tests are usually negative. In early stages of disease, surgery may preserve fertility. Additional treatment may use chemotherapy or radiation therapy.
Endodermal sinus tumor	Second most common. Occurs mostly in teens and young adults. Most common symptom is abdominal pain. hCG test is usually negative, but AFP is often increased. Women who have whole tumor surgically removed have a better prognosis. After surgery, combination chemotherapy is given. Radiation therapy is not effective.
Embryonal carcinoma	4% of germ cell cancers. Occurs mostly in teens. Usually found as a mass in the abdomen or pelvis. Other symptoms include those resembling puberty (in a prepuberty girl), irregular vaginal bleeding, lack of menstrual periods, and abnormal patterns of hair growth. hCG and AFP are positive. Treatment consists of removing the cancerous fallopian tube and ovary and combination chemotherapy. Radiation therapy is not effective.
Choriocarcinoma	Mixed germ cell tumors. Occurs mostly in girls before puberty and young women. Symptoms involve unexpected signs of puberty—pubic and axillary hair, uterine bleeding. Adult women have signs of ectopic pregnancy. hCG can be found in blood and urine. Gestational choriocarcinoma is treated with surgery and combination chemotherapy. Nongestational choriocarcinoma is treated with surgery.
Teratoma	Usually occurs before age 20 and often involves only one ovary. Symptoms include pelvic mass, abnormal uterine bleeding. Pain may or may not be noticed. hCG and AFP are negative. Treatment involves surgery to remove the affected ovary and fallopian tube followed by chemotherapy. Radiation is not usually useful.
Mixed germ cell tumors	Contain at least two germ cell types. Success of treatment depends on the size of the tumor and the cell types it contains. Treatment includes surgery followed by chemotherapy.

Cancer of the Ovary

tures include the fallopian tubes, uterus, bladder, rectum, lower colon, and the **peritoneum** (the sac lining inside the abdomen). **Peritoneal seeding,** tumor cells in the peritoneum, is the most common route of spread.

Peritoneal seeding allows cancer cells to lodge on the surfaces of the liver, diaphragm, bladder, and large and small bowel. The resulting irritation inside the peritoneum causes the formation of fluid called **ascites,** which causes the abdomen to swell.

The lymph channels and nodes around the ovaries provide another pathway for the spread of ovarian cancer cells. Lymph nodes most likely to hold cancer cells are those that surround the aorta (the body's major blood vessel that leads away from the heart) and those in the pelvis.

Blood vessels can and do carry cancer cells, but blood circulation is the least common method of spread for ovarian cancer. Cancer cells that are carried in blood vessels are likely to lodge in the liver, lung, pleura of the lung (tissue surrounding the outside of the lungs), kidney, bone, adrenal glands, bladder, and spleen.

Death from untreated ovarian cancer is usually the result of large amounts of cancer cells in the abdomen. Cancer cells in the bowel and the tissues that attach abdominal organs to the abdominal wall—the **mesentery**—cause these organs to stop working. The failure of these organs to function creates more problems, including bowel obstruction, liver failure, and altered fluid balance. Widespread cancer can cause sepsis (infection and bacteria carried in the blood), heart failure, and collapse of blood vessels. These combined problems are fatal.

WHO GETS CANCER OF THE OVARY?

The most important known risk factor for ovarian cancer is genetic predisposition, with up to 10 percent of epithelial types relating to genetics and the BRCA1 or BRCA2 genes that are also linked to breast cancer. Other risk factors for ovarian cancer include advancing age, menopause, diet, environment, never having children (nulliparity), not having children until later in life, history of another kind of cancer (particularly colon, endometrial, or breast cancer), and a family history of ovarian cancer. Women of Jewish descent also have an increased risk. Some experts believe the risks might be different between lesbian and heterosexual women, resulting in higher rates of ovarian cancer among lesbians. This has yet to be proven. (For more information about lesbians and breast and ovarian cancer issues, see the website www.annieappleseedproject.org/lesandbreasta.html.) The increasing use of fertility drugs and their potential link to ovarian cancer poses many unanswered questions. Since risk has not been ruled out, it is included in the informed consent for women who take fertility drugs. Other suspected but unproven risks associated with ovarian cancer include smoking, high

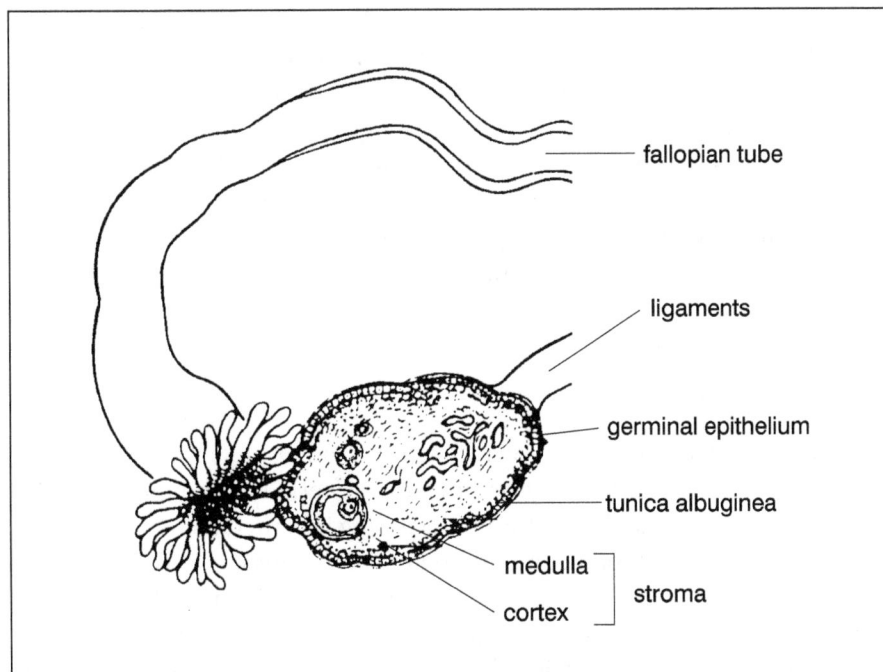

The normal ovary
(courtesy of National Cancer Institute)

dietary galactose intake, and antidepressant use. Although a cause–effect relationship has not been proven, there is some indication that the use of talc-containing powder in the genital area increases a woman's risk of epithelial-type ovarian cancer. Still, most women who develop ovarian cancer have no known risk factors.

Breastfeeding and use of oral contraceptives (birth-control pills) both seem to offer some protection against development of ovarian cancer. The longer total time a woman breastfeeds, the more protected she seems to be. The potential risk linked to use of hormone replacement therapy is unknown at this time.

Overall, ovarian cancer is more common in industrialized Western countries such as Switzerland, the United States, and Scandinavia than anywhere else in the world. In the United States, ovarian cancer is more common among older Caucasian women with a Northern European family history. This trend probably relates to diet and environmental factors, not heredity. Some studies suggest that diets rich in vitamin A and fiber reduce the risk of ovarian cancer, while diets high in saturated fats might increase the risk.

The risk for non-germ cell ovarian cancer increases as women age. Most ovarian cancer occurs in women fifty-five to fifty-nine years of age; fewer than 10 percent occur in women younger than thirty-five. This increased risk relates to the number of ovulations over time. Pregnancy before age twenty-five, early menopause, and use of birth-control pills all reduce the number and frequency of ovulations throughout a woman's lifespan and seem to offer some protection against ovarian cancer. Women with more than forty years ovulating, women who enter menopause later in life, women who have their first pregnancy after age thirty, and women over forty-five who have never been pregnant are all at higher risk for ovarian cancer.

Genetic Factors

Although ovarian cancer is known to run in families, less than 10 percent of ovarian cancers can actually be linked to genetic factors. Increased risk may be related to a number of things, including inherited factors, sharing of a similar environment, or a combination of these things.

A woman's chance of developing ovarian cancer is much higher if her mother, sister, or daughter has had it. The inherited mutations of the BRCA1 (Breast Cancer 1) and BRCA2 genes are probably responsible for almost all cases of familial ovarian cancer, or about 5 percent of all ovarian cancers occurring in women younger than seventy. These genes produce a chemical that helps the body fight off cancer. Most women have two copies of these genes. A defect in one of them limits the production of the cancer-fighting chemical and makes the woman much more likely to develop breast or ovarian cancer at some time during her life. Knowing their BRCA1 and BRCA2 status may be useful to some women in making decisions about health care. BRCA1 and 2 statuses also provide some insight into a woman's prognosis after an ovarian-cancer diagnosis: Women with a BRCA defect seem to have more positive medical outcomes than women without it.

In some treatment centers, women with a strong family history of ovarian cancer are offered the option of having their ovaries removed—**prophylactic oophorectomy**—when they decide not to have any more children. This procedure can be done on an outpatient basis by a skilled gynecologic surgeon using a laparoscope. Some doctors believe that since the ovary is no longer "needed," removal of the ovary *before* cancer develops is a method of preventing cancer. Not all cancer experts endorse this preventive surgery. Some studies suggest that it does not prevent the development of cancer. In fact, women who have had oophorectomy should continue to see their doctor every six months and have the CA125 blood test. There are also questions about the value and function of ovaries even after menopause, with most experts now of the opinion that they do continue to produce low levels of estrogen.

A History of Other Forms of Cancer

A woman who has already had breast or colon cancer has a higher risk of developing ovarian cancer. Cancer of the ovary sometimes occurs at or about the same time as cancers of the breast, colon, and uterus. This suggests that these cancers may have a common cause. Lynch syndrome II is a condition in which a family is more likely to develop ovarian and endometrial cancers, urinary system and kidney cancers, and colon and other cancers of the digestive system. The initial workup for any of these cancers must include testing for the others.

PREVENTIVE MEASURES

We do not know what causes ovarian cancer, so specific preventive measures are impossible to define. But protective factors are known: more than one full-term pregnancy, use of birth-control pills for even as few as three months (though studies point to five years as offering the most protection), and breastfeeding. Tubal ligation may also offer some protection. While women with a strong family history may consider prophylactic oophorectomy as a preventive measure, many find the side effects of removing ovaries and ovarian function—side effects like those of menopause—to be very difficult. A 1994 National Institutes of Health Consensus Statement suggested estrogen replacement therapy for both pre- and postmenopausal women after prophylactic oophorectomy. Without estrogen replacement, a woman who opts for oophorectomy places herself at risk for cardiovascular disease and osteoporosis. In addition, any surgery has risks. A decision to have prophylactic oophorectomy needs to be carefully thought through, with all the pros and cons weighed.

Dietary therapies are often promoted as a preventive measure for cancers. Even though the relationship of diet—vitamins, fiber, and fat—to ovarian cancer is not clear, the benefits of a healthful diet go beyond simply reducing the risk of ovarian cancer.

EARLY DETECTION

Why isn't there a way to screen for ovarian cancer as there is for cervical cancer? The development of screening tests is based on three major factors: (1) the disease must affect a great number of people and cause a great number of deaths, (2) there must be a precancerous or early phase of disease that is simple to detect, and (3) the disease must be one that responds to treatment. In addition, the test itself must clearly point to one disease and it must be relatively inexpensive. So far, no single test meets all three of these criteria for screening women for ovarian cancer, and screening is generally not offered as part of routine checkups for women presumed to be at "normal" risk.

CA125 is an antibody developed by the body in response to some cancers, and it can be detected by a blood test. When CA125 testing is positive, it does not always indicate ovarian cancer, so this is a "nonspecific" test. The CA125 level is increased in only 80 percent of epithelial ovarian cancers, and only half of the women with early stage ovarian cancer have increased levels of CA125. After testing finds abnormal levels of CA125 (normal is below 30 units per milliliter) and a review of the woman's medical history for evidence of risk and symptoms, additional testing generally includes transvaginal ultrasound (also called transvaginal sonography or TVS) and perhaps surgery.

New screening techniques being explored include color Doppler imaging (CDI) studies of ovarian blood vessels, new blood tests, and transabdominal ultrasound. A chemical called **lysophosphatidic acid** (LPA) is a recently discovered tumor marker that some experts believe holds promise in ovarian-cancer screening, but further testing in larger studies is needed before its value is truly known. Another tumor marker that might be useful in early detection is **serine protease**. Its presence in the prostate gland has been known for some time, but it has also been isolated in serum samples from a small number of women with ovarian cancer. Again, more study is needed before we can know for sure that it will be useful.

A new diagnostic test that identifies protein patterns in blood that are unique to ovarian cancer was first described in the cancer literature in 2002. This initial report was in the British medical journal *Lancet*, describing a study that screened blood samples from 116 women—50 who had cancer and 66 who had other noncancerous conditions. The test identified all 50 women with cancer, even those with early stage disease. More trials are needed, of course, but this test may well be available for general use within five years.

There has been no defined screening strategy even for women who have known risks. Still, experts usually recommend that women who have two or more immediate family members (mother, sister, daughter) with a history of ovarian cancer employ a combined approach. A screening strategy that combines CDI, transvaginal ultrasound, CA125, and manual pelvic examinations at regular intervals—**multimodality screening** (the use of several methods)—probably offers the most potential for success in detecting early ovarian cancer.

But even for women who may be at higher risk, the value of screening is not proven. Routine pelvic examinations done with an annual checkup will find one ovarian cancer in ten thousand women examined. The number of ovarian cancers found in this way would increase if the women being examined had developed symptoms. A doctor should assess further if a postmenopausal woman's ovary is large enough to be felt during the pelvic examination.

Several centers have established registry programs that focus on clinical research in early detection, public education about family history, and the importance of diagnostic tests and genetic counseling. The Gilda Radner Familial Ovarian Cancer Registry at the Roswell Park Cancer Institute in Buffalo, New York, is one of the best known of these programs. This center has a toll-free number, (800) 682-7426, and also supports a website at (www.ovariancancer.com).

In women *without* a family history, ovarian cancer is likely to be detected at a later, more difficult to control stage. Early signs and symptoms of ovarian tumors are often vague, if they exist at all. In more than three out of four cases, the cancer has spread outside of the ovary at the time of diagnosis.

Signs and Symptoms

The signs and symptoms of ovarian cancer are usually vague and can easily be attributed to other causes. See a doctor or nurse practitioner if you have the following problems and they persist over a period of time:

+ abdominal swelling or bloating

+ discomfort in the lower abdomen

+ feeling full after a light meal

+ nausea or vomiting

+ not feeling hungry

+ gas, bloating, indigestion

+ weight loss without dieting

+ a constant need to urinate

+ diarrhea or constipation

+ bleeding that is not part of a normal menstrual period

Cancer of the Ovary

Other Symptoms

Ascites causes swelling of the abdomen. Jane noticed that despite not gaining weight, she could not zip her jeans: This was the first symptom of her ovarian cancer. Gilda Radner described abdominal swelling, fatigue, and pain in her thighs and legs. If the cancer spreads to the muscle under the lung that controls breathing (the diaphragm), fluid may build up under the lungs, causing shortness of breath.

A woman must demand attention when she has persistent, unexplained digestive system symptoms, especially if she is over thirty-five and has a personal or family history of problems related to ovarian function.

Differences Between Ovarian and Other Abdominal Masses

Most ovarian tumors are benign; only one in five—20 percent—of all ovarian **neoplasms,** or growths, are cancerous. After a woman notices symptoms, additional tests will determine whether the neoplasm is benign or malignant. The diagnosis is made only after complete microscopic examination of the tumor mass by a pathologist. Ovarian neoplasms are either solid or cystic (fluid-filled).

Endometriosis is a condition in which endometrial tissues are found outside their normal place inside the uterus, such as in various sites throughout the pelvis or in the abdominal wall. The most common sites include the ovaries and the ligaments that support the uterus, peritoneum, and bladder. It occurs most often in women thirty-five to forty-five years of age. Endometriosis can also increase CA125 levels.

Masses in the fallopian tubes usually result from inflammation or tubal (ectopic) pregnancy. Actual neoplasms of the fallopian tubes are rare. Other masses in this area can be tissues "left over" from fetal development. The most common mass found in the abdomen is stool in the lower colon. Examinations after cleaning out the bowel with enemas will confirm or rule out stool as a cause of symptoms of an abdominal mass.

Inflammatory diseases of the small and large intestine may cause symptoms like those of ovarian cancer, such as diarrhea, nausea and vomiting, lack of appetite, and sometimes passage of blood or mucus from the rectum. Abscesses may form. Pain may or may not be noticed. Diverticulitis and other forms of inflammatory bowel disease are examples of conditions that can cause these symptoms.

Tumors of the intestine and kidney may also cause symptoms that can be confused with those of ovarian cancer. Description of the symptoms and X-ray studies are used to find the correct location of the tumor.

DIAGNOSIS

The diagnostic process is likely to take several trips to the doctor's office or the hospital for X rays and other imaging and laboratory tests. Some lab tests require days to complete and report, while staging tests take more time. Still, all of this testing is very necessary. A complete and accurate picture of the problem, cancer or not, is crucial for planning the right treatment. All the while, the woman and those who care about her are forced to wait and wonder. Uncertainty is often the most difficult part of the diagnostic process.

The diagnostic procedure starts with a complete history. This is a series of questions and discussions about the woman's family, past health experience, and pregnancies—including abortion, miscarriage, or stillbirth. A complete history should cover the following areas:

✦ Has any female family member ever had cancer of the ovary?

✦ Description of diet: vitamin supplements, fat content, fiber content

✦ Bowel habits
  - frequency of bowel movements
  - any diarrhea?
  - any constipation?
  - any gas pains?
  - changes in bowel habits; when was a change noticed?

✦ Bladder habits
  - number of times the woman passes water each day
  - color of urine
  - changes in bladder habits; when was a change noticed?

✦ Menstrual history
  - age when menstrual periods began (menarche)
  - age when menstrual periods stopped (menopause)
  - are or were periods regular?
  - are menstrual cramps usual?
  - has there been a change in periods? Describe these changes.

✦ Pregnancies
  - number of pregnancies
  - number of live births
  - any difficulties becoming pregnant?
  - possibility of pregnancy now?

After the history, a physical examination will include a Pap smear and a manual examination of the rectum and vagina. The doctor is looking for lumps or changes in the shape of the pelvic organs.

Because ovarian cancer usually does not show up in a Pap smear, the pelvic examination is the best method for finding ovarian tumors at an early stage. It is best if the bladder is empty, and sometimes laxatives, enemas, or both are used to empty the colon and rectum before the exam. The exam can reveal the size, shape, and location of a mass in the abdomen. Benign tumors usually feel smooth and are fluid-filled. They are movable, usually only involve one side, and are smaller than a tennis ball. Malignant tumors will most likely feel solid, have irregular walls, and are not movable. Ascites is usually found with malignant tumors.

The rest of the workup leading to a diagnosis is tailored to the woman's age, her symptoms, and her general condition. Blood and urine tests will assess liver, kidney, and other body functions. Depending upon the type of tumor suspected, levels of CA125 and other tumor markers in the blood might be tested. Alpha-fetoprotein (AFP) and human chorionic gonadotropin (hCG) tests might be ordered if a germ cell tumor is suspected. The hormone hCG is the hormone detected in some pregnancy tests, but it also shows up in some cancers. AFP is usually found in the human fetus, but it is also present in people who have cancers of the liver, testicle, lung, pancreas, and ovary. CA125 is also elevated (above 35 U/ml) in 80 percent of women with epithelial ovarian tumors.

Usually, this part of the workup takes place in the doctor's office. Some tests require that blood or urine samples be sent to outside laboratories.

After a complete physical exam and history, tests in the diagnostic process are likely to include some or all of the following:

+ **chest X ray** to look for fluid around the lungs and other tumors in the chest

+ **abdominal X ray**

+ **uterine sounding** to outline abnormalities in the uterus and abdomen

+ **Abdominal, pelvic, and/or transvaginal ultrasound** to outline characteristics of a mass and the ovaries, and information about the presence of ascites and involvement of other organs; pelvic ultrasound might be used to rule out pregnancy

+ **barium enema or colonoscopy** to rule out tumors in the rectum and lower (sigmoid) colon if there are symptoms involving the intestines or digestive function

- ✦ **mammography** might be used to rule out breast cancer

- ✦ **CAT** or **CT scan** might be used to define the size and location of a mass

- ✦ **Magnetic Resonance Imaging** (MRI) might be used during diagnosis but is more useful to monitor effects of cancer therapy

- ✦ **laparoscopy** to assess the internal organs of the abdomen using a laparoscope

- ✦ **laparotomy** to define the exact location and appearance of the mass and remove as much of the tumor as possible; this surgery is almost always necessary in the end, if a mass is present

Positron emission tomography (PET) scanning has yet to have much clinical use in the diagnosis of ovarian tumors, but its use is being explored in ongoing studies. At the moment, it is felt to add information to that discovered with more conventional imaging tests like CT and MRI, especially in the setting of recurrent ovarian cancer or follow-up of women who are at risk for recurrence.

After diagnosing cancer, it is important that the pathologist determines the exact kind of cancer. There are nearly forty different types of ovarian cancer, even though almost 90 percent arise from the epithelial surface of the ovary. But there are variations in treatment recommendations depending on how these different cancers behave.

STAGING

After making a cancer diagnosis, staging tests will be completed to find out if the cancer has spread to other parts of the body. The exact definition of the stage of disease is needed so that the best treatment can be planned.

Laparoscopy permits the doctor to see directly inside the abdomen and pelvis. Usually, a **laparotomy**—a surgery to open the abdomen and examine the organs directly—is required to accurately stage the cancer. During the laparotomy, the surgeon looks at all the abdominal organs and does a biopsy of the tumor. Microscopic examination will reveal the presence (or absence) of cell changes that make up what we know as cancer or "malignant changes." Some laboratory techniques can be done immediately, so the rest of the surgical procedure depends on what is seen through the microscope. If an organ is found to contain cancer cells, the surgeon will remove the whole organ or at least as much of the cancer as is possible.

Cancer of the Ovary

285

Diagnostic Imaging Techniques
Used for Ovarian Cancer

Exam	Information about the exam
Barium enema	Restrict diet beforehand to clear fluids, e.g., apple and cranberry juices, water, coffee, tea. Laxatives and enemas are given to clean out the bowel. The enema will feel cool and may cause cramps. The exam takes 30–60 minutes.
Ultrasound	There may be diet restrictions. The bladder should be full unless the doctor asks that the bladder be empty. A gel will be applied to the skin of the area being examined. A transducer, which makes sound waves, is passed over the skin. The woman may feel pressure, but no pain. The exam takes about 30 minutes.
CT scan	Be prepared to lie very still on a hard table for 30–60 minutes. The body is passed through a tunnel in which X rays are taken at precise intervals to make a computerized three-dimensional image.
MRI	Might be used to look for small tumors but is most use-ful in checking for the effectiveness of treatment. The body is placed in a tunnel in which X rays are taken to make a three-dimensional image.

The staging surgery is also the first treatment. Since most women with epithelial cancers already have some cancer spread, more therapy is almost always needed. Adjuvant therapy decisions are based on the stage, size, and location of any tumor that was not removed, presence or absence of ascites, and tumor cells in the ascitic fluid.

Stages of Ovarian Cancer

The International Federation of Gynecology and Obstetrics (FIGO) has outlined a staging system for cancers of the ovary, which offers physicians and other health-care providers a sort of common language for discussing ovarian cancer. In its basic form, the FIGO staging system flows from the earliest, most limited stage, Stage I, to advanced disease with involvement of other organs, Stage IV. It differs from the TNM staging system described in the discussion of breast cancer in Part Two. Some doctors use the TNM system, while others prefer the FIGO. The accompanying table on page 288 describes this staging system.

TREATMENT

Treatment for ovarian cancer is changing so rapidly that it would serve no useful purpose to precisely outline specific treatment protocols here: They might change before this book gets to the printer. For example, there are some very early but exciting developments in the possible use of vaccines against ovarian cancer.

Every person with cancer is encouraged to find the absolute most up-to-date treatment information possible—and that up-to-date information is most likely going to be available on the websites of major cancer centers and the National Cancer Institute (www.cancer.gov). If you are not at ease with computers, get help—a friend, a resource center, a nurse or social worker, a librarian . . . anyone with a bit of computer savvy can help with the search for information.

Before any decision is made with regard to treatment, young women especially may be interested in knowing that new technology and surgical techniques can preserve fertility. All of these techniques can only be used prior to the start of any treatment. Preservation of fertilized embryos is a possibility for women who do have a partner at the time of diagnosis. Assisted reproductive technology now includes the preservation of slices of ovarian tissue. The harvesting of ovarian tissue preserves oocytes, and the tissue can later be reimplanted. Another technique under study is the use of follicles from fetal ovaries. Ask the doctor, nurse, sex educator, or counselor about the options for preserving fertility and sexuality. An Internet search can start with the site offered by the American Society for Reproductive Medicine (www.asrm.org), the Society of Reproductive Surgeons (www.-reprodsurgery.org), or the Society for Assisted Reproductive Technology (www.sart.org).

Treatment plans do usually follow a more or less similar path, so we include a general overview here. Surgery is still the first line of treatment for ovarian cancer. The most positive outcomes are most likely to occur when a qualified and experienced gynecologic oncology surgeon performs the operation. During the operation, the surgeon will assess the fluid volume in the abdomen and samples of the fluid will be analyzed for the presence of cancer cells. When a woman seems to have early stage disease, biopsies should be taken from several areas inside the abdomen and underneath the diaphragm. The surgeon will also carefully inspect the bowel. Lymph nodes in the pelvis and around the aorta will be sampled for the presence of cancer cells. The surgeon will make every effort to remove all or as much of the tumor as possible. The fewer cancer cells left behind, the more likely it is that the woman will be cured.

FIGO Staging System for Cancer of the Ovary

Stage	Description
I	Growth limited to the ovaries
IA	Growth limited to one ovary; no ascites; no tumor on the external surface; capsules intact
IB	Growth limited to both ovaries; no ascites; no tumor on the external surfaces; capsules intact
IC	Tumor either Stage IA or IB but located on the surface of one or both ovaries; or with capsule ruptured; or with ascites present containing malignant cells; or with positive peritoneal washings
II	Growth involving one or both ovaries with pelvic extension
IIA	Extension and/or metastases to the uterus and/or tubes
IIB	Extension to other pelvic tissues
IIC	Tumor either Stage IIA or IIB, but located on surface of one or both ovaries; or with capsule(s) ruptured; or with ascites present containing malignant cells; or with positive peritoneal washings
III	Tumor involving one or both ovaries with peritoneal implants outside the pelvis and/or positive retroperitoneal or inguinal nodes; superficial liver metastasis equals Stage III; tumor limited to the true pelvis but with histologically proven malignant extension to small bowel or omentum
IIIA	Tumor grossly limited to true pelvis with negative nodes but with histologically confirmed microscopic seeding of abdominal peritoneal surfaces
IIIB	Tumor of one or both ovaries with histologically confirmed implants of abdominal peritoneal surfaces, none exceeding 2 cm in diameter; nodes negative
IIIC	Abdominal implants greater than 2 cm in diameter and/or positive retroperitoneal or inguinal nodes
IV	Growth involving one or both ovaries with distant metastases; if pleural effusion present, there must be positive cytology to allot a case to Stage IV; parenchymal liver metastasis equals Stage IV

After surgery, and depending on the cell type and the surgical staging, many women are offered a course of systemic chemotherapy. The drugs most often included in ovarian cancer treatment plans include cisplatin or carboplatin, paclitaxel (Taxol), and cyclophosphamide (Cytoxan). Some protocols only use one of these drugs—"**monotherapy**"—and others use two or more in what is called "**combination chemotherapy**."

Taxol was one of the most important new cancer drugs of the 1990s, and it is responsible for recent advances in the treatment of ovarian cancer. Taxol has side effects that can be at least as toxic as those of other anticancer drugs. Early reports about Taxol's anticancer effects pitted many factions against each other: women who thought Taxol was their best chance for survival, doctors, the drug industry, and environmentalists.

Environmentalists were concerned because, when Taxol was first developed, one Western yew tree (*Taxus brevifolia*) was destroyed to produce two to three doses. Newer formulations of Taxol use the leaves of the tree instead of the bark, a process that allows the tree to survive and produce more leaves. A partly synthetic version of Taxol called Taxotere has been approved for use in the treatment of breast cancer. Taxol and other drugs already in use, new drugs being developed, and more refined surgical techniques offer women more hope for successful treatment of ovarian cancer.

If the surgeon and pathologist determine that it is likely that some cancer is left behind after surgery, radiation therapy might also recommended. Some protocols call for the use of total abdominal and pelvic radiation therapy. Others use intraperitoneal radioactive phosphorus (^{32}P), though not often; its use is associated with later bowel complications.

Ovarian Low Malignant Potential Tumors

Tumors that are described as **low malignant potential tumors** make up about 15 percent of all epithelial ovarian cancers. Most ovarian low malignant potential tumors, nearly three-quarters of them, are in very early stages at diagnosis. The way these tumors behave is quite different from the other, invasive ovarian cancers, and they can be treated and managed much less aggressively.

In early stages—Stage I and Stage II—experts agree that total hysterectomy (TAH) and the removal of both fallopian tubes and ovaries (TAH/BSO) is all the treatment that is likely to be needed. If a woman wants to have children after treatment, it might be possible to remove only a part of the ovary or, in some cases, only the one involved ovary and fallopian tube. However, if her childbearing is not an issue to her, most physicians recommend removing remaining ovarian tissue, as it might put the woman at risk for recurrent tumor. Women with later stage disease will most likely go through TAH/BSO and additional treatment with chemotherapy and/or radiation.

Ovarian Germ Cell Tumors

Fewer than 5 percent of all ovarian cancers are **germ cell tumors**. Again, research findings lead to frequent changes in treatment recommendations, so women with germ cell ovarian cancers are strongly urged to seek up-to-date information and, whenever possible, to participate in a clinical trial that will offer them the most current treatment available. Since these tumors are so uncommon, it is especially important that women who have them take part in clinical trials that will help answer the questions this disease presents.

Treatment plans follow the same general outline as is used in other forms of ovarian cancer—surgery followed by chemotherapy and radiation therapy. At this writing, some of the chemotherapy drugs used in the treatment of germ cell tumors are the same as those used in other forms of ovarian cancer—cisplatin and cyclophosphamide, for example. For germ cell ovarian cancers, other drugs in current chemotherapy protocols include bleomycin, dactinomycin, etoposide, ifosfamide, and vinblastine.

In early stages, ovarian germ cell tumors are usually considered "curable." Again, surgery is the first line of treatment. In Stage I, removal of the affected ovary and fallopian tube (salpingo-oophorectomy) is the treatment of choice, particularly for a young woman who wishes to maintain her ability to bear children. If, after careful and complete staging and successful surgery, the woman is found to be free of tumor, no further treatment is thought to be needed. On the other hand, if staging was for any reason incomplete, or it is decided that the cancer is of a higher, more advanced stage, treatment with chemotherapy or radiation therapy will be recommended. Though cancer recurs in 25 percent of these women, even those with early stage disease, it can be treated with a good chance of cure.

Women with Stage II germ cell tumors might have a limited, fertility-sparing operation in which the affected ovary and fallopian tube are removed, but the uterus and the opposite ovary and fallopian tube are left intact. For women who are not concerned about fertility, total hysterectomy is the treatment of choice. However, women with Stage II disease can expect to go through chemotherapy, and possibly radiation therapy, following surgery.

There is some controversy about the value of what is called "second-look surgery" following initial treatment for Stage II disease. At this time, most experts agree that second-look surgery is not helpful when a woman's tumor is thought to be totally removed during surgery and she has gone through cisplatin-based chemotherapy treatment.

Stage III ovarian germ cell tumors require more aggressive initial treatment. In Stage III, TAH/BSO are recommended, along with removal of as much tumor from the abdominal cavity and pelvis as is possible. If there is any hint of disease remaining after surgery, and fertility is not an issue, radiation therapy will be given after surgery. A very small number of women, under very specific conditions, may be given the chance to preserve fertility by having only the affected ovary and fallopian tube removed—followed without exception by chemotherapy. Here again, second-look surgery is not believed to offer useful information when the tumor is believed to have been totally removed during the initial surgery and the woman has had cisplatin-based chemotherapy.

For Stage IV germ cell tumors, TAH/BSO, along with removal of as much tumor in the abdomen and pelvis as is safely possible, is recommended. As with other stages, fertility can be preserved with careful treatment planning for some women. Chemotherapy following surgery can still cure most women with advanced ovarian germ cell tumors. Radiation therapy is not usually used to treat Stage IV tumors. Second-look operations are not thought to be useful.

Stage I Ovarian Cancer

More than 90 percent of all ovarian cancers are epithelial. The remainder of this treatment review relates strictly to ovarian epithelial cancers.

About 25 percent of women with a newly diagnosed ovarian cancer have early stage (Stage I) disease and the best chance for cure. Total hysterectomy is the treatment of choice for women with Stage I ovarian cancer. This surgery also includes the removal of the **omentum,** a fold of the peritoneum. During the operation, the surgeon will look for signs of cancer cells inside the abdomen. About one-quarter of these women will have lymph nodes in the area removed. For women with Stage I cancer who want to become pregnant later, removal of only one ovary and fallopian tube might be possible. This decision is made based on the stage of cancer—the subsets of Stage I—and grade of the cancer cells (see Chapter 4).

Surgery alone does not always cure even this early stage cancer: The cancer reappears in about 20 percent of women. There is no agreement among experts about what might be the best adjuvant therapy for Stage I ovarian cancer; recommendations are based on the grade, stage subset, and type of the cancer cells. For example, women with grade 3 tumors, those with clear cell carcinoma, and many with Stage IC will require additional, or adjuvant, therapy.

Adjuvant therapy after surgery for women with Stage I disease might consist of radioactive phosphorus (^{32}P) or chromic phosphate placed into the abdomen, systemic chemotherapy, and radiation therapy of the abdomen and pelvis. Chemotherapy often prescribed for early stage ovarian cancer includes Taxol and cisplatin or carboplatin and usually continues for three to six months.

After treatment ends, a woman with Stage I ovarian cancer must continue to see her doctor for monitoring. Current recommendations are that visits to the doctor occur every three months for the first year, every four months for the second year, and then every six months for the next three years. A complete blood count (CBC) and a CA125 test will be taken every visit if the CA125 level was elevated at the time of diagnosis.

If CA125 is found to be increasing during follow-up, experts might recommend another surgery, on the assumption that the cancer has recurred. Other experts might advise waiting until there is clear evidence that the cancer has recurred. This question is heavily debated.

Stage II Ovarian Cancer

The surgery offered for Stage I ovarian cancer is also the surgery of choice for Stage II. Some surgeons will wash the abdomen out during surgery with radioactive phosphorus. Women with Stage II ovarian cancer will be offered chemotherapy regimens using a combination of Taxol and cisplatin or carboplatin, or cyclophosphamide and cisplatin. External radiation therapy may be used, or intraperitoneal phosphorus radiation. Recommendations for follow-up are the same as for Stage I disease. Since so few women are diagnosed at this stage, very little is really known about Stage II ovarian cancer.

Stage III and Stage IV Ovarian Cancer

Stage III and Stage IV ovarian cancer are not cured by surgery alone. In fact, some doctors believe that women with advanced ovarian cancer should not have surgery at all. To make matters even more confusing, no single form of treatment is recognized by doctors as the best, and there is controversy about what might be the best type of surgery. Some surgeons give women with advanced ovarian cancer one or more doses of chemotherapy before surgery, contending that chemotherapy shrinks the tumor and makes cancer cells less likely to escape during surgery. Other surgeons prefer to delay surgery until after a full course of chemotherapy. Sometimes radiation therapy is given directly into the abdomen during surgery.

At this time, the National Cancer Institute recommends treatment with total abdominal hysterectomy, including removal of the fallopian tubes and omentum. As much tumor as possible should be removed. NCI also recommends that surgery be followed by either a chemotherapy program or total abdominal and pelvic radiation therapy.

Side Effects Related to Drugs As Used in the Treatment of Ovarian Cancer

Side Effect	Carboplatin (Paraplatin)	Cisplatin (Platinol)	Cyclophosphamide (Cytoxan)	Paclitaxel (Taxol)	Topotecan (Hycamtin)
Hair loss	X	X	X	X	X
Diarrhea			X	X	X
Shortness of breath					X
Allergic reaction	unusual	X		X	
Mouth sores				X	
Low blood counts	X	X	X	X	X
Nausea and Vomiting	X	X	X	unusual	moderate
Nerve damage	uncommon	X		X	Headache, numbness, tingling sensations
Kidney damage	mild	X			

(adapted from Ovarian Cancer: Diagnosis, Treatment, and Nursing Interventions, Medical Education Systems, Inc., 1996)

Side Effects of Chemotherapy for Ovarian Cancer

The chemotherapy drugs used to treat ovarian cancer are powerful and more effective than ever before; they also cause side effects that can make treatment difficult for most women. Knowing that side effects are likely to occur and being prepared to deal with them are vital to a woman's overall ability to cope with the cancer and its treatment.

The doctor and nurse should prepare the woman for the possible side effects of the drugs proposed in the treatment plan. If this information is not offered, a woman should ask the doctor and nurse what side effects she can expect, and what actions she might take to minimize them.

Cancer of the Ovary

Specific Treatments

Second-look surgery after a chemotherapy program is the most accurate way to find tumors and cancer cells that were not destroyed by chemotherapy. Even though many doctors recommend second-look surgery, its value is debatable.

No study has actually shown an advantage in terms of survival for women who have a second-look operation. The NCI recommends that it be done *only* by a surgeon trained in gynecologic oncology and as part of a clinical trial when a new treatment strategy is being considered.

The benefits of second-look surgery are thought to include (1) allowing therapy to end if no disease is found, (2) pointing to the need to continue therapy if disease is present, and (3) gaining added information that will point to the overall prognosis. During second-look surgery, the surgeon evaluates the same areas that were assessed at the first surgery and makes an extensive sampling of all possible places where the cancer might spread. If a tumor is detected, the surgeon makes every attempt to remove as much of it as possible. **Intraperitoneal chemotherapy** (IP chemotherapy)—chemotherapy that is placed directly into the peritoneal cavity—is sometimes used to treat both early and advanced ovarian cancer. Since ovarian cancer usually spreads to the peritoneum, placing anticancer drugs directly into the peritoneal cavity makes sense. Levels of the drugs that spread out to the systemic circulation are kept low. Most often, women are asked to go through intraperitoneal chemotherapy *after* surgery and *after* they have completed a course of systemic chemotherapy.

IP chemotherapy is given through a tube, or catheter, that is inserted through the abdomen into the peritoneal cavity. If only one or two doses are planned, a temporary catheter might be used instead of a port. These catheters, such as the Tenckhoff and Trocar catheters, are similar to those used for kidney dialysis and require quite a bit of care and attention while they are in place. For this reason, many women and their doctors prefer ports.

A port provides easier access to the peritoneal cavity than other types of access devices and is usually recommended when therapy is likely to involve several IP procedures. The IP port is similar to the port used for vascular access (see the chart "Devices Used to Access a Central Vein" on page 105). The port limits the discomfort and bother related to using temporary access devices. Once the port is in place and the surgical incision has healed, it requires little or no care. There are many kinds of ports, and their care differs. Although a port can stay in place for several years, it will be removed when it is no longer needed. (This requires a minor operation.)

A doctor or nurse can help the woman learn the kind of care a port might require and can discuss what sort of access device is best. The woman should ask questions about where it will be located and whether it will be visible, what will be needed to care for the skin around the port, and whether the catheter requires any special care.

During IP chemotherapy, one to two quarts of fluid with anticancer drugs are allowed to flow into the peritoneal cavity and remain there for up to twenty-four hours. After the prescribed amount of time, the fluid is allowed to drain out. Some of it might stay in the peritoneal cavity; this will be absorbed by the body and is not a serious problem.

Women who have IP chemotherapy experience many different types of sensations while the fluid is in place. Pain is not usually a problem. If discomfort is felt, it is usually compared to gas pains, feeling full or bloated, or having cramps. In practice, I have noticed two things that make a difference. First, most women report that it is more comfortable if the solution is warmed to about body temperature before it is used. The bag of solution can be placed in a microwave oven for a minute or so to take the chill off. Cramps are often the result of letting the solution flow in too fast; slowing the drip rate can help relieve this. Just changing positions in the bed—turning slightly to one side—might also increase comfort.

There are concerns about the use of IP chemotherapy. There is no guarantee that the drugs placed into the peritoneum will come into contact with cancer cells. The techniques used to access the abdomen must be absolutely sterile, as bacteria entering the body through the IP catheter can cause serious infections. And, even after IP chemotherapy has ended, bowel obstruction and bowel adhesions can occur as a late reaction. Other concerns center on the fact that no one has identified the best drug or combination of drugs to use. Of course, the biggest question of all is: Can IP chemotherapy offer a woman more hope for cure, or at least control, of her cancer?

Radiation therapy is not widely used in the United States to cure ovarian cancer but it does have a place in combined modality protocols: It might be used before or after a chemotherapy regimen. Radioactive phosphorus and gold have been used to treat early stage ovarian cancer. Radioactive phosphorus is infused into the peritoneal cavity in a half quart of fluid in much the same way as IP chemotherapy. The woman is asked to change her position every ten to fifteen minutes to allow the fluid to distribute throughout the abdomen.

Radiation can be used to treat specific unpleasant symptoms caused by the cancer. It can reduce tumors or masses that cause pain, bleeding, or other distressing symptoms. Sometimes radiation can be used to slow down the formation of ascites. In these situations, radiation therapy might take only one or two treatments, but it can provide a great deal of comfort.

WHEN OVARIAN CANCER RECURS

Most women who have been diagnosed with advanced ovarian cancer will experience a recurrence of their cancer. Quite often, these women can be treated with chemotherapy again. Treatment for recurrent disease might also involve surgery to remove as much tumor as possible, and chemotherapy with a regimen that contains paclitaxel (Taxol) and cisplatin or carboplatin, especially if these drugs were effective in treating the woman's cancer before.

The chances of a positive response to therapy are good, and they increase as the length of time from initial treatment to recurrence increases; in other words, the more time from treatment to recurrence, the better. New chemotherapy drugs like topotecan, Taxol, and ifosfamide offer increased chances of controlling recurrent and advanced ovarian cancer. Other drugs that might be used include etoposide and altretamine. Hormonal therapy with tamoxifen, megestrol acetate, and leuprolide acetate have also resulted in remission for a few women. External radiation therapy of the abdominal and pelvic areas might be considered.

THE FUTURE

At the moment, there is no way to routinely test for defective BRCA1 genes—but such a test could very well be available soon. Women with a strong family history are well advised to consider registering with a registry such as the Gilda Radner Familial Ovarian Cancer Registry (www.ovarian-cancer.com). Participation in such a system can help women be aware of the latest developments in genetic tests and screening recommendations so that ovarian cancer can be managed much more successfully than in the past.

Biologic therapy may soon be a fourth form of therapy for ovarian cancer. In general, ovarian cancer seems to be very sensitive to the effects of the immune system, and scientists are exploring ways to take advantage of this trait. Experimental studies are being done that use interferon alone and in combination with chemotherapy to treat women with small amounts of tumor left after surgery. Other studies are examining IP interferon.

Monoclonal antibodies also offer hope for new treatments for ovarian cancer. The hope is that agents that are similar to the trastuzumab (Herceptin) that has increased survival for women with breast cancer, and the rituximab (Rituxan) used to treat lymphoma, might be developed to treat ovarian cancer. A monoclonal antibody called "Oregovomab" has been observed to stimulate an immune response that targets ovarian tumors, with the result being increased time between treatment and relapse.

Advances in the study of molecules and biotechnology have led to **gene therapy**, a form of treatment many experts believe holds promise in the treatment of ovarian cancer. Gene therapy is likely to be most helpful for women who have just minimal disease after initial surgery and when combined with other conventional forms of treatment like chemotherapy and radiation. In gene therapy, healthy genes replace damaged or mutated genes that are responsible for causing the development of cancer cells. Genes are transferred that cause conversion of "**prodrugs**" into enzymes that destroy cancer cells. Only the cancer cells are susceptible to the effect of these enzymes, so normal cell damage is avoided. So far, clinical trials using gene therapy for ovarian cancer have documented the safety of this form of treatment, but have not documented a great deal of value in actually affecting the cancer. Nevertheless, experts believe gene therapy definitely holds promise in the treatment of ovarian cancer.

Second-look surgery may be replaced by the use of antibodies that are combined with radioactive substances to pinpoint cancer cells. Tumor-associated antigens or tumor markers such as CA125 and CA 19-9 might eventually be more useful in finding ovarian cancers early. If these measurements are perfected, they could negate the need for second-look surgery.

A new class of chemotherapy drugs called camptothecins is being studied for their value in the treatment of ovarian cancer. Though early results seem promising, the experts think these drugs will expand the effectiveness of the existing drugs rather than work well alone. In 1996, the FDA approved one of these drugs, topotecan (Hycamtin), for use in women with advanced ovarian cancer or those for whom initial therapy was not successful.

As has already been mentioned, treatment for ovarian cancer is changing very quickly. The National Cancer Institute encourages all women with ovarian cancer to consider taking part in a clinical trial, available through cooperative study groups such as the Gynecologic Oncology Group (GOG), in treatment centers throughout the United States. A doctor or oncology nurse should be able to help locate a clinical trial that might be appropriate. More information is available through NCI's Cancer Information Service (see Resources).

It is most important that women facing ovarian cancer demand they get care from physicians who specialize in the treatment of women's cancers. The 'Gilda Radner Familial Ovarian Cancer Registry also offers the

Ovarian Cancer Help-line (1-800-OVARIAN) (682-7426) with a nation-wide listing of gynecologic oncologists. New York's Columbia-Presbyterian hospital offers a second-opinion service especially for women facing ovarian cancer. For more information, see www.secondmedopinion.com.

✦

Ovarian cancer is a frightening disease. Despite some progress in treatment, it is a leading cause of death for American women. Like all kinds of cancer, the best defense against ovarian cancer is to *find it early,* and this requires that every woman really know her body well. Each woman has to be watchful for symptoms that "just do not feel right." All women should have some idea of individual risk factors—especially those that relate to personal and family history. Every woman has to be open in her talks with her doctor or nurse practitioner and share her concerns and her unique history. Lastly, every woman has to be her own best friend. If ovarian cancer is a possibility, a woman's best chance for long-term survival is her demand for the right diagnostic tests.

— *Pamela Haylock*

CHAPTER **16**

CANCER OF THE UTERUS (ENDOMETRIAL CANCER)

The uterus—the womb—lies between the bladder and the rectum. It is usually the shape and size of an upside-down pear, but during pregnancy it expands as the fetus grows.

Cancer of the uterus—endometrial cancer—is the most common gynecologic cancer in the United States. It accounts for about 6 percent of all new women's cancers, affecting about thirty-nine thousand American women each year. The occurrence of cancer of the uterus has increased in the United States and other countries including Norway, Japan, England, and the Czech Republic.

Even though endometrial cancer affects so many women, few die from it. Early diagnosis is the major reason: Most cases are discovered before the cancer spreads outside of the uterus. Most women with endometrial cancer, at least those who have prompt access to good care, can look forward to complete cure of their disease.

The uterus is made up of two layers of tissue: a muscular, outer layer called the **myometrium** and an inner layer called the **endometrium**. The upper portion of the uterus is the **fundus,** the central portion is the body or **corpus,** and the lower end is the **cervix**. The fallopian tubes attach to both sides of the fundus and extend to each ovary.

Like all human tissue, uterine cells normally wear out, die, and are replaced by new cells. Sometimes, abnormal growth takes place and tumors are formed, which can be benign or malignant.

FIBROID TUMORS

Fibroid tumors, or leiomyomas, are benign. They are lumps of smooth muscle cells and connective tissue that develop in the wall of the uterus. Uterine fibroids vary in size from very small—the size of a pinhead—to melon-size. Fibroids are fairly common in women over thirty-five—even those not yet at menopause. Fibroid growth is related to the hormone estrogen, but the exact cause is not yet known. As estrogen production declines at menopause, fibroids can shrink and the problems they cause can go away. Most fibroids do not cause serious symptoms. Some cause no symptoms at all and require no treatment. Fibroids are seldom painful, but large fibroids can press on the bladder or rectum and be uncomfortable, and some may cause heavy bleeding during menstruation. If fibroids cause pain or heavy bleeding, it is a good idea to be assessed for possible treatment. Treatment options depend on many factors, including the kinds of problems the fibroids are causing, the size and location of the fibroids, the woman's age, and her wish to have children. Some doctors will prescribe drugs called GnRH agonists that actually mimic menopausal symptoms. These drugs can shrink fibroids and decrease bleeding and symptoms of anemia that relate to heavy bleeding. GnRH agonists are usually prescribed for a maximum of four to six months. If the fibroids and related symptoms are still present after this time, other treatment may be considered.

The most effective treatment is to remove the uterus—**hysterectomy**. Hysterectomy for noncancerous conditions is a treatment that is accepted by most doctors, but is no longer the first choice for many women, who may feel strongly about keeping their uterus. There are many questions and concerns about the way the uterus is involved in sexual response. Many women believe that orgasm is not as easy to achieve after the uterus is removed; others deny that this is a problem. If women are still of childbearing age, other options may be more suitable.

A procedure called **myomectomy** has become popular for women who do not want hysterectomy. In myomectomy, the surgeon removes only the fibroid tumor, entering the uterus through either the vagina or abdomen, depending on where the fibroid is located. With myomectomy, there is a chance of increased bleeding problems and the fibroids can grow back.

Uterine artery embolization (UAE) has been available for over twenty years, but its use was first limited to controlling severe bleeding problems. The first U.S. study documenting use of UAE to treat symptomatic fibroids was reported in 1996, and it is now thought of as a primary form of treatment for this condition. Basically, the blood vessels that supply nutrients and oxygen to the fibroid are blocked, causing the cells that compose the fibroid to degenerate, the formation of scar tissue, the shrinking of the fibroids, and a decrease in the woman's symptoms—a decrease that is usually dramatic. The procedure is performed by an **interventional radiologist**, a person skilled in performing procedures using radiologic (X-ray) imaging guidance, who inserts a small tube into the uterus through an artery in the groin area. The tube is filled with plastic particles to block the blood supply to the fibroids, causing them to shrink. The procedure is done under local anesthesia and usually does not require a hospital stay beyond twenty-three hours. There are questions about how the procedure might affect fertility, and thus UAE is not performed on women who wish to become pregnant. UAE, like all surgical procedures, is not without risk. The more common adverse reactions include allergic reactions to the contrast material (used to outline the fibroid's vascular supply during the procedure) and other medications used during the procedure. Potential postoperative problems include bleeding at the catheter's insertion site, pain, cramping, nausea, and fever. Women generally go home with prescriptions for pain medicines and antibiotics, but can resume a normal diet and activities fairly quickly. Most resume a normal work schedule within a week of the procedure. There are a few more serious complications, including failure to embolize the fibroid—all of which must be discussed with the radiologist prior to the procedure. Overall, UAE is a fairly safe procedure with high success rates.

ENDOMETRIAL HYPERPLASIA

Endometrial hyperplasia is an abnormal increase in endometrial and stromal cells that can affect all women, even teenagers. Some experts believe endometrial hyperplasia is a precancerous condition (it can be compared to cervical intraepithelial neoplasia, CIN). Sometimes, areas of hyperplasia can revert to normal, with or without medical treatment. Other times, hyperplasia persists or, if untreated, it can go through phases of increasing abnormality until it becomes a true cancer. There is no way to predict which will happen. Most endometrial hyperplasia is thought to be caused by ongoing estrogen stimulation. The most common cause is several menstrual cycles in which an egg is *not* produced.

Heavy uterine bleeding is the main symptom of hyperplasia. Other symptoms might include a history of skipped or delayed periods, or long intervals between periods.

The development of hyperplasia into cancer seems to be fairly slow, taking five years or more.

Treatment for Endometrial Hyperplasia

It is important for women diagnosed with endometrial hyperplasia to have a full workup, because hyperplasia and cancer can be present in a woman's uterus at the same time. What follows are general treatment guidelines; actual recommendations vary according to the woman's age and the cell pattern of the tissues involved.

Teenage girls and older women who want to preserve fertility and who have either "simple" or "complex" hyperplasia can be given hormone therapy—estrogen-progestin pills, such as low-dose birth control pills, given for three to six months—in an attempt to stimulate menstrual cycles. Tissue samples from the uterus will be tested three months after hormone therapy is completed. If they are normal, the woman will be followed for signs that normal menstruation and ovulation are occurring. Additional hormonal therapy is used if ovulation does not occur.

Women with "atypical" hyperplasia risk the hyperplasia turning into, or progressing to, cancer. Dilatation and curettage, or D&C (see Chapter 4), is recommended because atypical hyperplasia often occurs at the same time as uterine cancer, and a D&C offers a way to detect uterine cancer. Women who wish to keep their fertility and women who cannot go through surgery should be prescribed high-dose progestins and have uterine biopsies regularly.

The childbearing-age woman is treated with hormone therapy for three months, and tissue sampling is done right after this is completed. Hormone therapy to induce ovulation can be prescribed when the tissue samples are normal, or, if the woman is not interested in becoming pregnant, she can continue to use the estrogen-progestin hormones to induce normal, though artificial, menstrual cycles. Follow-up will include endometrial biopsy and a transvaginal sonogram. A D&C may be done when therapy is finished. As long as the uterus is present, progestin therapy should be continued since the risk of further hyperplasia developing remains. The uterus should be assessed regularly.

The woman nearing or in menopause may be treated with a hysterectomy or low doses of progestin. The need for hysterectomy is determined by the severity of the hyperplasia, the woman's wish for sterilization, and the presence of such symptoms as severe uterine bleeding. In some cases, hysterectomy may be recommended if a uterine tumor is suspected.

For the postmenopausal woman, unless she is not physically able, hysterectomy is usually recommended since the risk of developing cancer is quite high. Women who have not had a period for at least two years and have hyperplasia may very often have endometrial or ovarian cancers too. Progestin therapy might be offered to a woman whose physical condition will not allow her to go through an operation.

RISK FACTORS FOR UTERINE CANCER

As with most other cancers, age is the most important risk factor for the development of uterine cancer. Most women who develop uterine cancer are fifty to fifty-nine years old, and the average age is sixty-one years. Twenty-five percent are diagnosed before menopause, and 5 percent of these cancers occur in women younger than forty years.

Another risk factor for endometrial cancer is the use of "unopposed" estrogen replacement therapy for menopausal symptoms. The risk of developing cancer increases with the length of use and the dose of estrogens. It increases after two to four years of use and is greatest with large doses. So far, it is not known if or when the risk drops to that of a "nonuser" after estrogen is stopped. When estrogen used in replacement therapy is given in combination with (or "opposed by") a progesterone, the added risk of endometrial cancer associated with HRT disappears. The doctor or nurse will recommend the dose and schedule that maximizes benefits and minimizes risks.

Women who are obese produce more estrogen than women who are near average weight. An obese woman's risk of developing endometrial cancer is similar to that of a woman who takes estrogen replacements. Even a woman who is 30 pounds over her ideal weight has an increased risk of developing uterine cancer. Women with polycystic ovary syndrome, a condition in which cysts form on the ovary resulting in abnormal estrogen production, and some ovarian tumors are also more prone to develop endometrial cancer. The combined effects of hypertension (high blood pressure), diabetes, and obesity cause more women to develop uterine cancer. It is not clear why hypertension has an effect on the uterus; it may be that hypertension is caused by the diabetes and obesity and is not directly related to uterine cancer.

Women who begin menstruation early and women who go into menopause late are more prone to develop uterine cancer. Women who have never been pregnant are at slightly higher risk than women who have. Caucasian women, women of higher social and economic status, those who live in cities, and those of Jewish descent seem to be more at risk for uterine cancer. Black women have nearly double the death rate from uterine cancer as compared to white women.

Women who have had external radiation therapy to the pelvis are at higher risk of developing uterine cancer. A history of pelvic radiation therapy seems to be related to the development of cancer in 10 percent to 25 percent of women with this form of cancer; these women may have received radiation therapy anywhere from five to twenty-five years before the development of uterine cancer.

Women who have already had breast and ovarian cancers also have an increased risk of developing uterine cancer. The hormonal changes that go with other conditions, such as polycystic ovaries, menstrual problems, and inability to produce or release eggs (called **anovulation**), increase the risk of developing endometrial hyperplasia or uterine cancer. There is an increased risk of uterine cancer linked to tamoxifen treatment of breast cancer. Women who are on tamoxifen should have regular pelvic exams and should be examined right away if there is bleeding between menstrual periods.

The increase in the number of women with uterine cancers throughout the world suggests that environmental or dietary factors might also be involved.

PREVENTION

As strange as it seems, cigarette smoking has been linked to a *reduced* risk of uterine cancer—especially in women over fifty and those who are postmenopausal. This may be because smoking reduces estrogen production. However, *no one* should take up smoking to counteract the possibility of getting uterine cancer: Both active and passive smoking have so many more serious—and less treatable—health hazards for women!

The use of progestins (another female hormone) as part of estrogen replacement therapy also seems to either remove the risk or at least delay its onset. Birth-control pills that combine estrogen and progesterone in the same pill used for at least twelve months seem to offer some protection, with this protective effect lasting for at least fifteen years after the birth-control pills have been stopped.

EARLY DETECTION

Endometrial cancer is unique among most women's cancers in that it produces symptoms very early. Any new onset of heavy uterine or vaginal bleeding is a warning signal—even abnormally heavy bleeding in a premenopausal woman. Although this symptom is frightening, it does cause most women to seek medical care immediately. For some women, spotting or a blood-streaked, watery vaginal discharge that is either constant or seems to come and go might be a first symptom. Very rarely, low back pain is noticed by women who have advanced disease.

On the other hand, vaginal bleeding is not always a sign of endometrial cancer. Other cancers, like cancer of the cervix, vulva, and vagina, might cause similar symptoms. Vaginal infection can also cause vaginal bleeding. Sometimes bleeding from inflammatory bowel disease, hemorrhoids, and kidney and urinary tract problems can be confused with bleeding from the vagina.

DIAGNOSIS

Endometrial cancer is diagnosed using the same process as other gynecologic cancers. The nurse and/or doctor will take a complete history. The physical exam will include an examination of the vagina and genitals, looking especially for the presence of bleeding. The bimanual exam helps define the size, position, and shape of the uterus. The doctor or nurse practitioner uses two hands. In this "bimanual" exam, two fingers of one hand are used to examine the inside of the vagina. The other hand is used to apply pressure from the outside to compress the ovaries and the uterus between the hands. The Pap smear that is so useful in the diagnosis of cervical cancer is not as valuable in the diagnosis and workup of endometrial cancer. Still, it is likely to be included in a full workup since it might pick up some endometrial cells as well as cells from the cervix. Endocervical curettage provides tissue samples from the endocervical canal and is done *before* samples are taken from the endometrium. Endometrial sampling can be done by aspiration, biopsy, or a D&C. Any suspicious area on the cervix should also be biopsied in order to rule out cervical cancer.

Transvaginal ultrasound can help assess postmenopausal bleeding by measuring the thickness of the uterine lining. A thicker lining is more common in cancers than is a thinner (less than 5 mm) lining. This test is helpful when pelvic examination is difficult, such as in obese women. It may also help define which women should have a D&C, an especially helpful piece of information when considering the possible risks of anesthesia and D&C.

Chest X rays evaluate the status of the lungs and possible metastasis to the lungs. A **urogram** (X ray of the urinary tract) and a barium enema are used to look for tumors blocking or pressing on the ureters or bowel. Cystoscopy, sigmoidoscopy, or colonoscopy help the doctor decide whether the tumor has spread to the bladder or rectum. Ultrasound and a CT scan may be used to determine the extent of disease.

TYPES OF UTERINE CANCER

The most common form of uterine cancer, **endometrioid carcinoma** or **adenocarcinoma,** starts in the gland-filled lining of the uterus. There are four main types of adenocarcinoma: Ciliated adenocarcinoma, secretory adenocarcinoma, papillary or villoglandular adenocarcinoma, and adenocarcinoma with squamous differentiation—adenoacanthoma and adenosquamous. Together, the various forms of adenocarcinoma make up 75 percent to 80 percent of all uterine cancers. Other less common types of uterine cancer are uterine papillary serous (less than 10 percent), **clear cell** (4 percent),

Staging of Endometrial Carcinoma (FIGO System)

Stage	Characteristics
0	Abnormal hyperplasia or carcinoma in situ
IA	Tumor is limited to the endometrium
IB	Tumor invades less than halfway through myometrium
IC	Tumor invades more than halfway through myometrium
IIA	Endocervical glandular involvement only
IIB	Cervical stromal invasion
IIIA	Tumor invades serosa (the membrane that surrounds the outer wall of the uterus), adnexa (the organs connected to the uterus—the fallopian tubes and ovaries), and/or positive peritoneal cytology (cells present in peritoneal fluid)
IIIB	Vaginal metastases
IIIC	Metastases to pelvic and/or lymph nodes around the aorta
IVA	Tumor invades bladder and/or bowel
IVB	Metastases to distant organs, into the abdomen or inguinal (groin) lymph nodes

mucinous (1 percent), **squamous** (less than 1 percent), and with the remainder classified as **undifferentiated**. The clear cell and papillary types grow and spread more quickly and require more aggressive treatment.

Uterine sarcoma is very rare. It originates in the muscle or supporting tissues of the uterus and makes up less than 5 percent of all uterine cancers and less than 1 percent of all the gynecologic cancers. It has two distinct forms: leiomyosarcoma—arising from the uterine muscle—and mesodermal or mullerian and stromal sarcomas that start in endometrial epithelium. The only known risk factor for endometrial sarcomas is a history of radiation to the pelvis—usually radiation given from five to twenty-five years earlier as a treatment for uterine bleeding.

TREATMENT

The selection of treatment for uterine cancer depends on the type of cancer and the stage of disease. Early stage endometrial cancer—when the cancer has not penetrated through the two layers of the uterus—can usually be cured with removal of the cervix, uterus, ovaries, and fallopian tubes (hysterectomy and bilateral salpingo-oophorectomy). In cases where the tumor has gone through the wall of the uterus, or is thought to be an especially virulent cancer, surgery can be combined with radiation therapy. For women whose cancers have spread outside the uterus, hormonal therapy might be added to the treatment plan.

During surgery, it is important that the surgeon have tissue samples sent to the pathologist to test for the presence of hormonal receptors for progesterone and estrogen. For women who are unable to have surgery because of other health conditions, treatment can consist of radiation therapy alone, though cure rates are not as high as for those who have surgery. The combination of surgery plus chemotherapy is being studied at the National Cancer Institute and other research groups for both adenocarcinomas and sarcomas that have spread outside of the uterus (Stage III and above). Chemotherapy drugs used in clinical trials so far include ifosfamide, cisplatin, and doxorubicin.

Women who have early stage and limited disease are usually thought to be curable with removal of the uterus, ovaries, and fallopian tubes—hysterectomy and bilateral salpingo-oophorectomy. If the tumor has invaded deep into the muscle layer—myometrial muscle—additional treatment with radiation therapy is usually recommended. Some experts advocate the brachytherapy technique—using the vaginal candle or cylinder—that delivers radiation directly to the vaginal cuff as a way to reduce the risk of recurrence in the vagina.

The progestational hormones—hydroxyprogesterone (Delalutin), medroxyprogesterone (Provera), and megestrol (Megace)—are most commonly prescribed as a way to manage later stage disease or cancers in women who are unable to tolerate other, more aggressive, forms of therapy.

Advanced or Recurrent Disease

Treatment for advanced and recurrent uterine cancer varies according to how much or how far the cancer has spread and which organs and body systems are affected.

When there is a large tumor, both internal (radiation sources placed inside the uterus) and external radiation might be used. Hormonal therapy is useful when there is evidence that the tumor has spread, or metastasized. In advanced sarcoma, clinical trials currently combine two or more chemotherapy drugs.

Recurrent sarcoma and carcinoma are not generally considered curable. Instead, therapy can offer hope for controlling the disease and managing such distressing symptoms as pain, bleeding, and feelings of abdominal pressure. Treatment goals are guided by the extent and location of the cancer and its symptoms. Women with recurrent sarcoma can be offered chemotherapy.

Doctors sometimes adopt treatment plans from clinical trials even though the patient is not enrolled. Sarcoma trials are currently underway that look at the effects of various combinations of chemotherapy drugs that are individually known to have some positive effect on sarcoma. Some sarcomas have responded to radiation therapy, and progesterone hormone therapy can be helpful for women with some recurrent sarcomas.

Recurrent endometrial carcinoma can sometimes respond to radiation therapy. When recurrence is limited to the vagina, radiation has provided a cure for a few women. Women who test positive for estrogen and progesterone receptors respond better to progestin therapy. Negative receptor status usually means that a woman will not get much benefit from hormonal therapy. On the other hand, it sometimes predicts a better response to chemotherapy. Tamoxifen, the drug often used to treat postmenopausal women with breast cancer, is sometimes useful in the treatment of endometrial carcinoma—especially with those for whom progesterone therapy did not work.

In some women, even though other organs seem to be negative for cancer cells, there is evidence that the cancer has probably spread outside of the uterus. During surgery, fluid from inside the abdomen (peritoneal fluid) is collected and examined for cancer cells. The presence of these cells might mean that the cancer is more advanced than was previously thought, and treatment plans are likely to be changed in light of these findings. The chemotherapy drug doxorubicin seems to have some affect against uterine cancers and is combined with other drugs to treat advanced and recurrent disease. Clinical trials are being developed to find the most effective treatment for this situation.

Future Trends, Clinical Trials

Treatment for early cancer of the uterus is very effective and most women with early disease can be cured. However, there is no standard treatment— no treatment that is endorsed by a majority of doctors—for metastatic cancer of the uterus. Current studies are looking at ways to manage advanced disease more effectively. Most of these studies evaluate the effects—both positive and negative—of combining drugs, hormones, surgery, and radiation. The studies vary by the order in which these standard therapies are used and the doses given.

Some experts advocate the use of intraperitoneal radioactive phosphorus when cancer cells are found in the peritoneal fluid during surgery. (Radioactive material in a fluid is allowed to flow into the abdomen in much the same way as when intraperitoneal chemotherapy is given.) Other approaches include external radiation given to the whole abdomen. Other studies are testing the effect of systemic chemotherapy versus no chemo-therapy for women who have cancer cells in the peritoneal fluid.

After Treatment

After hysterectomy and removal of the ovaries, women are at high risk for **osteoporosis** (brittle bones). These women can prevent or at least diminish the problem by increasing their dietary intake of calcium to 1,500 mg/day (by taking supplements, eating dairy products, and so on). A vitamin D supplement improves the body's ability to use calcium. Weight-bearing exercises like walking, step aerobics, and swimming can minimize and even stop bone loss. Large amounts of caffeine and fiber can reduce the amount of calcium that is absorbed.

After treatment, a woman still needs an annual Pap smear and a general exam of the uterus, cervix, ovaries, and/or vagina (depending on the type of treatment). Although many women forego annual gynecologic exams and/or general medical exams after hysterectomy, for some (especially older women) the lack of regular medical checkups results in the development of other problems. For example, elderly women who have had hysterectomies are found to have more advanced vaginal or vulvar cancers than women who continue to get annual or regular gynecologic checkups.

QUESTIONS TO ASK YOUR PHYSICIAN

1. Should I get a prescription for a progestin along with estrogen replacement therapy?

2. What will be the long-term side effects of each of the treatment options I have been offered?
   — surgery (see the information about hysterectomy and surgical treatment for cervical cancer in Chapter 17)
   — radiation therapy
     - will there be changes in sexual function?
     - what can I do to prevent or at least decrease side effects?
   — chemotherapy
     - what are the side effects of each drug?
     - what can I do to prevent or at least decrease these side effects?
   — hormone therapy
     - will there be changes in sexual function?
   — what are the side effects of each drug?

- what can I do to prevent or at least decrease these side effects?

3. Will the surgeon request hormone receptor testing on surgical specimens? If not, why?

4. What is the schedule for follow-up examinations and what will be included in the exams?

HORMONE REPLACEMENT THERAPY

Hormone replacement therapy (HRT) has been used for over fifty years to treat postmenopausal symptoms and other conditions associated with and following menopause, and is often prescribed after a hysterectomy. In fact, it became more or less standard therapy before its actual effectiveness and safety were known. A major risk of hormone replacement therapy is that estrogens are linked to the development of endometrial hyperplasia, which is in turn related to the development of endometrial cancer. This association is very strong for postmenopausal women—the very group in which three-fourths of all endometrial cancer is found.

The Women's Health Initiative clinical trial studying hormone replacement therapy was abruptly ended in mid-2002 when data revealed that women using both estrogen and progestin actually experienced slightly higher rates of heart attacks, strokes, breast cancer, and blood clots. The entire rationale and strategies for hormone replacement therapy have finally come under close scrutiny. Dr. Susan Love, author of *Dr. Susan Love's Hormone Book* and adjunct professor of surgery at U.C.L.A. Medical School, in a *New York Times* editorial, says that we must take "the time to determine the safety and efficacy of a particular therapy before we embrace it." Since hormone replacement therapy has been offered as a preventive measure, she suggests that it is more important to focus on lifestyle changes—such as quitting smoking, eating a healthy diet, and exercising regularly. Finally, Dr. Love says that we need to demand that the practice of medicine be "based on solid evidence, not hunches or wishful thinking."

Other physicians will continue to offer women the choice to use HRT, but are likely to pay more attention to the real reasons women want HRT and to explore other or additional ways to achieve the same outcomes. Natural hormonal products—as opposed to synthetic products—are favored by many physicians. Routes of administration, such as via creams applied to the skin, diminish hormonal affects on the liver. Women who choose to use HRT need medical checkups every six to twelve months, which should include the following:

- blood pressure

- breast exam

- pelvic exam

- uterine tissue sampling (biopsy) if there is abnormal bleeding

Estrogen from any source can cause the development of hyperplasia. The role of estrogen in the development of endometrial cancer is receiving a great deal of attention in both the scientific and lay press. **Diethylstilbestrol** (DES), a synthetic estrogen, has been a known carcinogen since at least 1940, but it was used to prevent miscarriages from the mid-1940s right on into the 1980s and is blamed for an increased incidence in rare gynecologic cancers in daughters born to women who took it. Nevertheless, it is still used in HRT. (For more on DES, see Chapter 18).

In the past, a woman with a medical history that included uterine or breast cancer would not have been given hormone replacement therapy, but recent studies have demonstrated that uterine cancer does not absolutely rule out HRT.

How HRT Is Used

HRT is useful in the treatment of menopausal symptoms that affect quality of life—symptoms like the wretched hot flashes and night sweats, mood swings, forgetfulness, insomnia, and vaginal dryness. But since the relevations from the Women's Health Initiatve study have been made public, its actual risks and benefits are increasingly difficult to sort out. There is just one point on which experts seem to have some agreement: Shorter is better—taking HRT is not necessarily harmful, but taking hormones for the shortest time possible is best. There is no one best regimen. Instead, it is important that a woman and her doctor or nurse practitioner work out a hormone replacement plan that is highly individualized for that woman. Before a doctor prescribes HRT, the woman must go through a complete history and physical to identify her risk factors. If she has any history of abnormal uterine bleeding, she needs a more thorough evaluation that includes getting tissue samples from her uterus. The more common estrogen preparations and doses vary, but the effects are the same. Common doses are as follows:

Ethinyl estradiol	0.02 mg/day
Conjugated estrogens	0.625 mg/day
Estrone	1.25 mg/day

Medroxyprogesterone (Provera) 2.5 mg/day is an example of a progestin dose that might be prescribed. A woman might take an estrogen preparation that contains testosterone—such as the formulation called Estratest, in an attempt to counter other menopausal symptoms such as decreased sex drive or libido, nervous symptoms, and depression. A skin patch or "transdermal system" is available that delivers a controlled dose of estrogen and a progestin—over a time frame of a few days. These are convenient, eliminating the need to remember to take pills every day, but they have been known to cause skin irritation and discomfort. It's best to talk about routes of administration and drug delivery with the prescribing doctor or nurse.

The dose is likely to be much higher for a young woman who goes into early menopause after surgery or radiation therapy removes or destroys her ovaries. Doses should be increased *only* if symptoms are very severe and intolerable. Most doctors recommend that the estrogens be given in a cycle, with five to seven days each month off the drug. Some prefer including progestin therapy in the cycle—giving progestins the last ten days of each monthly cycle in addition to the estrogen. Progestin along with estrogen in the schedule of HRT seems to decrease the development of uterine hyperplasia and uterine cancers. This treatment schedule mimics the normal menstrual cycle and therefore might result in bleeding that resembles menstrual bleeding, even in women who are late postmenopausal. Some doctors prescribe estrogen and progestin doses daily—either continuously or on weekdays only with no drugs given on Saturday and Sunday. This schedule prevents bleeding.

In some situations, such as when a woman has had a form of cancer that is estrogen-dependent, estrogens cannot be given. Menopausal symptoms can be relieved to some extent by daily doses of progestins such as megestrol acetate (Megace) or medroxyprogesterone (Provera). These drugs reduce the hot flashes and sweating but may cause vaginal dryness, increased appetite, and weight gain.

If a woman cannot use or decides not to use HRT, is she just destined to endure the symptoms that bother so many perimenopausal and menopausal women? Not necessarily: There are measures that women can take on their own or with their doctors that might alleviate some of the more troublesome problems that accompany menopause and aging. These are outlined in the following table, and more details can be found in many good books currently available (see Resources).

— *Pamela Haylock*

Ways to Treat Menopausal Symptoms
Without the Use of HRT

Symptom	Action or Treatment	Comments
Hot flashes and night sweats	No intervention	Symptoms will decrease on their own over time
	Antidepressants such as Prozac and blood pressure medications may be helpful.	Prescription for antidepressants and antihypertensives and physician monitoring are required
	Avoid spicy foods	Dietary interventions can be done on your own
	Minimize alcohol and caffeine consumption	
	Try soy products	
	Black cohosh, a Native American herbal remedy	Available in over-the-counter medicines such as RemiFemin
	Try deep breathing when you feel a "hot flash" coming on	
	Wear natural fiber (cotton, linen, silk, hemp, for example) clothing in layers	Synthetic fibers like rayon, nylon, and polyester are not generally as breathable as natural fibers
	Sleep in the nude or wear a cotton, linen, or silk nightgown	Elastic in pajamas, panties, and bras can add to discomfort
	Use all-cotton bed linens instead of polyester or cotton/polyester blends	
Osteoporosis	Bisphosphonate drugs like Fosamax, the anti-estrogen Raloxifene, and calcitonin can be prescribed to slow down bone loss	Requires prescription and physician monitoring
	Make sure your daily diet has at least 1,000–1,200 mg of calcium—with calcium rich foods or calcium tablets. Supplement with Vitamin D to insure uptake of calcium	Dietary and exercise interventions can be done on your own
	Include weight-bearing exercises (such as walking and weight-lifting) in a regular exercise program	

Ways to Treat Menopausal Symptoms
Without the Use of HRT

Symptom	Action or Treatment	Comments
Insomnia	Over-the-counter sleep medications such as Sominex might be helpful	These medications are technically nonaddictive, but they can cause daytime drowsiness. Many contain the antihistamine diphenhydramine
	Herbal remedies such as Valerian and hops are helpful to some	
	Try the old fashioned "glass of warm milk" at bedtime	
	Try a warm shower or a soaking bath with scented bath salts	Consult with an aromatherapy expert for advice about soothing scents
Vaginal dryness	Try readily available lubricants like K-Y jelly and Replens	Lubricants—and the decision to engage in sexual activity—are choices that women can make on their own
	Regular sexual activity stimulates production and releases normal vaginal lubricants	
	Estrogen ointments and implantable rings help stimulate production and release of the body's normal lubricants	Ointments and rings require prescriptions
Mood swings and forgetfulness	Both symptoms might be related to sleep deprivation caused by hot flashes, night sweats. Try to improve the sleep problem as suggested above	All of these can be self-care measures women can undertake on their own.
	Black cohosh, the herb suggested to curb hot flashes, might also help stabilize emotions	Discuss use of herbal preparations and possible interactions with other prescription and over-the-counter medicines with your health-care provider
	St. John's wort has helped some women with mild anxiety and depression	
	Physical exercise can restore emotional stability	
	Engage the mind in mental exercises like word games, crossword puzzles, and stimulating conversations	

Ways to Treat Menopausal Symptoms
Without the Use of HRT

Symptom	Action or Treatment	Comments
Heart disease	Stop smoking	Smoking cessation, exercise and diet are all within a woman's own control. Expert help from smoking cessation professional, nutritionist, and physical therapist or trainer might be useful in starting a new self-care plan
	Moderate exercise may improve blood pressure and cholesterol levels	
	Choose a "heart-healthy" diet: low-fat, low-salt, and include plenty of vegetables, fruits and grains	
	Women with high cholesterol, family history of heart disease, and existing heart disease might consider lipid-lowering medicines.	Requires prescription and monitoring

CHAPTER 17

CANCER OF THE CERVIX AND CERVICAL DYSPLASIA (CIN)

Cancer of the cervix is, most often, a preventable disease. Nevertheless, it is the second most common cancer in women, and the leading cause of cancer deaths worldwide. Each year, 450,000 women are found to have cervical cancer and 240,000 die of this disease. Cervical cancer was the most common cause of cancer deaths in American women well into the 1930s, but introduction of the Papanicolaou (Pap) smear changed the picture dramatically. Since the introduction of the Pap, the death rate from cervical cancer has gone down by more than 40 percent. Now, cancer of the cervix is diagnosed in about 13,000 U.S. women each year, and the number of new cases has decreased over the past decade. Most recent statistics tell us that 4,000 women in the United States die from it annually.

There are ethnic and racial differences in the U.S. rates of cervical cancer, with Vietnamese women in America having the highest rate of cervical cancer and Japanese-American women the lowest. Most cases of cervical cancer should be found early through the use of the Pap smear, but the fact that 4,000 American women die from cervical cancer every year says that too many women do not get Pap smears. Despite the fact that the Pap smear has been endorsed by the American Cancer Society since 1957 as the screening test for cervical cancer, nearly one-third of all American women do not get Pap smears, and half of the women who are diagnosed with cervical cancer have never had a Pap smear.

Before cancer cells develop, some cells of the cervix go through abnormal changes called **dysplasia,** which may alter the size and shape of individual cervical cells, or the structure of the tissues made up of these cells. A Pap smear detects these abnormal cells. The right treatment during the dysplasia stage can prevent cells from going through more changes that would turn them into cancer cells. This is why an annual Pap smear is so important.

Eighty percent of all cervical cancers are diagnosed in developing countries. Women at greatest risk include those living in poverty, women over fifty years of age, and women who are illiterate. In developed countries, such as the United States, migrant and indigenous (Native American) women are also at high risk of developing cervical cancer.

NORMAL STRUCTURE OF THE CERVIX

At the lower end of the uterus, the tissue is squeezed together to form the cervix. The cervix, which is about one inch long, extends into the upper part of the vagina. The opening on the uterine side of the cervix is called the **internal cervical os** (*os* is the Latin word for "mouth"). Another small opening, the **external cervical os,** connects the inside of the uterus with the vagina. Normally the cervix is composed mainly of connective tissue lined with mucous membrane. Mucous membrane, a special form of epithelium, is the same type of tissue that lines the mouth, the entire digestive system, the reproductive organs, and the urinary tract. Connective tissue gives form and shape to organs. The mucous membrane of the cervix blends with the mucous membrane that lines the vagina; the area where cells of the cervix and cells of the vagina blend is the transformation zone, so called because the cells on one side are of one specialized type, and the cells on the other side are of another. These normal cells are constantly being shed, just like cells from the skin are shed. The Pap smear or Pap test (named after Dr. Papanicolaou, who discovered that cells from the cervix are shed into vaginal fluid) involves scraping some shed cells from the surface of the cervix and looking at them under the microscope.

DYSPLASIA OR CERVICAL INTRAEPITHELIAL NEOPLASIA (CIN)

Intraepithelial neoplasia is a premalignant (precancerous) change that can occur on the cervix, the vulva, and the vagina. Cervical intraepithelial neoplasia (CIN) affects more than fifty thousand American women each year. For some women, CIN will progress to cancer, but there is no way to predict whether CIN will or will not become cancer or the time frame in which the changes might take place.

When I was twenty-five years old, I worked on a study that involved women with early stage cervical cancer. While I was reading what seemed like volumes of books and articles about cervical cancer, I saw my gynecologist for a routine checkup. I was shocked when the doctor's office called to tell me that my "Pap smear wasn't quite normal" and asked that I schedule a biopsy. In the time between that phone call and my appointment, I read

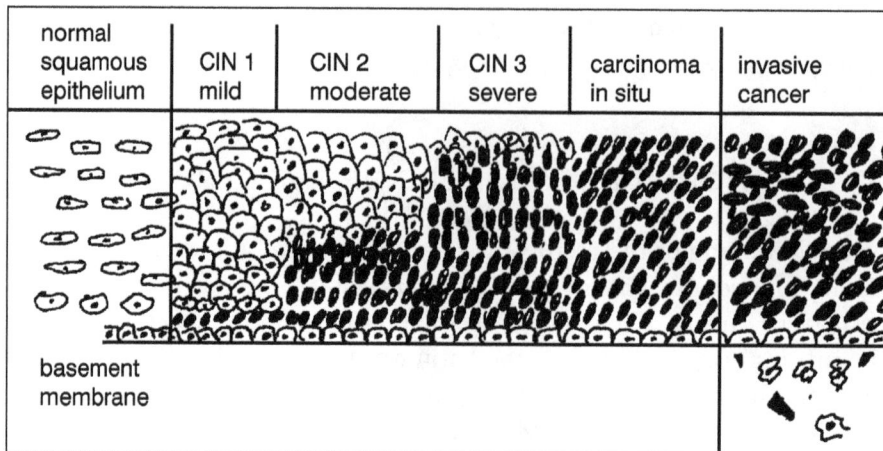

normal squamous epithelium	CIN 1 mild	CIN 2 moderate	CIN 3 severe	carcinoma in situ	invasive cancer

basement membrane

Precancerous lesions: CIN, carcinoma in situ, invasive cancer

everything else I could get my hands on about cervical cancer. By the time I had the biopsy, I was convinced that I had it. But I didn't bother to read much about dysplasia. I had the colposcopy and biopsy on a Thursday, and the pathology results would not be ready until the following Tuesday. In the five days I had to wait, I drove two hundred miles to Chicago to be with a friend for support. I was a basket case.

To make a long story short, the pathology report was encouraging: I did not have cervical cancer. I did, however, have severe dysplasia. The treatment of choice at that time was cryosurgery (destroying the abnormal cells with extreme cold), which I had without problem. There was a school of thought that birth-control pills were a factor in cervical dysplasia, so I was introduced to a diaphragm. (Newer forms of birth-control pills are not as likely to cause dysplasia.) It took almost two years for my Pap smear tests to revert to normal, but they did, and have remained so for over twenty-five years.

Cervical dysplasia, or CIN, can be scary. I knew enough to know that abnormal cells can be a sign of cancer. This experience showed me very early in my nursing career that even a slight chance of cancer is really frightening. The fact that my diagnosis was not cancer and that my Paps have remained normal is a positive comment on the value of routine check-ups and early treatment of CIN. The most important message is this: Do not be paralyzed with fear when you find you have CIN. Go through the diagnostic process and get the right treatment as soon as possible.

Dysplasia literally means "bad molding" and refers to abnormal tissue development. The degree of dysplasia is based on the proportion of normal cells that are replaced by abnormal cells and the severity of cell changes. CIN Grade I (mild dysplasia) involves less than one-third of the thickness of the cervical epithelium, CIN II (moderate dysplasia) involves one-third to two-thirds of the thickness of the epithelium, and CIN III (severe dysplasia and carcinoma in situ) represents two-thirds to full-thickness involvement of the cervical epithelium.

Who Gets Cervical Cancer and CIN?

The average age for women to have CIN is around twenty-eight. Over the past few years, more women in their late teens and early twenties have been found to have CIN. In one study involving eight hundred women with CIN, a third were twenty or younger at the time of diagnosis.

The risk factors for CIN and cervical cancer are the same: cigarette smoking, economic status, sexual activity, and viruses. Many of these factors are related, and sometimes it is not possible to identify any one specific risk. For example, African-American, Hispanic, and Native American women are at a higher risk for CIN and cervical cancer, but this is most likely related to factors caused by economic status, not genetic or hereditary factors.

Women who do not eat enough foods containing vitamin A (retinol) are at higher risk for CIN and cervical cancer. Women who have their first sexual experience at an early age and have several sexual partners over the years are more likely to develop CIN and cervical cancer. A problem in pinpointing any one of these risks as *the* cause of CIN is that women living in poverty often marry and have children earlier than do other women.

A woman with only one sexual partner is still at risk if her sexual partner has had many other partners. A woman who is married to a man whose previous wife had cervical cancer is at higher risk for developing CIN.

CIN does seem to be a venereal or sexually transmitted disease (STD), but until recently no single virus or bacteria had been proven to be the main cause. For a while, herpes simplex virus type II (HSV-2) was thought to be the culprit. HSV-2 is sexually transmitted, but research has shown that it cannot change normal cells to abnormal cells and it is no longer believed to cause CIN.

CIN and cervical cancer occur less often in Jewish women, which had led some to suspect that male circumcision has a protective effect. Actually, there had been suggestions since 1855 that circumcision might prevent sexually transmitted infections and reduce risks of penile cancer and urinary tract infections. Most authorities had discounted this theory, but a new international study published in 2002 in *The New England Journal of Medicine* seems to lend some credibility to the theory. Male circumcision in this study is indeed linked to a reduced risk of penile infection with the

*Cancer of
the Cervix
and
Cervical
Dysplasia
(CIN)*

319

human papilloma virus (HPV) and reduced risk of cervical cancer in the partners of these circumcised men.

It is now accepted as fact that nearly all (at least 95 percent) cases of cervical cancer are directly linked to infection by HPV. HPV is quite common: There are estimates that one-third of all American female college students are infected. About one in every ten men between the ages of fifteen and forty-nine is infected as well. A woman with HPV is fifteen times more likely to develop cervical cancer. If she is under twenty-one, her risk increases forty-fold. Several so-called high-risk types of HPV are linked to CIN and cervical cancer. Women with CIN and HPV are often seven to ten years younger than women with CIN who do not have HPV. Many experts believe that HPV is a cause of CIN and that HPV makes cells change over a shorter period of time. The virus causes cell functions to go awry, resulting in the mutation of the affected cells and, eventually, transformation into cancer cells. There is also some evidence that the herpes virus might weaken the immune system, which would allow a cancer to get started.

There is some contrary evidence. In one study, Native American women with dysplasia were found to have had fewer lifetime sex partners and fewer sexually transmitted diseases than women with normal Pap tests. In another survey of women with HPV, non-Hispanic white women had cervical HPV more often than did Hispanic and Native American women.

Women who smoke and those who inhale secondhand smoke have increased cervical cancer and CIN rates. Toxic chemicals formed by cigarette smoke have been found in cervical fluid and cervical cells. These chemicals weaken the immune status of the cervix. Younger women, especially teenagers, are even more likely to develop CIN and cervical cancer when they inhale cigarette smoke. This is because the cells of the cervix go through major changes during puberty that make them more likely to be damaged by toxic chemicals. The risk also seems to increase if the young female smoker is exposed to HPV through sexual contact.

PREVENTION

The human papilloma virus can rest on a cell's surface without causing infection or injury. If the cells are damaged with the tiny cuts or scrapes that occur during sexual intercourse, HPV can infect them and start to multiply. There are sixty-five known types of HPV. It is thought that 20 to 30 percent of adults are infected with one of these virus types, but most have no ill effects because the immune systems stop the virus. Only 3 to 4 percent of women who have the virus develop abnormal cervical cells, and most of these cells revert to normal after medical treatment or by themselves. In some women, however, the cells become cancerous. The most suspect types in relation to CIN and cervical cancer are HPV 16, 18, 31, 33, and 35. Despite new tests for HPV, its presence has not been a good predictor of cervical cell abnormalities. So far, widespread testing for HPV is not thought to be useful in routine CIN and cervical cancer screening.

Prevention of CIN and cervical cancer involves providing information to women—especially teens—about ways to decrease the chance of exposure to HPV and other carcinogens. The use of **barrier-type contraceptives,** such as condoms, during sexual intercourse is one way to decrease exposure to cancer-causing viruses.

One study found that women who did not have CIN or cervical cancer more often had male sexual partners who had had a vasectomy. Many researchers think that vasectomy done at an early enough age could be a protective factor. Likewise, there is once again interest in the protection offered by male circumcision. There are some indications that vitamin A, vitamin C, and beta-carotene offer some protection against the development of CIN and cervical cancer.

The risk of exposure increases with the number of sexual partners a woman has. Women should have regular pelvic exams and Pap smear screening. These should begin *before* a woman becomes sexually active. In several studies, teens who were sexually active before age seventeen were found to be more likely to develop CIN. Based on knowledge of how HPV works to cause cancer, researchers believe the development of a vaccine against the virus is possible and could prevent CIN.

DIAGNOSIS

Finding CIN and cancer of the cervix usually starts with an abnormal Pap smear. No single test can determine absence of cancer cells in all women, but several tests used together reduce the chances of missing cancer. Accurate diagnosis involves a step-by-step process that includes colposcopy, colposcopy-directed biopsy, endocervical curettage (ECC) or loop electrocautery excision procedure (LEEP), and pelvic examination.

Colposcopy, a simple process, is used to identify and determine the size of a suspicious area. The colposcope is an instrument that magnifies the image of the cervix. Cervical abnormalities cannot usually be seen by the naked eye; the colposcope allows them to be seen more easily. After a Pap test, the cervix is rinsed with weak acetic acid solution (similar to vinegar) to remove mucous and excess cells. The acetic acid also accents the difference between normal and abnormal tissues. The most abnormal-looking part is selected for biopsy.

*Cancer of
the Cervix
and
Cervical
Dysplasia
(CIN)*

321

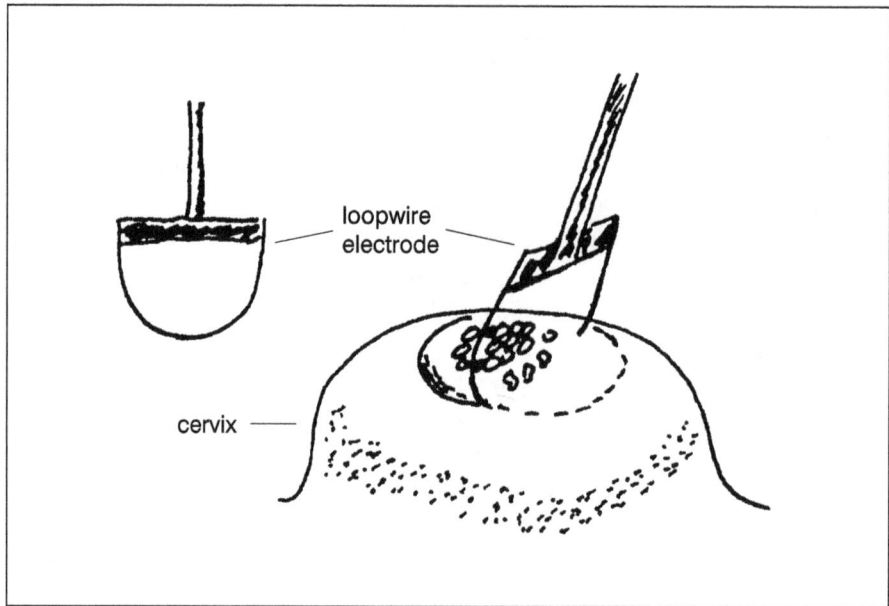

Loop Electrocautery Excision Procedure (LEEP):
The excision loop is used to remove area affected with CIN

Some respected authorities recommend that all women having colposcopy, unless they are pregnant, should also have **endocervical curettage** (ECC). In ECC, a large speculum is inserted into the vagina to gain access to the space between the internal os and the external os (the cervical canal). The whole surface of the cervical canal is scraped with a curette, a knife-like tool. This is done twice. Women usually feel some slight discomfort during ECC. After ECC, a punch biopsy of the cervix can be done, using the colposcopy findings as a guide. All of the tissue removed is collected and examined by a pathologist. ECC gives proof of the absence of cancer cells inside the cervical canal.

During **loop electrocautery excision procedure** (LEEP), the suspicious area is excised and the remaining tissue is cauterized. LEEP is both a diagnostic test and a treatment. Some diagnostic centers routinely use LEEP with ECC; others use one or the other. Tissues removed during LEEP are examined by a pathologist.

Sometimes **conization** is needed to rule out invasive, more advanced cancer. Women with positive ECCs need conization. It involves removal of part of the cervix with a scalpel or laser for examination by a pathologist. Conization is important in finding the extent of the cancer cells' invasion and, in turn, determining the best treatment plan (see figures on page 57).

Postmenopausal women with abnormal Pap smears often need conization because the cancer cells are usually located inside the cervical canal.

Some doctors ask women to put estrogen creams into the vagina for several days before colposcopy and biopsy to further highlight cervical tissue changes.

Conization is an outpatient surgery that is done under general anesthesia. After the woman wakes up from the anesthesia, she can expect to go home on the same day if bleeding is not severe. After four weeks, the woman is examined to check the healing process.

In general, use of a laser instead of a scalpel results in fewer bleeding and infection problems. The laser also reduces the chance of cervical stenosis after healing. **Stenosis** is a narrowing of the cervical opening that occurs as a result of scar tissue. A narrow cervical opening can block the path of sperm traveling from the vagina to the uterus, causing fertility problems.

For women who have abnormal Pap testing during pregnancy, colposcopy allows the doctor to see the cervix as clearly as possible. Conization is not often used during pregnancy except when the biopsy results suggest cancer. The cervix is filled with blood vessels during pregnancy, so avoiding the larger cone biopsy is in the pregnant woman's (and her baby's) best interests. A pregnant woman with a diagnosis of very early cervical cancer can deliver her baby vaginally, and then receive more complete therapy after delivery.

TREATMENT FOR CIN

The best treatment for CIN depends on the woman's age, her desire to have children in the future, the precise location of the abnormal cells, and the results of the colposcopy. Very simply, treatment involves destroying or removing abnormal cells. In a few instances, if the involved area is small and the abnormal cells are low grade, no immediate treatment is needed. If this is the case, the woman must return to her doctor for follow-up exams with Pap smear and colposcopy. The doctor or nurse practitioner should provide instructions as to the best plan for follow-up tests. Most of these small lesions will go away, or resolve, on their own, without treatment. This recommendation is usually made for pregnant women or women who are at high risk for infection (immunosuppressed).

Repeat exams at three and six months are sometimes recommended for women with CIN I. If a biopsy is done, the area removed may be the only area affected and biopsy alone might be the cure. For CIN II and CIN III, treatment is needed to stop the abnormal cells from turning into a cancer. Some doctors prefer that the Pap smear be repeated within two weeks of the initial Pap. During this two-week interval, suspected infections can be treated. If abnormal cells are still found, the woman should have a Pap

Cancer of the Cervix and Cervical Dysplasia (CIN)

323

smear every six months. Some doctors include colposcopy in the follow-up exams for CIN II. Others are more aggressive with CIN II and CIN III diagnoses and opt for immediate treatment. Some doctors will select from various outpatient treatments, including cryosurgery, laser vaporization, and LEEP. A more aggressive approach would use cervical conization or cone biopsy.

Excision (cutting out the abnormal cells) is used when the results of the colposcopy are uncertain, the ECC is positive, or the CIN is all or partly in the endocervix (the cervical canal). Excised tissue can be examined under the microscope so that an accurate diagnosis can be made.

Electrocautery, a method of "local destruction" of abnormal cells, has been used to treat CIN for many years. During electrocautery, electric current is passed through a metal rod that touches, burns, and destroys abnormal cells. It has been especially useful in the treatment of CIN I and II but is less effective for CIN III, and it does have some disadvantages. Some women have slight to moderate pain during and after the procedure. It causes scar tissue to form on the cervix, which reduces the ability of the cervix to stretch as it must during the delivery of a baby. For these reasons, electrocautery has fallen out of favor with many doctors, and fewer women choose this treatment option.

Cryosurgery, another form of local destruction, is as effective as electrocautery. Cryosurgery involves freezing the abnormal cells and tissue with carbon dioxide or nitrous oxide, which are applied using a probe called a **cryoprobe**. As the "frozen" cells die off, they are replaced by normal cells. Cryosurgery can be done in the doctor's office or at an outpatient clinic. Most women report cramps during the procedure but have few problems afterward. Women have a watery vaginal discharge for several weeks after cryosurgery. They should not use tampons, douche, or have sexual intercourse for four weeks after cryosurgery; this "pelvic rest" period is needed to reduce the chance of infection. Pap smear and colposcopy should be repeated in about four months (Pap smears done before four months would still show evidence of the damage from freezing) and then every six months. It is not unusual for Pap smears to remain slightly abnormal for one to two years after cryosurgery.

The major advantage of cryosurgery is that it does not cause as much scarring as electrocautery. On the negative side, the cryoprobe may be either too large or too small for the area to be treated, and some women may be "overtreated" and others "undertreated." The doctor's ability to detect recurrent or remaining disease is affected by the location of the abnormal area. Detection is more difficult if the abnormal area is located within the internal os; abnormalities outside the external os are easier to find and follow. Separate studies report failure-to-cure rates for cryosurgery of 5 percent, 7 percent, and 12 percent for CIN I, II, and III, respectively.

Laser vaporization is a popular and effective treatment for CIN. Laser vaporization can destroy most CIN of all grades; the procedure can be done in the doctor's office and does not require sedation or anesthesia. Women say they feel cramps during the procedure. Vaginal discharge and bleeding usually last for about two weeks. Like electrocautery and cryosurgery, four weeks of "pelvic rest" is advised. A Pap smear and colposcopy should be done after four months and then every six months.

Laser vaporization is as effective as electrocautery and cryosurgery for treatment of CIN, but is usually more expensive. Vaginal discharge continues for a shorter period of time than with electrocautery and cryosurgery. Bleeding and pain are more common with laser vaporization than with cryosurgery. Laser vaporization offers precise destruction of small areas and does not damage normal tissue. It can also reach and treat areas of the cervix that cannot be reached by cryosurgery and electrocautery. For these reasons, it may prevent the development of cancer. Some doctors reserve laser treatment for cases in which CIN involves a larger area or extends into the external os. It might also be used if cryosurgery or electrocautery has failed to destroy the CIN.

Conization may be used as a treatment for CIN as well as a diagnostic procedure.

Hysterectomy, removal of the cervix and uterus, was once the most common treatment for CIN. Even today, women who are beyond childbearing years may be offered hysterectomy. Of course, the choice of hysterectomy should be left up to the woman. She should know about other treatment alternatives, be familiar with the risks of hysterectomy, and have a clear idea of its benefits. Follow-up of hysterectomy is the same as for the other, more local forms of treatment. Postmenopausal women with a history of CIN have a higher chance of developing CIN of the vulva and vagina.

CARCINOMA IN SITU

Carcinoma in situ is a preinvasive cancer. Carcinoma in situ of the cervix is also called CIN III and Stage 0 carcinoma. Without treatment, carcinoma in situ usually turns into invasive carcinoma. It can be treated with the methods described for CIN, including vaginal hysterectomy (removing the cervix, the uterus, and part of the vagina). CIN treatments such as electrocautery, laser vaporization, and cryosurgery are options for CIN III, as long

*Cancer of
the Cervix
and
Cervical
Dysplasia
(CIN)*

325

as the woman knows that there is a higher risk of treatment failure. During hysterectomy, removal of the upper part of the vagina is not necessary when there is no sign of cancer in the vagina. (Cervical carcinoma in situ extends into the vagina in fewer than 5 percent of all cases.) In the United States, hysterectomy (removal of the entire uterus and cervix) has been the treatment of choice for women whose childbearing years are over or women who are interested in permanent sterilization. It is very important for all women, even those who have had their uteruses and cervixes removed, to continue to have regular pelvic examinations that include Pap smears.

CANCER OF THE CERVIX

Most cancers of the cervix start in the transformation zone. **Squamous carcinoma** is the most common and usually occurs in older women. **Adenocarcinoma** occurs in younger women, is often more aggressive, and does not respond as well to treatment. The natural history of cervical cancer—the course it would take if left untreated—involves spread to other pelvic structures first and then to the lymph nodes. Eventually the cancer metastasizes to the lungs, liver, and bones.

Early-stage cervical cancer, like CIN and carcinoma in situ, may not cause symptoms. As the cancer continues to grow without treatment, the first symptom might be a watery, blood-tinged vaginal discharge that the woman might not even notice. The woman may notice some painless bleeding that occurs at times other than during her normal period. She may notice spotting after sexual intercourse or douching. As the cancer grows, the bleeding might get heavier, grow more frequent, and last longer. Some women notice that their periods also last longer or that the blood flow is heavier than normal. Eventually, the bleeding is constant. Women past menopause are likely to notice these changes, since for them, bleeding is more likely to be seen as abnormal.

Symptoms of more advanced disease include pain in the flank or leg. This pain is related to pressure from the tumor on the ureters, the pelvic wall, and nerves. Many women with advanced disease describe pain on urination and notice blood in their urine. Advanced disease may block the urinary tract or the bowel. Blocked lymph channels and blood vessels can result in swelling of one or both legs.

Because of routine Pap smears, most women with cervical cancer are diagnosed at earlier, more treatable stages of disease. Usually these early stages of disease have no symptoms. After an abnormal Pap smear, a woman must have additional tests to define the problem—CIN versus actual cancer—and the extent of the disease.

FIGO Staging and Classification
of Cancer of the Cervix

Stage	Description
Stage 0	Carcinoma in situ
Stage I	Carcinoma confined to the cervix
Stage IA	Carcinomas not visible to the eye but seen with microscope
Stage IA1	Minimal microscopic evidence of stromal invasion
Stage IA2	Carcinoma detected microscopically that can be measured, is not deeper than 5 mm, and is not larger horizontally than 7 mm
Stage IB	Lesions larger than in IA2
Stage II	Involves the upper vagina, but not the lower third of the vagina, or some invasion into the parametria—the outer layer of the uterus
Stage IIA	Involves the vagina but not the parametria
Stage IIB	Involves the inner layer parametria
Stage III	Involves the lower third of the vagina or extends to the pelvic walls; obstruction of one or both ureters without involvement of the vagina or parametria
Stage IIIA	Involves the lower third of the vagina but does not extend to the pelvic walls
Stage IIIB	Involves one or both parametria and extends to the pelvic walls
Stage IV	Extends outside of the reproductive tract
Stage IVA	Involves the bladder or rectum
Stage IVB	Cancer spread outside of the pelvis—for example, to lungs, bones, or liver

Staging

The extent of the cancer is determined through several tests. HIV testing is generally performed in young, at-risk women: cervical cancer in HIV-infected women is often a more aggressive and difficult to treat cancer, and HIV status can change the treatment picture. The bladder is assessed by cystoscopy, done under general anesthesia or local anesthesia with sedation. If there are suspicious areas, biopsy can be done during cystoscopy. Intravenous pyelogram (IVP) is a special imaging study to measure the size of the kidneys, detect blockages, and evaluate suspicious masses. The large intestine (colon) and the rectum are assessed through sigmoidoscopy and proctoscopy. Barium enema examination is usually reserved for patients who are having bowel symptoms. Other imaging studies that might be used to evaluate the extent of the cancer include a chest X ray, CT scan, ultrasound, or magnetic resonance imaging (MRI). Positron emission tomography (PET) scanning is being used as a way to predict spread of cervical cancer. Blood tests check the function of the liver and kidneys, the presence or absence of anemia or blood loss, and the likelihood of an inflammatory reaction or infection.

As with all kinds of cancer, a classification system gives doctors and the health-care team a common language for discussion of cervical cancer. This is outlined in the chart above.

TREATMENTS FOR CERVICAL CANCER

Treatment options for invasive cancer depend on the woman's age, her general physical condition (including any unintended weight loss), the amount of cancer present, and her wish to save ovarian function. *The extent of the disease is the most important clue to the chance of cure.* The cure rate is nearly 100 percent in Stages 0 and IA and falls to 5 percent in Stage IV. Staging also determines the choice of treatment. Treatment is likely to include surgery, radiation therapy, or both. Chemotherapy has not been very useful in the treatment of cervical cancer.

In early cervical cancer, cure rates are exactly the same with either radical hysterectomy (removal of the uterus, cervix, supporting ligaments and tissues, upper part of the vagina, and pelvic lymph nodes) or radiation therapy. The choice of treatment is based on the size of the tumor on the cervix and evidence of the tumor extending into the vagina.

Surgery

Surgery can effectively remove small tumors. If a tumor is larger, radiation will probably be selected because it offers fewer problems than an extensive surgical procedure. In general, women under seventy are more likely to have surgery, though this is not a hard and fast rule. Many older women are in good health and are able to tolerate surgery. The woman who has surgery needs to be in generally good condition. If she has other medical problems—for example, lung or heart problems—radiation therapy may be easier for her. If the woman has distorted pelvic anatomy, perhaps from other earlier surgery, she may be better served by surgery since the success of radiation depends upon the even and predictable dispersal of radiation through tissues. A past history of pelvic inflammatory disease or inflammatory bowel disease increases the risks of bowel problems with radiation therapy.

In general, surgery is used for all cervical cancers Stage 0 through IIA. Women with Stage IIB and III are more likely to be treated with radiation therapy.

Early-stage cervical cancer includes cancers that have not invaded the cervix deeper than 3 millimeters (a little less than one-eighth inch). Some experts call this *microinvasive carcinoma* or *microcarcinoma*. The pathologist uses a microscope to decide whether the cancer cells have spread beyond the 3 mm limit and whether there are cancer cells in nearby lymph channels or blood vessels. Early-stage disease also includes the category *early stromal invasion,* in which a few isolated cancer cells are seen with signs of early spreading.

The woman with early-stage disease can be treated with conization (for women who may not be able to endure surgery or who wish to preserve fertility) or simple hysterectomy. If there is evidence of deeper spread, the woman might have a radical hysterectomy—removal of the uterus, upper third of the vagina, supporting tissues and ligaments, and pelvic lymph nodes. Removal of the ovaries and fallopian tubes (salpingo-oophorectomy) might also be recommended, particularly if the woman is over forty and postmenopausal. Keep in mind that the cure rates are exactly the same for women who have hysterectomy and those who have other forms of treatment with radiation therapy.

For invasive carcinoma, the treatment is much more aggressive. In Stage I and II, surgical removal of the cancer is possible. The surgery should include removal of the lymph nodes for any woman with cancer staged greater than IA1. Some surgeons prefer to do a vaginal hysterectomy and remove lymph nodes in the area. Removal of the ovaries is not entirely necessary in women who have not yet reached menopause since spread of the cancer from the cervix to the ovaries is rare. Modern surgical techniques allow the surgeon to move the ovaries outside of the pelvis so that they will not be exposed to radiation used postoperatively. Stage IB and IIA cancers can be treated with radical hysterectomy and one or two intracavitary radiation treatments. Lymph nodes removed during surgery are examined under a microscope for cancer cells. The presence or absence of tumor cells is an important predictor of the chance of cure. Women who have "positive" lymph nodes will usually need external radiation therapy to the entire pelvis after surgery. Radical surgery is indicated only for women who are considered healthy enough to go through surgery. Women with disease staged at IIB and beyond are usually treated with high doses of external pelvic radiation and intracavitary radiation. This means placing radioactive materials directly into the space inside the uterus.

The advantages of radical hysterectomy over traditional pelvic radiation therapy are as follows:

✦ young women can keep ovarian function

- sexual function is less affected by surgical techniques (though some might debate this)

- there is less chance of bowel complications

On the other hand, during radical hysterectomy the vagina may be shortened. Some of the most common complications of surgery include bladder problems and formation of fistulas, or open passages, in the tissue. The decision to have surgery may not rule out the need for radiation. During surgery, if lymph nodes are found to contain cancer cells, postoperative radiation therapy will be recommended.

Delayed complications of surgery do happen, though rarely. For example, 3 percent of all women who have radical hysterectomies experience bladder problems. These include problems beginning urination, increased need to urinate, and decreased bladder capacity. Most women describe some decrease in sensations related to the need to urinate that lasts up to six months after surgery. Because of these problems, women are more prone to urinary tract infections during the immediate postoperative period.

Radiation Therapy

Early and advanced disease can be treated with radiation. Radiation may be used alone as the major treatment or in combination with surgery. Radiation can be from an external radioactive source (a machine) or given internally by inserting radioactive substances directly into the area affected by cancer (brachytherapy). Brachytherapy, as discussed in Chapter 7, allows a high dose of radiation to target known cancer cells while sparing normal tissues that surround the cancer. Protection of the normal tissue reduces overall damage, side effects, and complications. Intracavitary implants can be used before or after external radiation therapy.

Brachytherapy can be done either with a vaginal applicator or by placing small hollow steel needles into the connective tissue surrounding the uterus, or parametrium; these are "afterloaded" with seed-shaped bits of radioactive material. This interstitial (meaning "between tissues") method might be used when the cancer is advanced. Advanced cancer may have changed the vagina's size and shape, making the use of the applicators difficult or impossible. Interstitial implants do cause more problems and complications than other applicators. Still, interstitial therapy is being used more often and is under study in many cancer research centers.

Specific information about the implant procedure needs to be provided by the radiation oncologist and/or the radiation oncology nurse. Radiation therapy affects organs that lie in the path of the beam; side effects that occur soon after radiation therapy ends—or perhaps during treatment—can

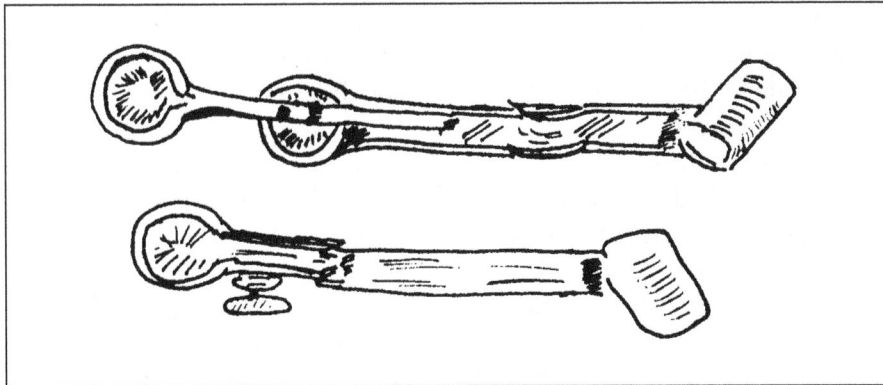

This pair of stainless steel **ovoids** is placed into the top of the vagina while a woman is under general anesthesia. The oval cylinders at the ends are hollow and hold a radioactive source. The ovoids rest against the cervix. After the applicators are in place, the vagina can be packed with gauze to prevent the applicators from being dislodged during the implant procedure.

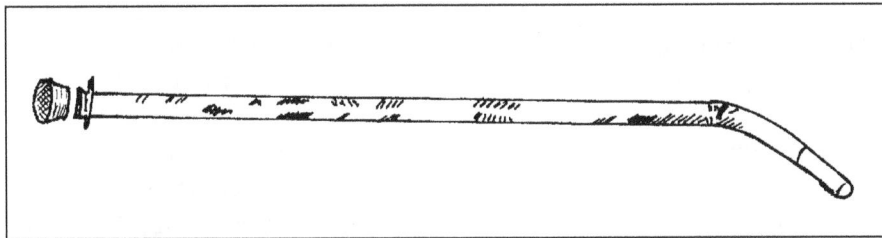

A hollow stainless steel **tandem** is placed into the uterus through the vagina. It is sometimes used with ovoids in the treatment of cervical, vaginal, and uterine cancers. A radioactive source like radium or cesium is placed inside the tandem during an afterloading procedure and left in place for a prescribed time period—usually 48–72 hours. The tandem is about 8–10 inches long and ¼ inch in diameter.

include skin reactions and inflammation of the bladder, bowel, and rectum. Side effects that reveal themselves six to twenty-four months after treatment has ended include vaginal changes (dryness, fibrosis, loss of ability to stretch), vaginal shrinkage (stenosis), and discomfort or pain with sexual intercourse.

The effects of radiation on sexual function depend on the body area in the radiation field and the total dose of radiation. Most sexual changes caused by radiation relate to the effects on the ovaries and the vagina. The ovaries can be surgically moved to a higher location outside the field of pelvic radiation, thereby preserving fertility and hormone production. When the ovaries are in the radiation treatment field in a premenopausal woman, ovarian function stops permanently and the woman will go into menopause. The symptoms and sexual changes in this woman will be similar

Cancer of the Cervix and Cervical Dysplasia (CIN)

331

to those of older women who go through menopause naturally. She might experience hot flashes, mood swings, decreased lubrication of the vagina, and thinning of the vaginal tissues. Any of these symptoms can interfere with sexual function.

If the vagina is included in the radiation field, the vaginal canal shrinks and becomes rigid. The woman will have a loss of lubrication and vaginal sensation. To prevent these changes, a woman can take several actions, such as resuming sexual activity as soon as possible and using a vaginal dilator with a water-soluble lubricant (more about these in Chapter 18).

Short-term side effects from radiation to the pelvic area can include the following: diarrhea, nausea, vomiting, bladder irritation, weight loss, and fatigue. Any of these side effects can affect a woman's desire or physical ability to have sex.

ADVANCED AND RECURRENT CERVICAL CANCER

Cancer will recur in about one-third of all women with invasive cervical cancer. Most cervical cancers that recur do so within the first two years after therapy. The exact location where the cancer recurs relates to the type of therapy initially used. After hysterectomy, about one-fourth of the recurrences occur in the upper part of the vagina or the area where the cervix was located. After primary treatment with radiation therapy, recurrent cancers are usually found in the cervix, the uterus, the upper vagina, and the pelvic wall. The most common signs and symptoms of recurrent disease are the following:

+ weight loss

+ leg swelling, often involving only one leg

+ pain in the thigh or buttock area

+ bloody vaginal discharge

+ signs of blocked urinary tract

+ cough

+ chest pain

The prognosis for women with recurrent or advanced cervical cancer depends on where the cancer is found. The most favorable prognosis is for women with what is called "central" recurrence: cancer found in the pelvic area. The outlook is not as hopeful for women whose cancer is found in bone, the lungs, the liver, or other areas outside of the pelvis.

Radiation Therapy for Recurrent and Advanced Cancer

When cancer returns in areas outside the pelvis, radiation therapy by itself can offer relief of symptoms, but not cure. Pain from bone metastases can be controlled by radiation. In some cancer treatment centers, external radiation is used when cancer recurs in the cervical area. These women are treated with a second full course of external radiation.

Chemotherapy for Advanced Cervical Cancer

So far, chemotherapy for cervical cancer that has spread outside the pelvis has not been very effective. Some studies have reported a "good response" to some chemotherapy agents (mitomycin-C, vincristine, bleomycin, doxorubicin, methyl CCNU, cisplatin), but a good response is not a lasting response: The cancer is not completely destroyed. Although some women do live longer, these studies usually do not report on the quality of life women experience during this "good response" time. Chemotherapy using the drugs fluorouracil with or without mitomycin is sometimes being used in combination with radiation therapy. Chemotherapy is increasingly being used as a palliative measure—useful in controlling the distressing symptoms that accompany advanced disease.

Surgery for Advanced Cervical Cancer

For women with only central recurrence—no cancer found in areas outside of the pelvis—a major surgical procedure called **pelvic exenteration** may offer hope for cure. Pelvic exenteration is an extensive operation. It involves removing most or all of the major organs in the pelvis. In addition to those removed in the radical hysterectomy (see next section), the bladder, rectum, and colon might also be removed. Urine and stool then need to be "rerouted" to openings on the abdomen so that body wastes can still leave the body. The results of this type of surgery can have huge psychological effects. The woman who opts for this surgery must be emotionally stable and prepared to go through a long, difficult recovery process.

Nearly 10 percent of women who have pelvic exenteration die during or soon after the operation. Complications immediately after surgery are mostly caused by heart and lung problems. Infections of the pelvic wall cause severe problems, too. Bowel complications can occur for a period of time starting right after surgery to as long as eighteen months later. Urinary tract and kidney problems are likely to be lifelong issues. The surgery itself is lengthy: In one study, each woman's operation took over seven hours. Most women stayed in an intensive care unit for one to two weeks and were in the hospital between five and six weeks. More than one-third of women who have pelvic exenteration can be expected to live longer than five years after surgery.

Despite all the hardships and risks of pelvic exenteration, this radical and risky surgery may hold the only chance for cure. If pelvic exenteration is suggested, a woman must weigh her risks and what she hopes to achieve by having the surgery. Reconstruction of the vagina now affords some women the chance to preserve sexual function even after exenteration. She must have a very clear idea of the body changes involved with a urinary or bowel diversion—changes that will affect her for the rest of her life.

Hysterectomy

Hysterectomy is controversial. In the United States alone, nearly a million hysterectomies are performed each year, yet there are only a few *real* reasons to have a hysterectomy. More than one thousand women die each year from complications after hysterectomy. For many women, removal of the uterus or womb is disturbing, and many women describe drastic changes in their sexual response. A woman should seriously consider these issues before signing the consent form.

One reason hysterectomy has lost popularity is that younger women still wanting to have children are being diagnosed more often with CIN. This increases the need for treatment that preserves a woman's childbearing capacity.

WHAT KIND OF HYSTERECTOMY? There are two ways to remove the uterus. In an **abdominal hysterectomy,** the uterus is removed through an incision in the abdomen. In a **vaginal hysterectomy,** the uterus is removed through the vagina. A surgeon should recommend an approach based on the reason for the operation and what would be the easiest, safest approach. A vaginal hysterectomy leaves no visible scar and is recommended when there is no risk that the uterus is abnormally attached to the intestine or other structures, and when the uterus is small enough to be removed safely through the vagina. The abdominal approach should be used when there are more risks associated with a vaginal approach or when the surgeon needs to look closely at the other abdominal organs. Some surgeons suggest that a vaginal hysterectomy requires more effort and skill.

Hysterectomy operations are also categorized by what organs and structures are removed during the surgery. In a **radical hysterectomy,** the uterus, cervix, supporting ligaments and tissues, upper part of the vagina, and pelvic lymph nodes are removed. The ovaries and fallopian tubes might also be removed, but this is not part of the standard operation. A **simple**

hysterectomy removes the uterus and possibly the ovaries, fallopian tubes, and cervix. The doctor should explain the variations in hysterectomy; the exact details have much to do with the woman's future health-care plans.

In his book *Women and Doctors,* which is highly critical of his peers, John M. Smith, M.D., outlines the following indications for hysterectomy:

1. Cancer of the uterus, fallopian tubes, or ovaries

2. Menstrual bleeding that does not respond to treatment and that causes the woman to be anemic

3. Large, benign tumors of the uterus that block or will soon block the urinary tract, cause severe pain or uncontrollable bleeding, and cannot be treated or removed while leaving the uterus in place

4. Chronic pelvic inflammatory disease that causes pain and is not treatable by any other means

Noted surgical gynecologists Philip DiSaia, M.D., and William T. Creasman, M.D., have numerous medical journal papers and gynecologic oncology textbooks to their credit. In their textbook, *Clinical Gynecologic Oncology,* they generally advocate vaginal hysterectomy for women who have carcinoma in situ. They also indicate that hysterectomy might be the treatment of choice for CIN in women who have completed childbearing and want permanent sterilization. They warn that removing the upper part of the vagina is not indicated in either CIN or carcinoma in situ.

Dr. Smith warns that "*any* other situation requires that you get some specific answers to a few questions, weigh the risk versus the benefits, and decide for yourself." He suggests that women facing a decision about hysterectomy should get the following information in order to make a good decision:

1. What *exactly* is wrong, and what are all the possible treatment approaches?

2. What are the possible effects of doing nothing?

3. What complications or problems are connected with all possible treatments, including hysterectomy?

4. What are *all* the effects that any treatment, including hysterectomy, might have?

5. Is it necessary or recommended that the ovaries be removed?

6. Is it possible to use surgical techniques to preserve sexual function?

The side effects of a hysterectomy—barring surgical complications—should not be serious. Menstrual periods will stop. Hormonal cycles will continue if ovaries are left in place, but there is no uterine lining to shed and bleed. There is no risk of pregnancy and no need for birth-control measures. There will be no further risk of uterine or cervical cancer if all uterine and cervical tissues are removed. Estrogen replacement after menopause can be used without increasing the risk of uterine cancer.

Removal of the ovaries, however, presents several new issues. Many surgeons recommend removing the ovaries, especially if the woman is close to or past menopause. Unless a premenopausal woman has a family history of ovarian cancer, most experts recommend that her normal ovaries not be removed. Removing functioning ovaries puts a woman into "instant" menopause. Without the estrogen produced by ovaries, the woman is likely to have symptoms associated with menopause: hot flashes, mood swings, and decreased vaginal moisture. There is also evidence to suggest that small amounts of estrogen are produced by the ovaries even after menopause, and experts are not quite sure what function this estrogen has. All in all, the general advice is to avoid removing normal tissue.

COMPLICATIONS OF HYSTERECTOMY As with any major surgery, hysterectomy is not without risks, which must be weighed against the benefits. Risks can occur even when the surgeon performs the operation with great skill. Some relate to any surgery while others are specific to the area directly affected by the operation. For example, blood clots can form in the veins of the pelvis or legs when anyone is immobile for an extended period of time. These clots can break free and move to the lungs, causing sudden death. After surgery, hemorrhage or abnormal bleeding can occur which, if not dealt with quickly and successfully, can also result in death. Other general risks that can result in death include infection, anesthetic complications, reaction to drugs, surgical mistakes, and administration of a wrong medication.

Other risks are not fatal but still cause serious problems. Fistulas—abnormal connections between organs—occur only rarely, but can be the result of surgical error, nutritional deficits, and previous radiation therapy to the abdomen. The most common fistula related to hysterectomy is a "vesico-vaginal" fistula (connecting the bladder and the vagina), resulting in passage of urine into the vagina. A fistula repair surgery is difficult and may not be successful. During hysterectomy, a ureter (the tube that carries urine from the kidney to the bladder) might be accidentally tied off or blocked. If this is not corrected, it can cause the loss of a kidney.

After surgery, a woman can expect some discomfort and tiredness. It is important that she knows what level of discomfort is normal and what is not. Nurses often offer preoperative education. They might work with the surgeon in an office setting, a hospital, or a surgery or gynecology clinic. Knowledge is a real source of power. The more a woman knows about what to expect during and after the surgery, the less anxious she is likely to be.

The information a woman needs related to any surgery includes what will be expected of her immediately after she awakens from the anesthetic. Many women are surprised at how much seems to be expected of them and are not prepared to take an active role in the healing process—at least not quite so soon. For these women, the surgical nurse seems almost like a villain, ready to inflict all kinds of torture! Indeed, women are often surprised that they will be sitting in a bedside chair within a few hours of surgery. The routine coughing and deep breathing exercises might be painful or at least uncomfortable. It is hard for most women to believe that they may be expected to go home usually within three days!

Immediately after any operation, the major priorities for surgical nurses include the effective functioning of their patient's lungs, keeping the incision free of infection, keeping the normal skin in good condition, allowing the intestines and urinary system to return to normal, and helping the patient to be reasonably comfortable. Each of these nursing priorities involves the active cooperation of the woman, and they need to be discussed *before* the operation (see "Questions to Ask Your Physician" later in this chapter).

Overall, the death rate from hysterectomy is about twelve out of ten thousand operations. This might not seem a huge risk—unless you or the woman you care for is one of those twelve. There is no accurate predictor of any of the mentioned complications. In some cases, a hysterectomy may be the best answer for a woman's gynecologic problem. The horror is that at least a few of these twelve women did not need a hysterectomy. The bottom line is that each woman needs to fully understand the risks and benefits of whatever treatment option she selects.

SEXUALITY ISSUES AFTER HYSTERECTOMY   Changes in sexual behavior after hysterectomy have not been well documented. Sexual behavior includes both sexual function and sexual desire. Of all the phases of sexual activity, sexual desire is the least understood. In women who have had cervical cancer, almost half describe some degree of disruption in what had been their normal sexual behavior. In one study, one in three reported changes in desire, excitement, and orgasm. One in three women also reported pain or discomfort with sexual intercourse.

It is known that the uterus plays an important role in the stages of the female sexual response, so it is likely that a woman can expect some changes following hysterectomy. Almost half of the women who have hysterectomy where the ovaries are removed describe a decreased sexual response and a reduced desire for and frequency of intercourse. On the other hand, some women become sexually active or resume sexual activity after treatment. A decrease in sexual response may be caused by changes in hormone production (when ovarian hormones are no longer present) and removal of the cervix and uterus, which trigger orgasm for some women. Hormone replacement therapy can lessen dryness, but hormone replacement therapy may not be an option for women with hormonally dependent tumors. An option for some women is the local application of estrogen cream or use of an Estring, an estrogen-filled ring that is inserted into the vagina, releasing small amounts of estradiol.

Many woman describe their orgasms as "different"—not better or worse—than they were before hysterectomy. Most describe a temporary loss of sexual desire for anywhere up to six months after treatment, with desire returning later during the first year. Removing the upper part of the vagina and vaginal shortening causes pain for some women, and in fact many women report that pain with intercourse is a problem. Changes in sexual positions, relaxation techniques, and use of lubricants might diminish discomfort and enhance sexual pleasure.

Both body image and self-esteem are greatly affected by diagnosis and treatment for a gynecologic cancer. Women often fear rejection, isolation, and unacceptability. Women with a new diagnosis of gynecologic cancer describe a decrease in both sexual activity and sexual satisfaction. Sometimes the woman's sexual partner has fears or misconceptions about the cancer and its treatment.

Many women whose sexual adjustment after surgery is good credit their success to supportive sexual partners. A second major factor in successful adjustment is the ability to get accurate information about what to expect after surgery. A woman and her partner can better adjust to changes by exploring their feelings about sexual expression and satisfaction. It is important that the woman and her partner have a clear understanding of what her sexual functioning can be during and after therapy. Many women find that counseling that includes sexual information is a crucial part of successful adjustment.

Several studies report that even though doctors and nurses think discussing sexuality with their patients is important, less than half feel comfortable in actually initiating this conversation. There are often quite a number of resources available in a community—and just asking the question can open up possibilities. Many health-care professionals and settings prefer to designate someone as a "sexuality resource person"—someone with a good deal of expertise and understanding about issues surrounding sexuality and cancer survivorship. Certified sex educators and sex counselors are available in many communities.

There is a growing number of resources that offer guidance and help with sexuality issues. The American Cancer Society (ACS) offers the booklet (also available on the ACS website—www.cancer.org) *For the Woman Who Has Cancer and Her Partner* (and a similar booklet for men). The Sexual Health Network at www.sexualhealth.com offers resources for people with health-related problems. The American Association of Sex Educators, Counselors and Therapists (www.assect.org) offers a list of therapists for each state. His and Her Health (www.Hisandherhealth.com) is a medical and sexual health news website run by urologists. These are not the only resources available, but they do provide a good starting place when looking for help with sexuality issues.

QUESTIONS TO ASK YOUR PHYSICIAN

1. How long will I need to stay in the hospital or clinic?

2. How long can I expect to be off work?

3. What activities should I do and which should I avoid?

4. Should I expect bowel function changes, for how long, and what treatment is needed?

5. Should I expect urinary function changes, for how long, and what treatment is needed?

6. Regarding follow-up care:
   — How often do I need pelvic exams and Pap smears?
   — What is the plan and schedule for follow-up appointments?
   — Are there self-care activities to help prevent complications (for example, signs and symptoms of infection, whom to call, how to avoid infection)?
   — What medications will be needed, on what schedule, and what are their side effects?
   — Will I need other treatment modalities after surgery (for example, radiation therapy)?
   — What are signs and symptoms of recurrent disease that must be reported to the doctor or nurse?

7. What changes in sexual function can I expect?

8. Are there other lifestyle changes I need to know about (for example, quitting smoking and using barrier-type birth control devices such as diaphragms or condoms)?

9. What and where are the community resources to help meet the demands of treatment and survivorship?

Each woman facing treatment—whether a hysterectomy or another treatment option—must have a very clear understanding of what is expected of her: what her role is in the treatment process and the roles of the surgeon, the nurse, and any other member of the health-care team.

✦

The growing understanding of the way cervical cancers start and grow offers many opportunities for prevention and treatment. Preventive measures being explored include chemoprevention using retinoids (vitamin-A compounds). Given the importance of the virus HPV in the development of cervical cancer, it is logical to think that vaccination might someday offer some prevention. In fact, this is true; vaccines and immunotherapy are very popular and promising areas of research. Experts predict that this new century will bring prevention of cervical cancer via vaccination—an advance that would save hundreds of thousands of women worldwide from this preventable cancer.

— *Pamela Haylock*

CHAPTER 18

CANCER OF THE VAGINA

The vagina connects the cervix and the vulva. It is the passageway for fluid to leave the body during menstrual periods, the entry for sperm to reach an egg to create a baby, and the birth canal through which a baby travels during a normal vaginal delivery.

Cancer of the vagina is one of the rarest cancers in the human body. Primary cancer of the vagina accounts for less than 2 percent of all gynecologic cancers in the United States—around two thousand new cases each year. It is strange, but cancers affect the tissues on either side of the vagina—the cervix and the vulva—much more often than the vaginal tissues. It is more common for cancers to start in the cervix and spread down to the upper part of the vagina than it is for them to start in the vagina. Sometimes cancers that started in the uterus, urethra, ovary, bladder, and rectum spread to the vagina.

Most vaginal cancers occur in women fifty to seventy years of age. At least in the United States, it is usually found early and the cure rate is high. The exception is for the even more rare clear cell adenocarcinoma, which usually occurs in women who are between seventeen and twenty-one years old and have a history of being exposed to the hormone DES while being carried in their mothers' uterus.

Most (85 percent) vaginal cancers develop from the epithelial, or skin-like, tissues and are squamous cell carcinoma. Adenocarcinoma accounts for nearly all the remaining types of vaginal cancer, though it is so rare that other primary cancers should be ruled out before the diagnosis of vaginal adenocarcinoma is accepted. Vaginal malignant melanoma and sarcoma occur but are even more uncommon.

RISK FACTORS

Probably because these cancers are so rare, information about possible risk factors is scant. The cause of squamous cell carcinoma of the vagina is not known. Some experts suspect that fluids collect in the upper part of the vagina and cause irritation that eventually leads to cancer. Other factors linked to squamous cell carcinoma of the vagina include a past history of vaginal trauma, syphilis, use of a vaginal pessary (a device used to support a displaced uterus or prevent conception), prolapse of the vaginal wall, history of vaginal warts, and frequent episodes of vaginitis and other factors that irritate the vaginal wall. Women who live in poverty are more likely to develop vaginal cancer.

Clear cell adenocarcinoma of the vagina is linked to in utero exposure to the hormone diethylstilbestrol (DES). About one in one thousand women exposed to DES in utero go on to develop vaginal adenocarcinoma (discussed later in this chapter).

It is guessed that some factors that cause cancer of the cervix might also cause cancer of the vagina, including the human papillomavirus (HPV). Women who have had radiation therapy for a previous cervical cancer may be at higher risk of developing a second gynecologic cancer. After a hysterectomy, many women fail to have regular gynecologic exams, which allows a vaginal cancer to go undetected. Because this disease is so rare, proving these theories is difficult.

PREVENTION

Without knowing the true cause of primary vaginal cancer, preventive care is geared toward finding these cancers early. The most effective way to find vaginal cancers before symptoms develop is by having a clinical examination that includes a Pap smear. For this reason, Pap smears should still be used for every woman, including those who have had a hysterectomy. Vaginal cancer usually grows slowly, so most experts suggest that adequate screening consists of Pap smears every three to five years. If a woman has other risk factors, she should be screened more often.

BENIGN VAGINAL DISEASE

Vaginal carcinoma in situ, also called **vaginal intraepithelial neoplasia (VAIN)**, is less common than cervical and vulvar intraepithelial neoplasia and accounts for only 0.4 percent of all gynecologic cancers, but its incidence is increasing. VAIN is thought to be a precancerous condition.

Most of the time, a woman with VAIN will not have symptoms; occasionally she may have spotting after sexual intercourse. Routine Pap smears are crucial to finding VAIN early. After a Pap smear, vaginal colposcopy and biopsy establish the diagnosis. In women with VAIN, precancerous cells or actual cancer cells may be found in another part of the lower genital tract (cervix or vulva). Other tests need to be done to look for other problems.

Treatment for Benign Vaginal Disease

Surgical removal of the affected area has been the standard treatment for VAIN. For many women, curative treatment can be done during the biopsy. If there are several areas affected, partial or total removal of the vagina might be needed. Some surgeons try to create a new vagina during this surgery, but this has mixed results. Many women describe uncomfortable or painful sexual intercourse and other problems with sexual function after this surgery.

Radiation therapy has been used, but the structure of the vagina makes an even distribution of the radiation difficult. Radiation can cause **vaginal fibrosis**—thickening and loss of ability to stretch—and sometimes the formation of fistulas or abnormal connections between the vagina, rectum, and/or urethra. Radiation through intravaginal applicators is used in some treatment centers, but some experts do not advocate this treatment and warn that its use results in recurrence more often than other treatment methods do. The vaginal fibrosis and stenosis that can result from the treatment may make follow-up examination difficult.

Chemotherapy has been used directly in the vagina with 5-fluorouracil (5-FU), which seems to yield high cure rates with few side effects. Intravaginal chemotherapy can cause burning and shedding of the vaginal lining that is serious enough to keep this treatment from getting widespread approval. There has been no agreement on the optimal dose, length of treatment, or method of application.

The use of the laser has become accepted in the treatment of VAIN. Some physicians use only local anesthesia and a sedative medication, but usually laser treatment of VAIN is done under general anesthesia. Pain and bleeding are the major problems associated with laser therapy, relating to the depth of treatment and the power of the laser. Healing is complete in four to six weeks, and most women can be cured with a single treatment. Sexual function is not thought to be altered, although there is no real research to verify what surgeons believe to be the case.

Following laser surgery, a woman may need mild pain medications. "Vaginal rest"—no intercourse, baths, swimming, or douching—for four weeks is important to promote healing. If a woman has needed extensive laser treatment, she might use a vaginal dilator from three times a week to once a day as a way to minimize scarring of the vagina and keep it open and flexible. Having intercourse on a regular and frequent basis has the same effect. The doctor or nurse can explain how to use the dilator correctly. Vaginal application of estrogen cream two or three times a week may be prescribed for postmenopausal women. Estrogen cream helps vaginal tissues heal. After two weeks, and again at two months, the doctor or nurse practitioner will need to assess the woman's healing status.

VAGINAL CANCER

Most vaginal cancers do not cause symptoms. However, signs of vaginal cancer include feeling the need to strain during urination or bowel movements (tenesmus), feelings of having to urinate often, pain with urination, bladder pain, vaginal discharge, and painless bleeding, especially after sexual intercourse. Some women might have a foul-smelling vaginal discharge.

Diagnosis and Staging

After making an initial diagnosis through a Pap smear, colposcopy, and/or biopsy, a woman's doctor will need other diagnostic tests to define the extent of the cancer. The tests, in addition to the history and physical, include chest X ray, intravenous pyelogram (IVP), cystoscopy, and proctosigmoidoscopy. Lymph nodes in the groin and the upper leg will be examined. Some doctors will also perform a **lymphangiogram,** in which the pelvic lymph system is injected with a dye and X-rayed, but this is commonly being replaced by MRIs. A barium enema is especially needed if the woman has had a recent episode of diverticulitis, since that will be a factor in planning for radiation therapy. The chart below outlines the FIGO stages of vaginal cancer.

FIGO Staging System for Vaginal Cancer

Stage	Characteristics
Stage 0	Intraepithelial carcinoma
Stage I	Cancer limited to the vaginal lining
Stage II	Cancer involves the tissue beneath the lining but does not extend to the pelvic wall
Stage III	Cancer extends onto the pelvic wall or pubic symphysis (pubic bone)
Stage IV	Cancer extends beyond the pelvis and involves the bladder or rectum

Treatment

Like all cancer treatment decisions, treatment recommendations are based on the stage, size, and location of the cancer. Other factors include the presence or absence of the uterus and whether or not the woman has had radiation therapy to the pelvis.

Historically, surgery has been the major treatment offered to women with vaginal cancer. Surgical choices vary from limited, local procedures to extensive, complicated operations:

+ *Laser surgery* uses laser to destroy cancer cells in Stage 0.

+ *Wide local excision* removes the cancer and some of the tissue around it. Skin grafts may be needed to repair the vagina.

+ *Vaginectomy* removes the entire vagina. It is used when the cancer has spread outside the vagina. It can be combined with radical hysterectomy. Lymph nodes in the pelvis are also likely to be removed.

+ *Pelvic exenteration* removes the lower colon, rectum, bladder, cervix, uterus, and vagina if the cancer has spread to other pelvic organs—the bladder and/or rectum.

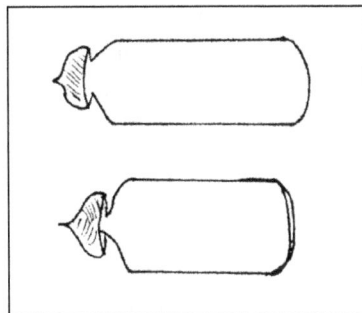

In many of these procedures, the surgeon can use skin grafts to reconstruct the vagina.

Radiation therapy is the treatment of choice for most vaginal cancers. External radiation therapy can treat cancers of the upper part of the vagina in a woman who has a uterus. After external radiation is completed, a "boost," or extra dosage, directed at the tumor with an intravaginal applicator, such as the cylinders depicted, is sometimes recommended. The intravaginal radiation can be done in two separate procedures spaced about two weeks apart.

Vaginal cylinders are made of stainless steel or lucite, are hollow, and hold a radioactive source. Some vaginal cylinders have lead shielding that protects certain parts of the vagina from radiation exposure. They are made in different shapes and sizes to conform to different vaginal contours.

If the woman has had her uterus removed, treatment plans can consist of intravaginal radiation therapy, external pelvic radiation therapy, and interstitial implants. Some cancer centers use a combined surgical procedure and radiation therapy called an **open implant**. During a laparotomy—an abdominal incision to provide access to the inside of the pelvis—a surgeon places radioactive needles into the affected area, and leaves them in place for the prescribed length of time—usually a few days. Other treatment plans combine external and interstitial radiation therapy.

TREATMENT FOR ADENOCARCINOMA Treatment recommendations for adenocarcinoma are different from those for squamous cell carcinoma. The differences are based on what is known about the natural history of the disease. Even for early Stage I cancer, surgery is fairly extensive, involving total vaginectomy, hysterectomy, and lymph-node dissection. Some women may opt for combined intracavitary, interstitial, and external radiation instead. Other women may receive a combination of surgery (wide local excision), lymph-node dissection and sampling, and interstitial therapy. Later, more advanced stages may require combinations of surgery and/or interstitial, intracavitary, and external radiation.

Recurrent Vaginal Cancer

If vaginal cancer does recur, it is most likely to reappear in the pelvic area and will do so within two years of initial therapy. Pelvic exenteration is the treatment of choice in recurrent disease, but it occurs so infrequently that not much is written about the surgery or its outcomes. Radiation therapy is also an option. Chemotherapy has not been effective in the treatment of vaginal cancer, or at least there is not enough data to make clear recommendations for its use.

After Treatment

Treatment can have side effects. Fistulas and damage to the normal vaginal tissues can be late side effects of radiation therapy. Vaginal fibrosis is also an effect of radiation therapy. Just as in other procedures that surgically disrupt lymph and blood flow, lymphedema can be a serious complication following surgery. The extensive surgical procedures, hysterectomy and pelvic exenteration, will have long-lasting and, in some cases, permanent consequences.

Vaginal reconstruction—creation of a new vagina—is done with skin and muscle flaps. Whole sections of skin and underlying muscle, usually from the inner thigh, are cut away and swung upward to create a new vagina. A tube is constructed and inverted into the pelvic cavity to replace the original vagina. Right after surgery, the new vagina will be packed with sterile gauze. A woman might wear a vaginal mold and/or a special support called a **stent** for several weeks during the healing process. She might use a vaginal dilator as soon as the incisions have healed, and will need to use it regularly for the rest of her life. She might insert estrogen cream into the vagina to increase blood vessel formation and the flexibility of the vagina. Skin grafts need special care, and the newly created vagina may require daily vinegar douching. The woman can resume sexual intercourse in about six to eight weeks and should use a water-soluble lubricant. Most women report that it takes up to a year or longer to achieve somewhat normal vaginal function, but that sexual satisfaction and orgasm are possible with vaginal grafts.

The sexuality issues, body image problems, and emotional responses to treatment are similar to those discussed in the previous chapter on cervical cancer and in the next chapter on vulvar cancer.

Posttreatment follow-up consists of regular Pap smears, pelvic examinations with colposcopy, and other exams as needed.

QUESTIONS TO ASK YOUR PHYSICIAN

1. What surgical procedure is the first choice in treatment, and what will be the short-term effects? What are the risks? What are the alternatives? Will there be skin grafts? What activities will I be able to do, and what will my limits be? What wound care will I need to do for myself? How long should healing take? What can I do to speed healing?

2. Should I plan for outside help when I get home? What resources are available to me (home-care nurses, home aides, physical therapy, and so on)?

3. What are the expected long-term effects of the surgical procedure? Should I expect changes in urinary function? Should I expect changes in sensations from my genitals? Will my clitoris be preserved? What about other aspects of sexual function—when can I resume sexual activity? Should I use vaginal dilators? How do I use a vaginal dilator? Where can I get one?

4. What is my chance for developing lymphedema? Will I have lymph-node dissection? What can the surgeon do to lessen my chances of developing lymphedema? What can I do to decrease my chances?

5. What are the local resources for counseling for me and my partner?

6. Will I need radiation therapy? Will it be external, intracavitary, or interstitial? When will this be scheduled, and how many treatments will I need? If I have intracavitary or interstitial radiation, how long will I stay in the hospital?

7. What side effects can I expect from the radiation therapy? Are there things I can do to decrease the chances of side effects or at least to minimize them?

8. What is the plan for after-treatment checkups and follow-up appointments for each specialist involved?

9. Will I need referrals to physical therapy or other rehabilitation services? If not, why?

DES (DIETHYLSTILBESTROL)

Diethylstilbestrol, or DES, was the first synthetic estrogen, developed in England in 1938. It was prescribed to mothers during pregnancy to reduce the chance of miscarriage. Many women who were exposed to DES in the womb or uterus during the 1940s and 1950s have been found to have a rare kind of cancer twenty years later. The Eli Lilly drug company produced and marketed DES as a drug with effects similar to those of naturally occurring feminine hormones. When the drug was first used for women, there had been no studies of its long-term effects. Historically, it has been prescribed

+ as hormone therapy for women in menopause or women whose ovaries had been removed or never developed

+ for prevention of postpartum breast engorgement in mothers who did not want to breastfeed their infants

+ for treatment of prostate cancer in men

+ for treatment of breast cancer

+ for prevention of miscarriage

The current *Physicians' Desk Reference* lists only two current indications for the use of diethylstilbestrol:

1. Treatment of advanced breast cancer (palliation only)

2. Treatment of prostate cancer (palliation only)

A report published in the *American Journal of Obstetrics and Gynecology* in 1948 indicated that DES might prevent miscarriage. It was based on a study of hundreds of pregnancies dating back to 1943 in which mothers thought to be in danger of miscarriage were given DES. From there, more studies led researchers to believe that normal pregnancies could be made "more normal" and could produce healthier, more "rugged" babies. As a result, even women who were not necessarily at risk for miscarriage were given DES. Prescription of DES continued unchecked until 1971, when the FDA issued a warning that DES was contraindicated in pregnancy. Even after the FDA warning, many doctors continued to prescribe DES during pregnancy and *it is still not banned*. A *Wall Street Journal* report (December 23, 1975) documented eleven thousand prescriptions written in 1974 for pregnant women. Use of DES continued until 1975 in England and the Netherlands, 1977 in France, 1981 in Spain and Italy, and 1983 in Hungary. The FDA finally acknowledged that DES could cause cancer in 1975, when other hormones were linked to cancer.

The DES Cancer Network estimates that approximately 4.8 million American children born between 1943 and 1970 were exposed to DES in utero. In 1966, a fifteen-year-old girl was found to have a rare cancer of the vagina. This type of cancer, clear cell adenocarcinoma, was so rare that only a few cases had ever been reported, and never in someone so young. Over the next few years, more young women were found to have this type of cancer. The common thread in all the cases was that the mothers of the girls had taken DES during pregnancy.

The rest of the DES story is a testament to government foul-ups and misguided medical research. Despite the fact that DES had been a known carcinogen since 1940, it was promoted as a useful drug. Despite the reported relationship between DES and clear cell adenocarcinoma, it continued to be prescribed for pregnant women. Despite studies showing that DES caused more stillbirths, doctors continued to give the drug to pregnant women. Despite the fact that the FDA had received information about the harmful effects of DES by 1971, the drug was not restricted. Recommendations to doctors to discontinue use of DES during pregnancy and to notify all women who had used the drug were finally published in 1974. *Despite these recommendations, many doctors continued to prescribe DES during pregnancy.*

DES has also been used as a "morning-after pill"—a pill designed to prevent a pregnancy after unprotected sex. The only problem is that the drug did not always work, and many women who took it became and remained pregnant while using high doses of DES during crucial fetal development.

For a period of twenty to thirty years, nearly every American woman who chose not to breastfeed was given DES (or other types of hormones) for several days after birth to "dry up" her breast milk. This practice was stopped after 1978 following an FDA recommendation.

The incidence of clear cell cancer peaked in 1975 and has been declining ever since. It is impossible to know exactly how many women took DES, how much DES they were given, and the exact time frame of the exposure. Total dose ranges varied widely. The worst time to have been exposed to DES (in terms of in utero exposure) was during the first three months of a pregnancy. It is during this time, the first trimester, that the fetus's reproductive system is forming. Many women were not provided information about drugs they were given during pregnancy. Many were told they were being given vitamins. For others, dose determinations cannot be made because old medical records are unavailable or have been destroyed. Some doctors fear legal action and are not willing to reveal information about patients for whom DES was prescribed.

The DES-exposed population includes:

+ DES mothers

+ DES daughters

+ DES sons

+ Third-generation children (children of DES-exposed offspring)
  (Braun, 1991)

The women who took DES—the DES mothers—have a higher risk for breast cancer than women who did not.

Clear cell cancer is still being diagnosed in women whose mothers took DES. In the United States, more than six hundred women have been diagnosed with clear cell cancer to date. The youngest was seven, but most clear cell cancers occur from the mid-teens to the mid-twenties. The upper age limit for the development of this cancer is not known. DES daughters have a higher rate of cervical and vaginal dysplasia and carcinoma in situ (at least double the rate) than do nonexposed women.

In utero exposure to DES causes birth defects, usually involving the reproductive tract. These defects can be cell abnormalities and malformations, resulting in changes in uterine tissue, blocked fallopian tubes, malformed uterus, incompetent cervix, and inability to ovulate. DES daughters who do become pregnant have a greater risk for tubal pregnancy, miscarriage or stillbirth, and premature labor and delivery. Premature babies are at risk for any of the problems encountered in premature delivery. In babies born to these mothers, the effects of DES extend to a third generation.

The limited research that has been conducted on DES sons has shown relatively few problems. Still, DES sons do have more reproductive tract abnormalities than sons who were not exposed. Abnormalities vary in severity but can include malfunction of the genitals, benign cysts inside the scrotal sacs, malformation of the penis, sterility due to low sperm count, and testicular problems.

Anyone who has been exposed to DES could suffer profound emotional effects. DES mothers live with tremendous guilt. DES sons and daughters live with the need for frequent medical examinations, knowledge of abnormalities and deformities, fear of developing cancer, and concerns about having a child who might be another victim of DES exposure.

By now, most DES daughters (and sons) in the United States are between twenty-five and fifty-five years old, with the majority in their early to mid-forties. It is estimated that one in every one thousand DES daughters will develop a clear cell adenocarcinoma. The good news is that the annual increase in the occurrence of DES-related clear cell adenocarcinoma that started thirty years ago began decreasing in the late 1980s. Also, the survival rate is actually better than the survival rates for some other gynecologic cancers, probably as a result of the close observation of women known to have been exposed.

So, how can women today best meet their health-care needs? First, women need to know whether they have been exposed to DES. Ask your mother, if you can, if she was given DES during her pregnancy with you. If she does not know, but perhaps was thought to be at risk for miscarriage, did she take any medication to prevent the miscarriage? If there is any suspicion, it should be discussed with a gynecologist who can include this information with a complete history and physical examination as well as follow-up exams.

The DES daughter should have a gynecologic examination yearly starting at age fourteen or when she starts to menstruate, whichever comes first. The purpose of early and regular exams is to detect abnormalities and cancer at earlier stages. Exams before puberty are not usually recommended, but might be needed if a young girl develops abnormal bleeding or discharge. In this case, the doctor might wish to perform the examination while the girl is under anesthesia or at least heavily sedated. Mothers can teach their daughters to use tampons during their periods, which will stretch the vagina and make examinations easier for both the doctor and the young girl. The annual exams should include the following:

+ visual inspection of the cervix and vagina

+ digital examination of the vagina

+ colposcopic examination during the first exam

+ Pap smear from the cervical os and the walls of the upper part of the vagina

+ colposcopy exam of suspicious areas

+ biopsy of suspicious areas

+ bimanual examination of the vagina and rectum

+ breast examination and mammography
(DiSaia and Creasman, 1989)

Treatment for abnormal, noncancerous findings are varied and there is no standard recommendation. Some doctors prescribe contraceptive jellies and foams that will lower the vaginal pH and promote normal growth of the mucous membrane. Progesterone has also been used in the vagina for therapy. Neither of these approaches is supported by published studies. In most cases, the abnormalities disappear on their own and no therapy is needed.

The DES Registry in the United States collects information about exposed daughters who have developed clear cell carcinoma. Studies were conducted at the University of Chicago beginning in 1951, and follow-up on these women is still being done. There is no registry in the United States that collects data on exposed mothers or their healthy sons and daughters. Registries do exist to some extent in the Netherlands, France, and Australia. However, there is a real possibility that funding for DES-related research will dry up. DES Action (a consumer group) and the Herbst Registry advocate further research into the effects of DES exposure.

During hearings in 1991 before the NIH Office of Research on Women's Health, the spokeswoman for the DES Cancer Network and DES Action stressed the continued research needs relating to DES. Further research is still imperative to resolve lingering questions:

- What is the effect of the dose of DES given? (There were wide variations in dosages given to pregnant women across the United States.)

- What other long-term effects will occur?

- What is the best way to treat people who get cancers associated with DES exposure?

- What effect will menopause have on exposed mothers and daughters?

DES Action continues to advocate on behalf of people affected by DES exposure. It offers information and referral services, informational publications, and a quarterly newsletter. DES Action is affiliated with the DES Cancer Network, created to meet the special needs of women who have had clear cell adenocarcinoma through meetings, telephone counseling, and a newsletter. These organizations have affiliates in twenty-two states. For more information contact:

DES Action
610 16th St., Ste. 301
Oakland CA 94612
(510) 465-4011

E-mail: desaction@earthlink.net
Website: www.desaction.org

DES Cancer Network
514 10th St. NW, Ste. 400
Washington DC 20004-1403
(800) DES-NET-4 (337-6384) or (202) 628-6330
E-mail: DESNETWRK@aol.com
Website: www.descancer.org

Laboratory studies demonstrate that the effects of DES continue throughout the life of those exposed. There are also growing concerns for effects of "the third generation"—the grandchildren of women who took DES. It is entirely possible that the age with the greatest health hazards has not yet arrived. DES Action and DES Cancer Network recommend that all DES-exposed individuals, men and women—and now, the third generation—be monitored by doctors with knowledge and expertise in DES-related problems. The DES Action website offers a nationwide physician referral list.

— *Pamela Haylock*

19

CANCER OF THE VULVA

The **vulva** is the outside skin or external part of a woman's vagina. It extends from the pubic mound to the rectal opening and surrounds the urethra, clitoris, and vaginal opening.

Cancer of the vulva is rare and accounts for only 4 percent of all gynecologic cancers and 1 percent of all cancers in American women. There are fewer than 3,500 new cases each year. Vulvar cancer occurs most often in women after menopause (85 percent), though it is becoming a little more common in women under forty and appears most often in women during their mid-sixties. In most Western countries, about half of all vulvar cancers are found when they are quite small (less than about ¾ inch, or 2 cm, in diameter) and are very curable. Routine self-examination of the vulva can increase a woman's chance of finding this cancer early.

RISK FACTORS

Little is known for certain about potential risk factors for vulvar cancer, though there are some factors that are suspect. A few studies suggest that diabetes is a risk factor. Cancer of the vulva also seems to be related to sexually transmitted diseases, including condyloma (wartlike growths) and especially human papillomavirus (HPV). A history of other gynecologic cancers places a woman at an increased risk for vulvar cancer. Nearly a third of all women who are diagnosed with vulvar cancer had in situ or squamous cancer of the cervix at least five years earlier. A history of inflammation of the vulva with itching and burning sensations and shrinkage and thickening of vulvar tissues (leukoplakia) increases the chance of developing vulvar cancer.

Smoking cigarettes and drinking more than two cups of coffee a day are risk factors. Women who work as maids or in laundries, drycleaning, or other garment services have an increased risk for vulvar cancer. Very overweight women are also at greater risk. Some experts guess that in obese women, moisture and warmth in the genital area may relate to the development of this cancer.

Lack of cleanliness around the genital area has been thought to be related to vulvitis and vulvar cancer for some time, but this has not been scientifically proven.

PREVENTION

The lack of a clear cause-and-effect relationship between any of the risk factors and the development of vulvar cancer makes hard and fast recommendations for preventive care impossible. Infection with HPV is the most seriously considered factor, so preventing infection with the virus by using condoms and limiting the number of sexual partners is one action any woman could consider. She could also consider using coffee in moderation, quitting smoking, and maintaining an appropriate weight. Having the doctor or nurse practitioner examine and treat vulvar irritation and genital warts as soon as possible is important to decreasing risks. Other preventive measures involve good hygiene of the vulva, including the following suggestions:

- ✦ wipe from front to back after urination or a bowel movement

- ✦ use white, unscented toilet tissue

- ✦ wear white panties or pantyhose with a 100 percent cotton crotch; avoid girdles

- ✦ avoid wearing tight jeans or slacks

- ✦ use mild detergent to wash clothes and rinse clothing well; avoid excessive bleach

- ✦ sleep without panties to allow air to reach the vulva

- ✦ use mild, unscented soap for bathing

- ✦ avoid using "feminine hygiene products"—sprays, wipes, deodorizers

- ✦ avoid scented tampons, sanitary pads, and panty liners
  (Sandella, 1987)

Other than these preventive measures, the best precautions a woman can take is to remember the early warning signs and practice regular vulvar self-examination so that early diagnosis gives her the best chance for cure.

Vulvar Self-Examination

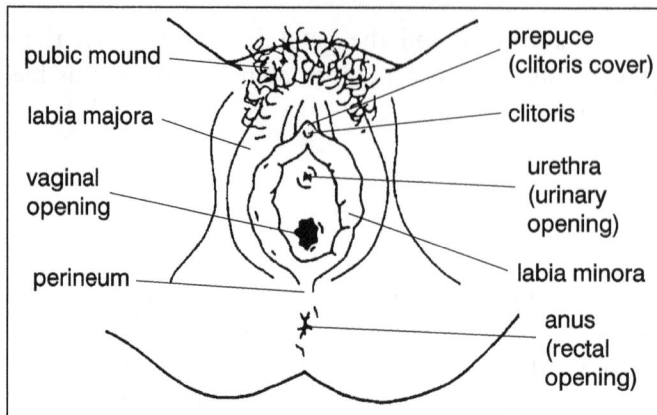

View of normal external female genitalia

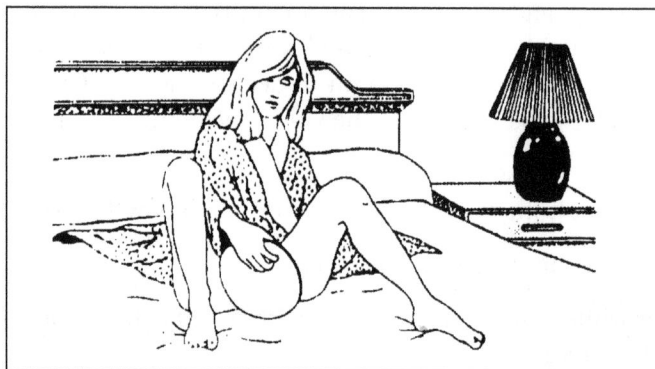

Perform **Vulvar Self-Exam (VSE)** during or after a bath. Use a mirror to make viewing easier; a flashlight can help you see certain areas more clearly.

(This series of illustrations on pages 356, 357, and 358 reprinted with permission from the Oncology Nursing Press, Inc. Sandella, Judy. "Vulvar self examination [VSE]." Oncology Nursing Forum 14[6]:71–73, 1987.)

A woman should perform vulvar self-examination once each month. As with breast self-exam, by practicing vulvar self-exam she grows familiar with the appearance of her vulva and can watch for changes and warning signs. Then she can consult her doctor or nurse practitioner if she notices a change.

BENIGN VULVAR DISEASE

Several noncancerous conditions can affect the vulva. They include the non-neoplastic epithelial disorders: **lichen sclerosis, squamous cell hyperpla-**

sia (formerly called hyperplastic dystrophy), **Paget's disease** of the vulva, and **vulvar intraepithelial neoplasia** (VIN).

Vulvar intraepithelial neoplasia, formerly known as Bowen's disease, may be a precancerous problem. Like cervical intraepithelial neoplasia, VIN is also classified as carcinoma in situ. Herpes simplex virus type II and HPV are viruses suspected of starting the mutation process that leads to cancer. When the immune system is compromised, women are thought to be more susceptible to the carcinogenic effects of viral infections.

Careful visual examination of the vulva during a routine gynecologic exam is a good screening method for VIN. If abnormal areas are noted, a biopsy (with or without colposcopy) that removes enough tissue must be done and will most likely require local anesthesia. A Pap smear and examination of the cervix and vagina with colposcopy should be included in the exam because of the increased chances of other gynecologic cancers with VIN.

Treatment for Vulvar Intraepithelial Neoplasia

Treatment recommendations for vulvar intraepithelial neoplasia are based on the extent and location of the disease. If the VIN is seen in only one area and is thought to be minimal, surgical removal of the abnormal area is the likely treatment. It allows all the abnormal tissues to be assessed under the microscope. Surgical excision performed by a competent surgeon will result in a fast, complete return to normal vulvar function and appearance. Topical chemotherapy using 5-fluorouracil (5-FU) used to be a common treatment for VIN, but it is no longer used because it causes large, painful skin sores.

Cryosurgery has been used, but has mostly been replaced by laser surgery. Healing after cryosurgery on the vulva is slow and the woman endures severe pain. Laser surgery has high cure rates, can be done under general anesthesia, and requires only a short hospital stay. The pain is most severe four to five days after laser surgery. Warm, soaking cleansing baths (sitz baths), oral

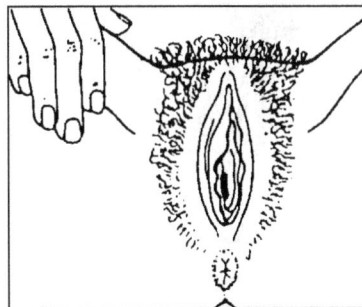

Inspect the vulva to look for any warning signs: Are both sides alike?

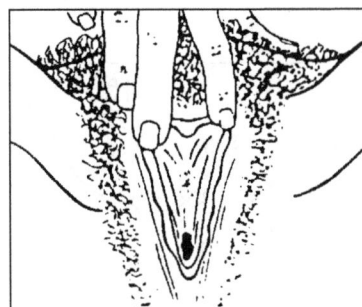

Push back the cover of the clitoris

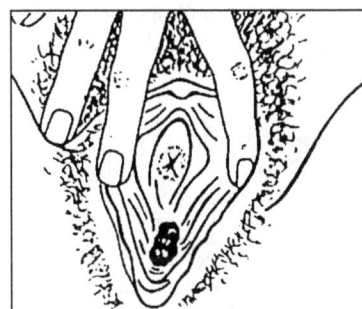

Separate the lips of the labia with your fingers and examine the inner parts: the urinary opening, the vagina, and the skin between the vagina and the anus

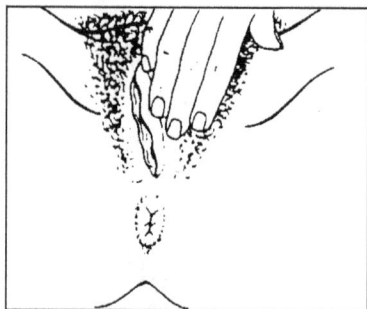

Feel the vulva for lumps or thickening; press all the areas of the vulva with the flat part of your fingers

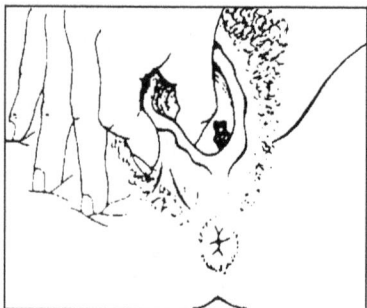

Circle the vaginal opening with your thumb and index fingers

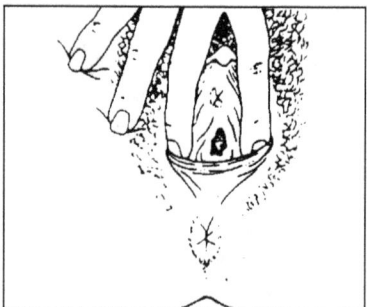

Compress the tissue; it should be soft, slightly moist, and not tender

pain pills, and complete pelvic rest (no douches, no sex, no tampons) increase comfort and help the healing processes.

Follow-up for the first two years after therapy consists of colposcopy and a Pap smear after three to four months, then at least every six months if the examination is normal.

For VIN that involves several areas of the vulva, vulvectomy used to be the treatment of choice. In 1968, surgeons started using a procedure called **skinning vulvectomy,** which offers high cure rates and a more normal postoperative appearance. This procedure involves the surgical removal of vulvar skin and replacement with a skin graft. The procedure can be done so that the clitoris is saved. Clearly, a skilled surgeon is needed to perform this operation. The woman needs to understand that she will be confined to bed rest for some time after surgery to allow the skin grafts to heal.

Today a surgeon might recommend laser vulvectomy instead of skinning vulvectomy. The laser vulvectomy eliminates the need for skin grafts, and it can be an outpatient procedure. The cure rate and appearance are similar to that of skinning vulvectomy with fewer postoperative problems.

Interferon, a biologic agent used in the treatment of several other cancers, is being used in several experimental treatments for VIN. It seems to be especially useful in treating VIN that is associated with HPV infection.

VULVAR CANCER

Signs and symptoms of vulvar cancer include

- ✦ constant itching of the vulva
- ✦ change in color of the skin of the vulva
- ✦ burning sensation in the vulva during urination
- ✦ change in a mole or birthmark on the vagina

✦ a lump or mass on the vulva, such as a wartlike lump or fleshy, white patches

In many cases of vulvar cancer, a woman has delayed getting medical attention or has been treated for vulvar problems not properly diagnosed as cancer. For these women, it is lucky that vulvar cancer grows slowly and usually does not spread until the disease is quite advanced. Without treatment, cancer of the vulva usually spreads to nearby organs (vagina, urethra, and anus) or through the lymph channels to lymph nodes in the groin and pelvis.

Diagnosis

Diagnosis of vulvar cancer is made after examination of biopsied tissues. A doctor might use cystoscopy, proctoscopy, intravenous urography, and X rays of the lungs and bones for staging purposes. Biopsy can confirm presence of bladder or rectal involvement.

Half of all vulvar cancers are found on the labia majora, though they can appear on the labia minora (15 to 20 percent), clitoris, Bartholin's glands, and perineum (the space between the vagina and the rectum). The most common cell type (nearly 90 percent) is squamous cell carcinoma, but melanoma, sarcoma, and basal cell cancers can also occur.

Treatment

The small or early vulvar cancers that make up half of all vulvar cancers are usually treated with surgery. More-advanced cancer is usually treated with a combination of surgery and external radiation therapy. Newer treatment plans that integrate surgery, radiation therapy, and chemotherapy are tailored to the type and extent of disease. Research is under way to study the effects of using chemotherapy and radiation *before* surgery in cases of advanced vulvar cancer.

Surgery is the most-common treatment used in all stages of cancer of the vulva. It can be a relatively minor operation in which only the tumor and the area immediately surrounding it are removed, or it can be extensive and remove the vulva and other organs that have become involved with cancer. The surgical procedures used for vulvar cancer are as follows:

✦ *Wide local excision* removes the cancer and some of the normal tissue around it; can be done in a doctor's office or outpatient surgery department

+ *Radical local excision* removes the cancer and a larger area of normal tissue around the tumor; lymph nodes may also be removed

+ *Skinning vulvectomy* removes the skin of the vulva that contains the cancer

+ *Partial vulvectomy* removes some but not all of the vulva

+ *Simple vulvectomy* removes the entire vulva, but no lymph nodes

+ *Radical vulvectomy* removes the entire vulva and surrounding lymph nodes

Stage 0 or carcinoma in situ, also called VIN, can be treated by local excision, laser therapy, or skinning vulvectomy (with or without skin grafts). The cure rate is essentially 100 percent. Topical chemotherapy using 5 percent fluorouracil cream has been used but it does not offer reliable results—sometimes it works well, sometimes it doesn't.

Women with Stage I vulvar carcinoma have a good chance for cure. There is no standard procedure that is right for every woman with this stage of disease. The three most important factors to be considered are

1. the woman's age

2. the condition of the noncancerous part of the vulva

3. the presence or absence of lymph-node involvement around the tumor

If the cancer involves one tumor on an otherwise normal vulva, and lymph nodes are not thought to be involved, radical local excision is the

FIGO Staging for Cancer of the Vulva

Stage	Characteristics
0	Carcinoma in situ, intraepithelial carcinoma
I	Tumor confined to vulva and/or perineum, and is less than 2 cm in diameter
II	Tumor confined to the vulva and/or perineum, and is more than 2 cm in diameter
III	Tumor of any size with spread to the lower urethra and/or vagina, or anus, and/or lymph nodes on one side
IVA	Tumor of any size with involvement of lymph nodes on both sides or tumor spreading to the bowel or bladder
IVB	Same as IVA but with metastasis to distant organs and/or pelvic lymph nodes

treatment of choice no matter what the woman's age. This procedure usually includes exploring the lymph nodes.

If the cancer in is an area that also has VIN or other abnormalities, the treatment choice could depend on the woman's age. Elderly women who have had long-standing, uncomfortable symptoms and are not sexually active might prefer a radical vulvectomy. For younger women, the primary tumor can be removed by radical local excision and the remainder of the vulva treated by more conservative surgical or medical treatment. For example, topical steroids might be used to treat benign disorders of the vulva, such as lichen sclerosis and squamous cell hyperplasia, with local excision or laser therapy used to treat the VIN. In any local excision, the lymph nodes in the groin and upper thigh should be explored. Radiation therapy can be used to treat women who have health problems that would make surgery more risky. In some centers, radiation has also been used to treat the groin for women who refuse surgery or have other conditions that would rule out surgery to explore the groin area.

Vulvar cancer that involves the clitoris presents a special problem. Surgical removal of the clitoris can have major emotional and sexual effects. Physically, surgery in this area can interfere with the lymph channels that supply the genital areas and can cause uncomfortable and serious swelling. Radiation therapy can be used to treat tumors involving the clitoris; it causes a quick skin reaction that may require treatments to be stopped for a week or two before completing therapy.

Radical local excision is used for vulvar tumors where preservation of the clitoris is possible. If there is a large perineal wound after surgery, skin and muscle flaps might be surgically created to close the wound.

Women with Stage II cancers will usually be treated with radical vulvectomy and lymph-node dissection. Radiation therapy might be used in cases where the tumor extends close to the edge of the tissues removed, if the tumor is more than 5 mm thick, or if lymph nodes are found to contain cancer cells. The five-year survival rate for women without lymph-node involvement ranges from 70 to 90 percent; the rate drops to 40 percent if nodes contain cancer cells. Again, radiation therapy can be used as a first-line treatment if the woman is physically unable to withstand surgery.

Stage III vulvar cancer is treated in much the same way as Stage II. If area lymph nodes are found to contain cancer cells, external radiation therapy will be recommended after surgical wounds have healed. Some women may be given radiation therapy before surgery. The rationale for preoperative radiation therapy is that it can decrease the tumor size and thus the extent of surgery required. As might be expected, the chances for cure are lower with more advanced cancer. The most important predictor of chances for cure is the absence or presence of cancer cells in the lymph nodes.

Treatment of Stage IV vulvar cancer can involve radical vulvectomy combined with pelvic exenteration. Other options might involve surgery followed by external radiation. Preoperative radiation might increase the surgeon's ability to remove large tumors. Radiation combined with chemotherapy using 5-fluorouracil is sometimes suggested.

Radiation therapy can also be used at this stage to treat women who are physically unable to go through surgery. In this case, too, the radiation might be combined with chemotherapy using 5-FU.

Recurrent Vulvar Cancer

Regular posttreatment follow-up is done so that recurrent disease will be spotted as early as possible. Eighty percent of all recurrences occur during the first two years after initial treatment, either in the vulva or another place. A woman's treatment options depend on the site and extent of the recurrence. Radical excision is used to remove a recurrent tumor that has not spread. Radiation can also be curative for women whose recurrent tumor is small and has not spread. When the tumor returns more than two years after it was first treated, a combination of radiation and surgery is the most likely treatment. Other surgical options include radical vulvectomy and pelvic exenteration. So far, no standard chemotherapy plan has been effective in the treatment of women with widespread or metastatic vulvar cancer.

After Treatment

In addition to general posttreatment examinations, Pap smears, and colposcopy, cancer of the vulva and its treatment have long-term physical and emotional effects. Immediately after surgery, most care strategies focus on preventing infection, maintaining blood and lymphatic circulation in the operative area, and adding to the body's own healing ability. Good nutrition is especially important to promote healing. Discomfort and pain can be controlled with medications.

One of the most distressing problems that can occur after lymph-node dissection and removal is lymphedema. This happens when lymph vessels or blood vessels are injured or disrupted, the flow of lymph fluid is blocked, and as a result an abnormal amount of lymph fluid collects in the tissues of the arms or legs. Lymphedema increases the woman's susceptibility to infection. It occurs as a result of any lymph-node dissection in vulvar cancer and affects nearly 60 percent of all women who have node dissection in varying degrees. Treatment of lymphedema is discussed in Chapter 25.

If surgery involves the loss of fat tissues around the perineum, long periods of sitting can be uncomfortable. Surgery can also create changes in the urinary system. For example, the urinary stream direction might change, or urine may "spray" instead of leaving the body in a stream. One nurse advises women with these problems to use a cone-shaped urinal that is made for women to use outdoors while camping. This product can be found in camping supply stores and mail-order catalogs.

Probably the most long-lasting, serious consequence of vulvar cancer is the psychological stress resulting from treatment. Sexual satisfaction is very low in women after vulvectomy. External pelvic radiation can cause scarring and the loss of the vagina's ability to stretch during intercourse. If the clitoris is removed during vulvectomy, the woman loses the organ that may be most important to her sexual response and satisfaction. Genital numbness can be a problem, and sexual intercourse may be painful after surgery. A woman may also fear rejection by her sexual partner. If a woman's self-image and body image are disturbed, it can also lower her sexual desire and pleasure.

As in other cancer diagnoses, the fear of recurrence or metastasis is always a concern. Surgeons are looking for less radical forms of treatment—perhaps combinations of surgery, radiation, and chemotherapy—that offer improved emotional and sexual outcomes.

Some women feel that allowing a sexual partner to help in postoperative wound care was partly to blame for ending or changing their sexual relations. Each couple is wise to carefully consider the choice to use a husband or lover as caregiver.

Vulvar cancer does leave obvious effects. Some degree of disfigurement and change in function will be a part of the woman's life forever. Husbands and partners are affected too, and both the woman and her partner need to make adjustments throughout the years. Using vaginal dilators, which are available by prescription, and having regular sexual intercourse can stretch the vaginal tissues. Using water-soluble lubricants and changing sexual positions (for example, to a side-lying position) can also reduce discomfort during intercourse. Some women find comfort from counseling that helps couples explore alternatives to vaginal intercourse, and that allows a woman to express her feelings of grief over the loss of her normal sexual function.

Vulvar self-examination is critically important after initial therapy because recurrent vulvar cancer is always a possibility. But there is effective treatment for recurrent disease if it is found early. Other gynecologic cancers can affect women after treatment for vulvar cancer, and early detection is always the key to long-term survival or cure.

QUESTIONS TO ASK YOUR PHYSICIAN

1. What surgical procedure is the best choice for treatment, and what are the short-term effects? What are the risks? What are the alternatives? Will there be skin grafts? What activities can I do? What wound care will I need to do for myself? How long should healing take? What can I do to speed healing? Should I plan for outside help when I get home?

2. What will be the long-term effects of this surgical procedure? For example, should I expect changes in urination? Will there be numbness in my genital organs? Will my clitoris be preserved? What about other aspects of sexual function—when can I resume sexual activity? Should I use vaginal dilators?

3. What are my chances of developing lymphedema? Will I have lymph-node dissection? Are special surgical precautions being used to prevent lymphedema? What can I do to decrease my chances of developing lymphedema?

4. What are the local resources for counseling for myself and my partner?

5. What additional treatment will I need after initial therapy? Will I need radiation or chemotherapy? When will this adjuvant therapy start? How do I select a doctor? (Or, how does the doctor decide who will become my other doctors?)

6. What is the plan for follow-up appointments with the surgeon? With the gynecologist? With the radiation oncologist?

7. Will I need referrals to physical therapy or other rehabilitation services?

— *Pamela Haylock*

CHAPTER **20**

RARE GYNECOLOGIC CANCERS

CANCER OF THE FALLOPIAN TUBE

Cancer starting in the fallopian tube is one of the least common of all gynecologic cancers (less than 1 percent). Only about 1,500 cases have been reported since the first report in 1847, and most are single case reports. Most cancers affecting the fallopian tubes are actually metastases from cancers of the ovary or uterus rather than a primary fallopian tube cancer. Therefore, experience with this cancer is very limited and, as a result, diagnosis usually happens as a result of exploratory surgery. Experts think that cancer of the fallopian tube is very much like ovarian cancer, and the treatments for these two cancers can be similar. One major difference between them, though, is that fallopian tube cancers are usually diagnosed in an earlier stage than ovarian cancers are—probably due to more symptoms, including abdominal pain, resulting from tubal dilation and abnormal bloody-watery vaginal discharge.

Who Gets Cancer of the Fallopian Tube?

Because experience with this disease is limited, hard evidence for risk factors is not available. Still, cancer of the fallopian tube seems to be found more often in women who have had few or no pregnancies and women who have had several tubal infections and pelvic inflammatory disease. Most women found to have this cancer are in their fifties. There is one reported case in a teenager, but there is absolutely no information about the girl, her treatment, or the outcome of her treatment.

Recent studies indicate that women with fallopian tube cancer might also be at slightly higher risk to have ovarian and breast cancers, leading to the suspicion that it might be associated with the BRCA1 and BRCA2 mutations. Experts recommend that genetic assessment be offered to women who are diagnosed with fallopian tube cancer, and also that these links be considered when a woman requests prophylactic oophorectomy for ovarian cancer.

Signs and Symptoms

Most women who have cancer of the fallopian tube have symptoms including vaginal bleeding and/or a bloody-watery discharge, colic-type pain especially in the lower abdomen, distension, and feelings of pressure in the abdomen. Each symptom can occur by itself or in combination with one or two others. For example, a woman might have both pain and a bloody vaginal discharge.

During physical examination, particularly if performed at the time of the symptoms, the doctor or nurse practitioner may be able to feel a pelvic mass. This is likely to be fluid-filled; if it ruptures, the discharge will increase. As the mass decreases, so does the pain, but the cancer will continue to grow.

Diagnosis

Diagnosis before surgery is rare. Women are examined for symptoms, which usually mimic other gynecologic or intestinal problems. Some women may have a dilatation and curettage (D&C). If the D&C is negative and symptoms continue, the doctor should explore the possibility of cancer of the ovary or fallopian tube.

X rays, ultrasound, and CT scans of the pelvis may or may not confirm the presence of a tumor. Transvaginal sonography (TVS) might be used. Even after surgery in which a mass is found, it is difficult to tell benign from malignant cells. If the mass is near or includes the ovary, it may be hard to determine whether the tumor started in the tube or in the ovary. This is a very important call for the pathologist to make, since the prognosis for each situation may be quite different. Some cancer centers use the tumor marker CA-125 in diagnosis and follow-up.

Of the limited cases available for study, it seems that most women diagnosed with this cancer have early-stage, curable disease.

Treatment

The minimum treatment for cancer of the fallopian tube is a total abdominal hysterectomy that includes removal of both ovaries and both fallopian tubes. During surgery, it is important that samples of the fluid from the abdomen be examined for cancer cells. The presence or absence of cancer cells in this fluid gives the oncologist an important indication of prognosis and guidance in selecting therapy.

Postoperative therapy is indicated regardless of the extent of the cancer found during surgery. It may include the instillation of radioactive fluid directly into the abdomen (intraperitoneal radioactive chromic phosphate). External radiation therapy following surgery is often recommended. The use of chemotherapy and hormones are not well-defined at this time, but for women whose cancer has spread beyond the tube, oncologists routinely advise chemotherapy, primarily protocols that use cisplatin. Other drugs being studied for possible use in fallopian tube cancers include paclitaxel and topotecan. A second-look laparotomy—having a second operation after chemotherapy has ended—is often advised for women whose tumor has spread to other areas in the pelvis.

Survival statistics for fallopian tube cancers mimic those of ovarian cancer. The five-year survival rate of women with early stage cancer is 60 to 90 percent, depending on the exact stage of disease, the use of adjuvant therapy, the success of surgical removal, and other factors.

GESTATIONAL TROPHOBLASTIC NEOPLASIA

Gestational trophoblastic neoplasia (GTN), also called **gestational trophoblastic tumors** (GTT), is a relatively new term for a group of related tumors. In the year 4 B.C., Hippocrates described one form of GTN, the hydatidiform mole, as "dropsy of the uterus" and blamed its formation on unhealthful water. Before the mid-1950s, the prognoses for these diseases were dismal; today, GTN is the most curable gynecologic cancer.

There are several classes of gestational trophoblastic tumors. They include hydatidiform moles (which can be complete or partial), chorioadenoma destruens (or invasive mole), choriocarcinoma, and placental-site trophoblastic tumor.

Hydatidiform Moles

A **hydatidiform mole** is formed when a sperm and ovum join in the uterus but there is no fetal development. The cystic tissue that forms resembles a clump of grapes. It does not spread to other parts of the body.

In the United States, the hydatidiform mole occurs in about 1 of every 1,200 pregnancies. In other parts of the world, it occurs much more often. In the Far East, it is reported in 1 of 120 pregnancies.

Most women who experience hydatidiform mole are fifty years old or older. The risk is lowest for women twenty to twenty-nine. Women fifteen

Rare Gynecologic Cancers

367

or younger and forty or older have an increased risk. Nutritional factors may play a role in the development of this form of neoplasia; carotene (vitamin A) deficiency and animal fat seem to be linked to higher rates of hydatidiform mole formation.

Women who develop hydatidiform mole during one pregnancy are more likely to develop it in subsequent pregnancies.

SYMPTOMS   Most if not all women with hydatidiform mole notice a delay in menstrual periods for several cycles; most think they are pregnant. Vaginal bleeding occurs, most often during the first three months of the suspected pregnancy. Vaginal bleeding may be profuse, resulting in serious loss of blood. About a third of the women report nausea and vomiting. Because of abnormal hormonal production, particularly human chorionic gonadotropin (HCG), the woman might have symptoms of overstimulation and function of the thyroid gland, or hyperthyroidism.

Nearly half of all women with hydatidiform mole have an increase in uterine size that is excessive for the believed length of the pregnancy or gestational age of the fetus. On the other hand, a third are found to have a smaller than expected uterus compared to gestational age.

DIAGNOSIS   A doctor might suspect a diagnosis of hydatidiform mole when a pregnant woman has vaginal bleeding or is toxic during her second trimester. The diagnostic process will likely include a pelvic exam; ultrasound; chest X ray; kidney, liver, and thyroid function tests; urinalysis; and blood tests, including a test for the hormone beta HCG. Although this hormone is expected to be present during a normal pregnancy, higher than normal levels, especially on repeated testing, might indicate hydatidiform mole.

Amniography can be used to make a definite diagnosis. During amniography, a procedure performed by an interventional radiologist, a needle is inserted into the uterus. Dye is injected through the needle and X rays highlight the distribution of the dye. The absence of amniotic fluid, or at least a very small amount it, is a characteristic pattern of the mole.

TREATMENT   The surgeon removes the hydatidiform mole either by D&C and suction evacuation, or by hysterectomy. The choice of therapy depends on the woman's desire for future pregnancy.

After surgery, the woman's blood and urine are monitored at one- to two-week intervals for levels of beta HCG until it reaches normal levels for two successive tests. The length of time varies for each woman but usually lasts for at least eight or nine weeks after removing the mole. After that, the HCG level is tested every other month for a year. The woman should use contraceptives for one year after treatment.

If the HCG level does not revert to normal or actually increases during the follow-up period, remaining or recurrent hydatidiform mole is suspected. At this time, the woman goes through more evaluation and will likely be started on chemotherapy.

Chorioadenoma Destruens (Invasive Mole)

Chorioadenoma destruens or an **invasive mole** is a hydatidiform mole that extends into the muscle layer of the uterus. It usually does not spread beyond the uterus. It is rarely diagnosed because most women are treated without actually removing the uterus and therefore the muscle layer is not closely examined. Instead, the invasive mole can be surgically removed or removed with suction D&C.

Choriocarcinoma

Most experts prefer to use the general term **GTN** rather than the older term **choriocarcinoma** to refer to this class of tumors. A GTN may have started as a hydatidiform mole or from tissue that remains in the uterus after an abortion or normal delivery of a baby. Malignant GTN can spread to other parts of the body, including the bowel and urinary systems, the liver, the lung, and the brain. Placental-site trophoblastic disease, an even more rare form of GTN, starts in the uterus where the placenta was attached.

DIAGNOSIS The symptoms and diagnostic workup are much the same as for hydatidiform mole. A positive beta HCG is diagnostic, but a negative test does not rule out the disease. A D&C might be useful and can provide tissue for microscopic exam and diagnosis. In some cases, a woman with GTN may have no disease in the uterus but have metastatic disease.

The prognosis for metastatic GTN is generally poor. This is especially true if any of these five factors are part of the woman's history or current status:

+ the last pregnancy was more than four months ago
+ the beta HCG blood level is high (more than 100,000 IU in a 24-hour urine sample or more than 40,000 mIU in a milliliter of blood)
+ the cancer has spread to the liver or brain
+ the woman has had chemotherapy and the cancer did not disappear
+ the tumor started after the completion of a normal pregnancy

TREATMENT Treatment decisions are based on the cell type, the stage of disease, the levels of beta HCG, the amount of time the disease has persisted, the sites of metastasis, and the type and extent of previous treatment.

As in the case of hydatidiform mole, treatment will most likely involve surgery and radiation. In general, the tumor is removed by D&C or hysterectomy: The placental-site gestational trophoblastic tumor is removed by hysterectomy. If disease has not spread outside the uterus, the woman is likely to be treated with chemotherapy. In this case, a single drug, usually methotrexate, is used for chemotherapy. Other drugs sometimes used to treat nonmetastatic GTN include 5-fluorouracil (5-FU), dactinomycin, and etoposide. Treatment with this type of regimen can be curative.

Even when the disease has spread to the brain or liver, some women still have a chance for long-term survival. Treatment can be the same as for nonmetastatic GTN; methotrexate is considered the drug of choice. Some women are placed on a multidrug program that includes methotrexate, dactinomycin, and chlorambucil. Etoposide, vincristine, and cyclophosphamide might be used in other plans for combination chemotherapy. Radiation therapy has only a limited role in the treatment of metastatic GTN.

✦

Some of the cancers that affect women are so rare that very few doctors have much experience or expertise in their management. There also is not much information available in the medical literature that could give a doctor—or a woman with one of these cancers—really good guidance. For these reasons, women might want to consider requesting information about participation in a clinical trial sponsored by the National Cancer Institute (NCI) or one of the cooperative clinical groups. NCI's Cooperative Group Program supports groups of researchers, cancer centers, and community-based doctors who conduct various phases of clinical trials around the United States, Canada, and Europe. One such cooperative group is the Gynecologic Oncology Group. NCI clinical trial information is available directly through its information line and on its website, www.cancer.gov. A woman can also ask her doctor, nurse practitioner, or clinical nurse specialist for information. At the very least, she should be able to talk to a gynecologic oncologist who can provide information about clinical trials that are studying her type of cancer.

— Pamela Haylock

PART FOUR

LUNG CANCER AND COLORECTAL CANCER

Lung and colorectal cancers affect both men and women. Even so, women need and want information about these very common cancers. Cancers of the lung, colon, and rectum affect more American women than breast, ovarian, cervical, and other gynecologic cancers combined, and lung cancer kills more American women than any other form of cancer. Including discussions about these cancers that are largely preventable but still kill so many women is critical, we believe, to making *Women's Cancers* a valuable resource for anyone concerned about cancers affecting women.

CHAPTER 21

LUNG CANCER

Lung cancer is *the* major cause of cancer deaths in American women: It causes more deaths than breast and ovarian cancers combined.

In the early 1900s, lung cancer was a rare disease; today, it is all too common. Since the 1950s, the number of cases of lung cancer in men has increased by more than 130 percent, but now the rate in men is actually falling. *In women, the number of lung cancers diagnosed has risen by more than 400 percent in the last thirty years and is still rising!* No other form of cancer has increased at such an alarming rate. The tragedy is that the overwhelming majority of these deaths are caused by smoking and are thus *preventable!*

WHO GETS LUNG CANCER?

Even though anyone can get lung cancer, people who smoke are much more likely to develop lung cancer at some point in their lives. Smoking is the single largest risk factor linked to this disease. Three-fourths of the women who do get lung cancer have a health history that includes smoking.

When nonsmokers are diagnosed with lung cancer, it is likely to be the **adenocarcinoma** variety—though adenocarcinoma can certainly be diagnosed in people who do smoke. Exposure to asbestos, even for as short a time as one month, increases the risk of cancer for up to twenty-five years after exposure. The combination of asbestos exposure and cigarette smoking acts to drastically increase the risk of lung cancer. **Mesothelioma**, cancer of the lung membranes, is usually associated with asbestos exposure. Exposure to low-level radiation from radon and its decay products is thought to cause about 5 percent of lung cancers in some locales, though the evidence for this is based on studies of miners who are exposed to radiation in their work.

The air pollutant most often linked to lung cancer is passive, or secondhand, tobacco smoke. Other air pollutants that are thought to increase risks are diesel exhaust, pitch and tar, dioxin, arsenic, chromium, cadmium, and nickel.

Lung cancer can start in scars in the lungs caused by tuberculosis. Longer exposure to risk factors—for example, the length of exposure to asbestos, the number of years smoked (with the highest risk of developing cancer occurring after twenty to forty years of smoking), and the number of cigarettes smoked over a lifetime, all increase the chances of developing lung cancer.

Most people who develop lung cancer are over fifty. The average age of women who develop cancer will most likely drop as women start smoking—exposing themselves to carcinogens—at an earlier age.

Women, Smoking, and Lung Cancer

Many people rightly ask the question, "Why isn't lung cancer a huge feminist issue?"

Consider the facts. Since 1987, more women die each year of lung cancer than breast cancer. In the United States alone, more than sixty-six thousand women die from lung cancer and another eighty thousand are diagnosed with lung cancer every year. The rate of lung cancer in women is soaring, mostly because smoking has become so common among girls and young women. At the start of the twentieth century, the few women who smoked cigarettes were either quite rich, with no need to worry about public opinion, or were considered vulgar. Tobacco companies did not market cigarettes to women for fear of societal backlash. By the 1920s, a growing number of female college students and women who liked to think of themselves as trendsetters were smoking. During and after World War II, many women took up cigarettes. Since then, women have become primary targets of cigarette advertising and promotion. Cigarette advertising ties smoking to women's freedom and equality with men as well as promoting it as an alternative to eating sweets and getting fat and unattractive.

Smoking causes lung cancer, and lung cancer is a killer. No ifs, ands, or buts about it. Smoking kills more people than AIDS, car accidents, alcohol, homicides, illegal drugs, suicides, and fires *combined*.

In addition to an increased risk of lung cancer, female smokers risk other medical problems including infertility, tubal pregnancy, miscarriage, abnormalities in babies they bear, early menopause, heart disease, stroke, osteoporosis, cervical intraepithelial neoplasia (CIN), and cancers of the cervix, bladder, kidney, endometrium, mouth, esophagus, larynx, and pancreas. There is evidence that smoking increases the risk of macular degeneration, a leading cause of blindness in people over sixty-five. Even though skin wrinkles hardly qualify as a health problem, it is established that smoking also causes the early appearance of facial wrinkles. (Smokeless tobacco, like chewing tobacco and snuff, is not harmless either—it causes oral cancers, tooth decay, and gum diseases.)

Secondhand Smoke

Exposure to secondhand smoke is also called "passive smoking," with good reason. The health problems created by secondhand smoke are the same as those experienced by smokers. It has been estimated that at least 1,500 nonsmoking American women (and 500 nonsmoking men) die each year as a result of cancers caused by passive smoking. Nonsmoking wives have an increased risk of lung cancer if their husbands smoke. As many as twenty thousand Americans die each year from heart disease related to passive smoking. Secondhand smoke alters blood flow to the heart and within the heart muscle itself, and increases a woman's risk of heart disease. A child's lung function can be permanently damaged by exposure to secondhand smoke. Smoke increases a child's risk of developing asthma. Once asthma occurs, the child will have more serious and lasting asthmatic problems.

PREVENTION

Although most cancers can be prevented by simply avoiding use of tobacco products, there is interest in finding measures that might counter the effects of tobacco and, in general, reduce the chances of developing lung cancer.

Chemoprevention

Research has recently been conducted at many cancer centers across the country on the use of a group of vitamins called **antioxidants** to prevent the development of cancers. Vitamin A, which contains beta-carotene, retinoic acid, and selenium is being studied for its potential in preventing the development of lung cancer in heavy smokers and the recurrence of cancer in people who have already had lung cancer. Fruits and vegetables rich in vitamin A and vitamin C might help decrease a woman's risk of lung cancer. At this time, however, researchers do not have enough solid information to make recommendations.

Reducing Smoking in Teenagers

If we can find ways to discourage kids from smoking, the lung cancer problem will almost disappear during their lifetimes: Most adults who smoke would be nonsmokers if they had never smoked as teenagers. Almost all adult smokers first tried smoking before they were twenty years old.

Every day, three thousand young people start smoking and become regular smokers; over half of these new smokers are girls. Kids start smoking for many reasons: Their parents smoke, they have low self-esteem, they underestimate the power of nicotine addiction, they see smoking as a way of self-expression or a show of independence, they are seduced by the desirable image of smokers projected in advertising, they succumb to peer pressure and a need to be like their friends, and they are simply curious. But, once smoking becomes habitual, it is a tough habit to break. Seven out of ten young people who smoke say they regret starting, and three out of four have tried to quit at least once and failed.

In the year 2000, over one-third of all U.S. high school seniors were current smokers—representing a decline in smoking rates since 1997. A report issued by the National Cancer Institute in 2002 documents a decline in the rates at which teen boys start smoking. There was no evidence of a similar decline among teen girls, and, in fact, the rates of smoking initiation for girls sixteen and older have increased since 1994. Smoking rates vary among different ethnic groups. Native-American and Alaskan-Native teens have the highest smoking rates and African-American teens, the lowest. The report suggests that protective influences on teens—factors that make teens less likely to smoke—include religious involvement and participation in high school sports. Higher smoking rates, on the other hand, are related to poverty.

The risk of lung cancer is an abstract idea for most teens. But aside from the perceived remote risk of lung cancer, there are other very real and immediate physical consequences of smoking. Cigarette smoking is linked to obstruction of the major airways and slower growth of lung function in teenagers. The risks of asthma and severe asthma attacks are much higher for teens who smoke. The normal functions of blood vessels are impaired even in healthy fifteen-year-old smokers. Teenage girls seem to be more vulnerable than boys to the effects of smoking on lung function. The risk of cervical dysplasia is higher for teenage girls who smoke, because nicotine and other cancer-causing chemicals from cigarette smoke make their way to cervical fluids and tissues.

A gift we can give to the next generation is to help our children get rid of the curse of nicotine addiction and tobacco-related illnesses. Dr. David Kessler, former director of the U.S. Food and Drug Administration, suggests "the solution to this epidemic lies in the next generation. By altering the smoking habits of young people, we could radically reduce the incidence of smoking-related death and disease, and the next generation would see nicotine addiction go the way of smallpox and poliomyelitis" (*New England Journal of Medicine* 333, no. 3: 186–89).

As a child nears the end of her teenage years, her attempts to stop smoking are likely to taper off. The sooner she can be helped to stop smoking, the better her chances of becoming a permanent nonsmoker.

School-based group programs that use peer leaders have a good track record. These programs use role-playing methods to teach young people how to cope with pressure, how to refuse peer suggestions, and how to be assertive. Efforts to curb teen smoking need to start early—way before children begin to experiment with cigarettes. Effective counseling programs can be designed by groups that include parents, teachers, school nurses, psychologists and psychiatrists, the kids themselves, and other community members who can help in these efforts.

Community, state, and federal governments are exploring other strategies to stop or limit smoking among children, including plans to prohibit tobacco sales to children, restrict advertising and promotion of tobacco products, and increase taxes on tobacco sales.

Smoking Cessation

Most lung cancers are preventable through two actions: Do not start smoking and avoid exposure to secondhand smoke. Those who already smoke can decrease their risks of lung cancer by quitting.

Quitting smoking improves lung function and decreases the risks of heart attack and stroke almost as soon as smoking stops, but it takes ten to fifteen years for the risk to drop to the same level as that of a person who has never smoked. Other long-term benefits of quitting include decreasing bone-calcium loss and lowering the chances of all the other threats to health that are linked to smoking.

To a person who has never smoked, quitting smoking might seem like an open and shut case—it's bad, and smokers should stop. Unfortunately, quitting is often not simple at all. Because the relapse rate is so high, quitting smoking has been described as more difficult than beating heroin addiction. The nicotine contained in cigarettes is addictive (a fact that tobacco researchers and tobacco company executives have known for decades).

There is evidence that smoking-cessation techniques that are especially for women—designed around the reasons women start smoking and using women's particular skills and strengths—are more successful than methods that ignore unique these female traits. Women start smoking for different reasons than men, and women stop smoking for different reasons than men, so taking into account these male–female differences increases a woman's chances of success in quitting.

In their book *How Women Can* Finally *Stop Smoking* (Alameda, CA: Hunter House, 1994), Klesges and DeBon review several studies that describe how men and women smokers differ. They point out that women say that smoking makes them feel good, that smoking is something they just do automatically without thinking, and that smoking sort of becomes a best friend by providing pleasure and comfort in many situations. They discuss the important fact that not everyone wants women to quit smoking. The tobacco industry and even other women smokers encourage women to smoke. But the most important difference between men and women smokers is that women are much more concerned about appearance and gaining weight. Appearance, "looking cool," and a desire to stay slim are key factors that encourage teenage girls to start smoking. Later, women are less inclined to try to quit because of a fear of weight gain.

There are several ways to increase the chances of quitting smoking for good. Some symptoms women experience when trying to quit are similar to those that occur during the menstrual cycle: irritability, anxiety, hunger, and inability to concentrate. Nicotine-withdrawal symptoms might be confused with those that occur normally in a woman's cycle, or withdrawal symptoms added to those of the menstrual cycle might seem too much to take.

For many women, withdrawal symptoms and menstrual symptoms both increase just before and during the menstrual period. Klesges and DeBon suggest that a woman make a special effort to time her stop-smoking attempt to start at the end of her period, or the beginning of her cycle.

Involvement in a smoking-cessation group increases the chances of success for many women. Enlisting the help of a friend who wants to quit can help too. Nicotine skin patches and nicotine gum can increase the chances of success when they are used along with other changes in behavior. However, *nicotine replacements do not increase the chances of success when they are used without changes in other habits and activities.* Even though nicotine replacements are available without a doctor's prescription, a doctor, nurse, or other health-care professional who is knowledgeable about smoking cessation can assist a woman in creating a plan that will help her stop smoking for good.

While she is quitting smoking is a time when a woman can take her health and well-being into her own hands. Though smokers cite a doctor's advice to quit as an important reason for trying to stop, only half of current smokers say their doctor suggested they quit or offered advice on how to do so successfully.

In 1996, the U.S. Agency for Health Care Policy and Research (AHCPR) released the *Smoking Cessation Clinical Practice Guideline* (see Bibliography). In it are suggestions for ways that health-care professionals can help people fight tobacco addiction. The advice offered in these guidelines is summarized here:

+ Get involved in individual or group counseling sessions that last at least 20 minutes each, with sessions running for several weeks.

+ Use nicotine replacements such as nicotine gum and nicotine patches.

+ Get help learning problem-solving strategies and new coping skills.

+ Get social support counseling.

+ Find a smoking-cessation program with staff members who have been specially trained in smoking-cessation strategies.

+ Some health insurance policies will pay for smoking-cessation treatment, so check your health plan for possible help in paying for treatment.

For specific help in quitting smoking, find allies—friends, a friend who wants to quit too, a knowledgeable health-care professional, a group specifically for women. Klesges and DeBon say, "When you do quit smoking, it will probably be one of the more difficult things you will ever do. It will also be one of the most important things you will ever do for you and the people around you." *How Women Can* Finally *Stop Smoking* is available from any bookstore or directly from the publisher, and it costs much less than a carton of cigarettes. As the authors say, "Start down that road today."

WEIGHT GAIN AFTER SMOKING CESSATION Women who try to stop smoking are often concerned about weight gain. It is true that most smokers who quit gain weight and that women tend to gain a little more than men, but most women gain fewer than 10 pounds (4.5 kg). African Americans, people less than fifty-five years of age, and heavy smokers (more than twenty-five cigarettes per day) are more prone to gain weight.

Despite these facts, the weight gain after quitting smoking is little if any health risk when compared to the risks of continuing to smoke. The weight gain is probably caused by eating more food, drinking more alcohol, and changes in the way the body uses food (body metabolism). There is some evidence that nicotine increases the body's use of calories and that nicotine replacement delays weight gain.

Lung Cancer

379

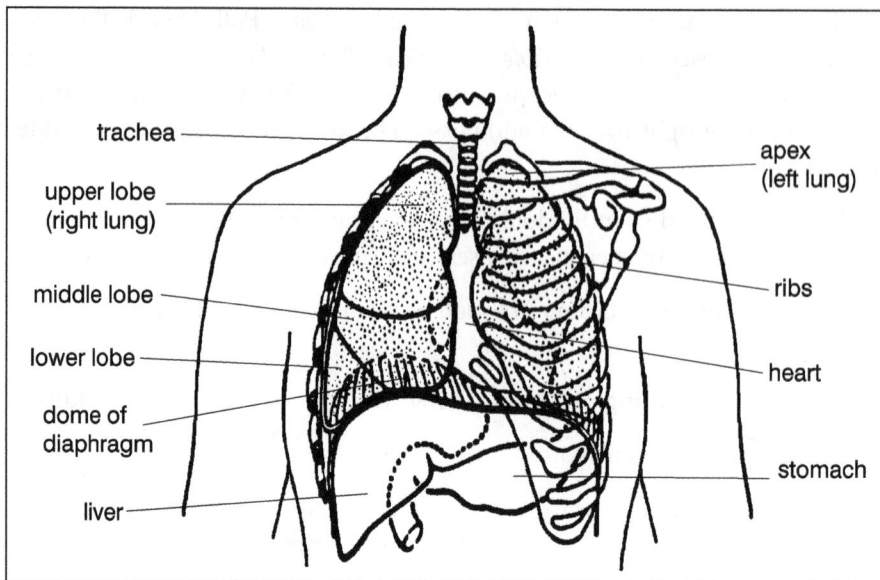

Position of lungs

(reprinted courtesy of the National Cancer Institute NIH Publication Number 90-526)

The AHCPR panel that devised the *Smoking Cessation Clinical Practice Guideline* offers these suggestions for someone who is trying to stop smoking and is concerned about weight gain:

+ Do not go on a strict diet when trying to quit. Instead, adopt a healthful lifestyle that includes moderate exercise, plenty of fruits and vegetables in the diet, and limited alcohol.

+ Wait until the urge to smoke is gone before trying to reduce weight.

NORMAL LUNG ANATOMY AND FUNCTION

The lungs are a pair of cone-shaped organs that are part of the **respiratory,** or breathing, **system.** They fill most of the chest cavity but are separated from each other by a space, the **mediastinum,** that contains the heart and its large blood vessels, the trachea or windpipe, the esophagus, lymph nodes, and the thymus gland. Each lung has a slit, the **hilus,** close to the mediastinum where the bronchi, blood vessels, and nerves enter and exit the lungs.

The work of the lungs is to exchange the oxygen in the air we breathe for the carbon dioxide we exhale. Air rich in oxygen enters the body through the nose and mouth and travels down the throat, or **pharynx.** It

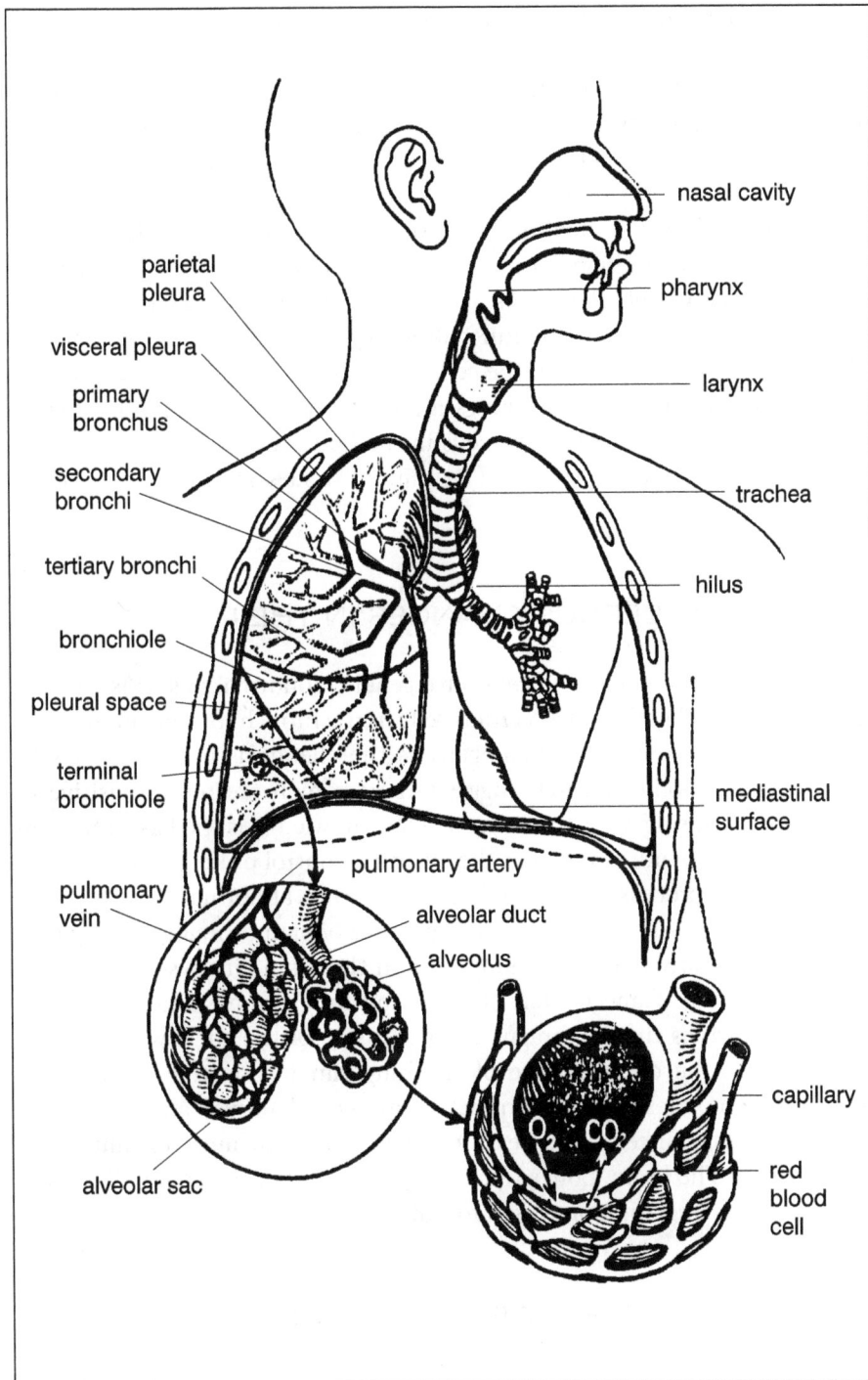

The respiratory system
(reprinted courtesy of the National Cancer Institute NIH Publication Number 90-526)

passes through the voicebox, or **larynx**, into the chest through the trachea and bronchi into the lungs.

The structure of the trachea and bronchi can be compared to an upside-down tree. The trunk is the trachea, and the two main branches off the trunk are the bronchi. One of the bronchi goes to the right lung and one goes to the left lung. Smaller branches, or **secondary bronchi**, lead to smaller and smaller bronchi and eventually divide into **bronchioles**. The bronchioles end in millions of tiny air sacs called **alveoli** that contain capillaries, or blood vessels. The walls of these vessels allow the exchange of carbon dioxide and oxygen. The lungs drive out the carbon dioxide, and red blood cells carry oxygen to all the cells in the body.

The trachea, bronchi, and lungs are made up of several kinds of cells. Normally, these cells, like all the cells in the body, divide and multiply in a controlled way to repair worn-out or injured tissues and allow for normal growth.

CANCEROUS CHANGES IN THE LUNG

Most types of cancerous lung cells have genetic abnormalities. It is thought that an abnormal gene makes certain cells in the bronchi or lung more likely to be damaged from such carcinogens as the chemicals in tobacco smoke and radiation. Some research suggests that women are more sensitive to these cancer-causing agents than men. This knowledge is the basis for exciting and hopeful studies aimed at the eventual control of lung cancer.

When the process of cell division goes astray, abnormal growth occurs and tumors form. These tumors can be either benign or malignant. Cancer can develop in any part of the lungs and in the main airways—the trachea and the bronchi. Cancers that start in the lung often spread to nearby structures such as the diaphragm and the inside of the chest wall. Cancers that start on the outer surface of the lung can invade the ribs and the nerves and muscles between the ribs (intercostal nerves and intercostal muscles). Lung cancer can spread, or metastasize, to more distant structures as well. The brain, bones (including the bones of the spine), liver, and adrenal glands are common places for lung cancer to metastasize.

TYPES OF LUNG CANCER

Lung cancers are divided into two major classes depending upon the type of cell that has become malignant: **small cell lung carcinoma** (SCLC) and **non–small cell lung carcinoma** (NSCLC). These two major types of lung cancer are further divided into subtypes. Each type acts in distinct ways, and treatment is based on what is known about each type of lung cancer. Small cell varieties, for example, are known to spread more quickly.

Small Cell Lung Carcinoma

Small cell lung carcinoma (SCLC), also known as oat-cell carcinoma, includes subclasses called "intermediate-cell carcinoma" and "combined oat-cell carcinoma." This class often shows rapid spread (metastasis) to the lymph nodes in the area of the tumor, the brain, the bones, the lung, the liver, the adrenal glands, and the skin. Because it spreads quickly, this class has often already metastasized to other organs at the time of diagnosis. Without treatment, the typical survival time is five to twelve weeks. Most people do not live past two years after diagnosis.

Non–Small Cell Lung Carcinoma

Non–small cell lung carcinoma (NSCLC), also known as epidermoid or squamous carcinoma, includes several subclasses:

+ adenocarcinoma (the most common type to affect women and nonsmokers)

+ large cell carcinoma

+ adenosquamous carcinoma

+ bronchial-gland carcinoma

+ mesothelioma

+ carcinosarcoma

+ pulmonary blastoma

+ malignant lymphoma

The pattern of spread is similar to that of the small cell lung cancers, but is usually slower. People with early stage disease generally have a 20- to 60-percent chance of being alive five years after diagnosis, depending on the stage and type of cancer. Half of all patients will not be candidates for surgery at the time of diagnosis because of their poor physical status and the spread of the cancer.

If the cancer is diagnosed early and the tumor can be safely removed, surgery is the treatment most likely to offer a cure. Diagnosis at a later stage cancer is likely to require radiation therapy, alone or combined with surgery and, possibly, chemotherapy. Radiation can be used to treat metastatic sites.

EARLY DETECTION

Unlike some other cancers, there has been no good way to find lung cancers early, and most lung cancers are found when a person is being examined for other medical conditions. Annual chest X rays are not very useful in detecting early lung cancers. Small-cell lung cancers grow quite quickly and can develop and spread in the time elapsed from one annual examination to the next. Early symptoms can resemble those of a cold or emphysema and are often ignored.

Lung cancer experts are now advocating for a combination of sputum cytology (testing sputum for cancer cells) and CT scan to be used to routinely screen people known to be at risk to develop lung cancer. A number of studies have shown that with these tests, cancer can be found in the early stages of disease, when chances of cure, or effective treatment, are higher. The effect of this strategy on survival needs to be fully evaluated before it is accepted as standard procedure.

Signs and Symptoms

A cough is the most common symptom of lung cancer. Finding blood in sputum (material coughed up from the lungs and spit out through the mouth) is common. Coughing up blood even once is reason enough to see a doctor and have a chest X ray and bronchoscopy, a test done using a special scope to examine the bronchi. The most common symptoms of lung cancer are

- ✦ cough

- ✦ coughing up blood (hemoptysis)

- ✦ shortness of breath

- ✦ wheezing

- ✦ hoarseness

- ✦ pneumonia

- ✦ chest, shoulder, or arm pain

- ✦ weight loss

- ✦ bone pain

- fatigue

- swelling in the face, neck, or upper chest

- headaches or seizures

- finger clubbing (thickening of the tissues at the base of the fingers)

DIAGNOSIS

If lung cancer is suspected, several tests are needed to confirm the diagnosis and determine whether or how far the cancer has spread. A physician, nurse practitioner, or physician assistant can take a thorough history, perform a complete physical examination, and order a chest X ray. Comparing an old chest X ray with a new one is important, so old medical records are helpful. Chest CT scans and MRI tests may also be used. If the X ray reveals signs of a tumor or mass, cells from the area must be examined under a microscope.

Looking for cancer cells in sputum is often the next step, but negative sputum tests alone do not rule out cancer. Further testing will be done if sputum tests are negative but an X ray reveals a mass. Cells can be retrieved using bronchoscopy, percutaneous needle biopsy, or mediastinoscopy—procedures most often performed by thoracic surgeons or at least by general surgeons skilled in these procedures. During **mediastinoscopy,** a scope is inserted through a small incision through the chest into the mediastinum, the area between the lungs. The scope allows a visual inspection of the area and is also a way for cells to be retrieved for examination under a microscope.

In some cases, the surgical procedure **thoracotomy** is the only way to obtain suspect cells, but this operation might be unacceptable to a woman who is already suffering from illness and to her doctor. A new technique called **video-assisted thorascopic surgery** (VATS) may eventually take the place of thoracotomy. The patient is put to sleep under general anesthesia. The surgeon makes three or four small incisions in the chest and inserts a special scope with a miniature video camera through them. Using the scope, the surgeon views the inside of the chest wall, diaphragm, lung, heart, and major blood vessels. Biopsies can also be done through the scope (see Chapters 3 and 4 for information about biopsy and other diagnostic tests).

If other tests have not been successful in confirming a diagnosis, the surgeon might do a biopsy of potential sites of spread—metastatic sites—of the cancer.

Staging Lung Cancer

Staging tests describe the extent, or stage, of the cancer and help the doctor determine the best options for treatment. Various kinds of tests will be used to determine whether the cancer has spread to other parts of the body. Specifically, the examining doctor will use various imaging tests (including CT and MRI) to examine the adrenal glands, liver, spleen, bones, and brain. Some cancer centers use SPECT (single photon emission computed tomog-

TNM Staging System for Lung Cancer

Primary tumor (T)

Stage	Description
TX	Cancer cells are found in sputum or washings, but tumor is not seen in X ray or bronchoscopy
T0	No sign of a primary tumor can be found
Tis	Carcinoma in situ
T1	A tumor is found that is smaller than 3 cm in diameter, with no evidence of spread to the bronchi or other lung tissues
T2	A tumor larger than 3 cm in diameter, or a tumor that is smaller but is spreading into one or both bronchi or other lung tissues
T3	A tumor of any size that is spreading into the chest wall and other nearby structures such as the diaphragm, the sac around the heart, the blood vessels around the heart, the trachea, the esophagus, or the vertebrae
T4	A tumor of any size that has spread into the chest or heart and other structures in the chest

Lymph node involvement (N)

Stage	Description
N0	No lymph nodes are thought to be involved
N1	There is spread to lymph nodes around the bronchi
N2	There is spread to lymph nodes around the bronchi and into the mediastinum
N3	There is spread to lymph nodes on the side of the chest opposite where the primary tumor is located and in nodes just below the clavicle (collarbone)

Distant metastasis (M)

Stage	Description
M0	There is no known spread (metastasis) to distant organs
M1	Distant metastasis is present in one or more distant sites or organs

Stages of Disease

Stage	TNM Groups
Occult stage	*TX N0 M0*
Stage 0	Tis N0 M0
Stage I	T1 N0 M0
	T2 N0 M0
Stage II	T1 N1 M0
	T2 N1 M0
Stage IIIA	T1 N2 M0
	T2 N2 M0
	T3 N0 M0
	T3 N1 M0
	T3 N2 M0
Stage IIIB	T(any) N3 M0
	T4 N(any) M0
Stage IV	T(any) N(any) M1

raphy) images that require monoclonal antibodies to be injected into the patient before a special X ray is taken. The places in the body where the antibodies collect may indicate spread of the cancer. PET (positron emission tomography) scanning is a similar X-ray test that might be used.

MRI (magnetic resonance imaging) of the chest can be helpful in checking the area of the heart and the major blood vessels leading to and away from the heart. MRI may also be used if a patient has a history of sensitivity to the injected dyes used in some CT scans.

Other tests use elements present in the blood. Carcinoembryonic antigen (CEA) is sometimes used as a tumor marker in lung cancer. Complete blood counts may provide useful information about body functions.

STAGING SMALL CELL LUNG CANCERS The staging system usually used for small-cell lung cancers divides cancers into two subgroups.

In the **limited stage,** the tumor is found only in the primary site, the mediastinum, and a few lymph nodes. All of the tumor sites in limited stage small cell lung cancer can fit into one reasonable radiation therapy treatment field. The TNM system is likely to be used for patients thought to be in the limited stage and who might be considered candidates for surgery to remove the cancer.

In the **extensive stage,** the tumor has spread beyond the area defined as the limited stage.

Lung Cancer

Stages of Lung Cancer

(adapted from American Cancer Society Textbook
of Clinical Oncology, *2nd edition, 1995)*

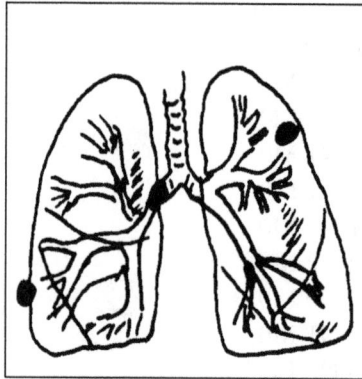

Stage I

Small, single tumor with
no lymph nodes involved

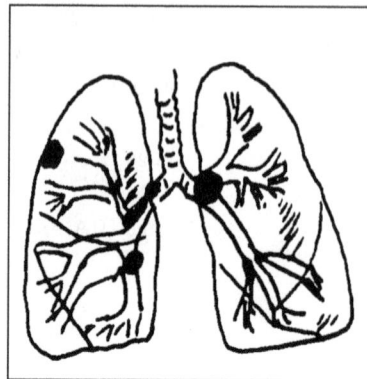

Stage II

Tumor can be in any place in one
lung or the other, and local lymph
nodes are involved

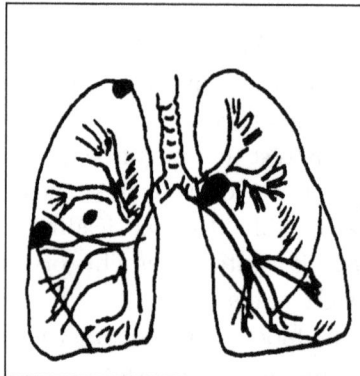

Stage IIIa

Tumor now involves both lungs,
and has spread to the chest wall
and lymph nodes

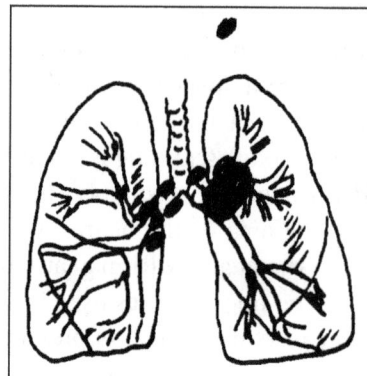

Stage IIIb

Tumor is large, involves other
structures in the chest, and has
spread to lymph nodes outside of
the chest

TREATMENT

Quit smoking after lung cancer? Hasn't the damage already been done?

Quitting smoking even after a diagnosis of lung cancer is helpful. In
study groups, people with lung cancer who stop smoking find that their
ability to breathe is improved, shortness of breath is decreased, they cough
less, and there is decreased production of sputum and phlegm.

Nicotine increases the body's use of energy and can actually drain off nutrients that would otherwise help the body heal. People who quit smoking report that their senses of smell and taste and their appetites improve. They feel more in control of their lives without a dependency on cigarettes and have a sense of pride in finding the will to break the smoking habit.

The most suitable treatment for lung cancer depends on many things: the woman's general state of health, her ability to tolerate treatment, the type of cancer, and the extent of the cancer's spread. A woman should make final treatment decisions only after honest and open talks with her doctors and family. The treatment can be difficult to tolerate and requires the full cooperation of the woman, an ability to work with her health-care team, and the support of her family and friends.

Surgery alone is an option only for people diagnosed with early stage disease. Since more than 70 percent of people diagnosed with lung cancer have advanced disease, treatment is likely to include surgery, radiation, chemotherapy, or combinations of two or all three treatment methods.

Treatment for Small Cell Lung Cancer

More than two-thirds of all people with small cell lung cancer have extensive disease at the time of diagnosis and, for them, chemotherapy is the first treatment choice. If there is no evidence of cancer spread and the person's physical condition allows her to go through a major operation, surgery to remove tumor is the treatment of choice. If surgery is not an option, or if surgery alone does not offer hope for cure or control of the cancer, chemotherapy and/or radiation therapy can be added to the treatment plan.

The most common treatment options for each stage of small cell lung cancers are outlined below. More precise and complete information can be provided by the doctors or nurses involved in the treatment.

In the **limited stage,** in which the tumor is confined to the area above the diaphragm and can all be included in a single radiation therapy field, the following treatments are the most common:

+ In the small subset of people whose tumor is limited to a small area on the lung surface, surgery to remove the primary tumor followed by chemotherapy

+ Chemotherapy with two to five different drugs for four to six months

+ Radiation to the chest along with chemotherapy, especially in people less than sixty-five years old

- In some cases, radiation therapy to the brain may be offered as a way to prevent development of brain metastases; there are risks of altered brain function

In the **extensive stage,** in which tumor has spread beyond the definition of limited stage, the following treatments are the most common:

- Chemotherapy using two to four different drugs for up to six months

- Radiation therapy for treating sites of metastatic spread

- In some cases, radiation therapy to the brain may be offered as a way to prevent development of brain metastases; there are risks of altered brain function

Treatment for Non–Small Cell Lung Cancer

The three major types of non–small cell lung cancer—**squamous** (or epidermoid) **carcinoma, adenocarcinoma,** and **large cell carcinoma**—all have the same chance of cure with surgery. Early in their history, these cancers usually spread to lymph nodes close to the primary tumor—what are called "regional lymph nodes." The next likely place for them to spread is to the nodes in the area between the lungs, the mediastinum.

Stage I and II cancers are considered curable with surgery alone or in combination with chemotherapy, and some of these early stage cancers might be cured with radiation therapy alone. Radiation is the option most often selected for people whose other health conditions prevent them from having surgery. Stage III and IV cancers are usually treated with radiation alone or radiation along with surgery and/or chemotherapy. People with metastases to other organs (those in the M1 group) are treated with chemotherapy or radiation to treat symptoms caused by the tumors.

The most common treatment options for each stage of non–small cell lung cancers are outlined below. More precise and complete information can be provided by the doctors or nurses involved in the staging procedures and treatment.

In **Stage 0,** in which the tumor cannot be seen by X ray though cells have been found in sputum, surgery is the most common treatment.

In **Stage I,** in which the tumor is about 3 cm in diameter but there is no sign that the cancer has spread to lymph nodes or other sites, the most common treatment options are

- surgery

- VATS (see page 385)

- radiation (if surgery is ruled out by the person's physical condition)

- chemotherapy (before or after surgery)

- photodynamic therapy (a form of laser therapy)

In **Stage II,** in which the tumor is at least 3 cm in diameter and there are signs of tumor spread to nearby lymph nodes on the same side as the original tumor, the most common treatment options are

- surgery

- radiation (if surgery is ruled out by the person's physical condition)

- surgery and radiation

- radiation and chemotherapy

- chemotherapy

In **Stage III,** in which a tumor of any size has spread to the chest wall and nearby lymph nodes, the most common treatment options are

- radiation

- chemotherapy

- surgery (for those in the IIIA group)

- combinations of radiation, chemotherapy, and surgery

- endobronchial laser therapy for obstructing tumors

In **Stage IV,** in which a tumor of any size has spread to the mediastinum, heart, major vessels, trachea, esophagus, or spine, or has produced fluid in the chest, the most common treatment options are

- radiation to relieve symptoms

- chemotherapy

- radiation and chemotherapy

- endobronchial laser therapy for obstructing tumors

Surgery

The surgeon selects a type of surgery depending on the stage of the disease, the location of the tumor, and the person's overall health, paying the greatest attention to the person's heart and lung condition. If lung function is impaired, such as by emphysema, surgery may be out of the question.

Operations for lung cancer

(adapted from American Cancer Society Textbook of Clinical Oncology, 2nd edition, 1995)

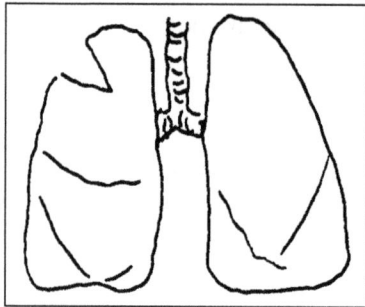

Wedge or segmental resection

The two are similar procedures except that in the segmental resection, more lung tissue is removed

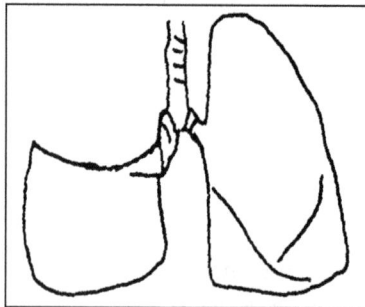

Lobectomy

Removes an entire lobe of the lung

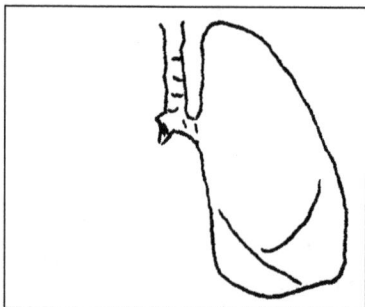

Pneumonectomy

The entire lung is removed

For Stage I or II non–small cell lung cancer, the tumor can be removed in a procedure called a **segmental** or **wedge resection**. In this operation, the chest is opened and the tumor is removed, along with a small section of surrounding lung tissue. This procedure preserves as much normal lung tissue as possible.

More often, the lobe or section of the lung that contains the tumor is removed (**lobectomy**) or the entire lung is removed (**pneumonectomy**). Lobectomy or pneumonectomy may also be recommended for Stage IIIA disease. In limited small cell lung cancers, in which the only known tumor is small and located on the lining of the lung, segmental or wedge resection might be recommended. Otherwise, surgery is not used in small cell lung cancer.

Whether to have surgery for lung cancer is a serious decision. Death as a result of surgical complications is always a risk. The larger the tumor, the more extensive the operation and the greater the risks of serious problems and death. A woman needs to openly discuss with the surgeon the potential for complications during and after surgery. In general, the discussion should cover infection, pneumonia, shortness of breath (**dyspnea**), pain, blood loss during surgery, and the use of chest tubes.

The woman needs thorough preparation for surgery. She will need to learn to do things that will improve her lung function during and after surgery. Techniques such as coughing and deep breathing will decrease the chances of lung congestion and of contracting pneumonia.

It is important to quit smoking at least two weeks before the operation, as smoking up until surgery contributes to the chances of postoperative problems. After surgery, a decision to stop smoking permanently will decrease the chances of developing a second lung cancer.

Pain and its management are important topics to discuss with the doctor. Even though pain is often present even before treatment starts, the woman and her health team need to consider pain in relationship to the planned surgery, and plan appropriate treatment.

Postoperative pain is best managed with strong opioids such as morphine, and many surgeons allow patients to use patient-controlled analgesia (PCA) after surgery. As pain dwindles, other medicines such as acetaminophen (Tylenol) and ibuprofen (Advil) can be used.

When pain is controlled, the necessary postoperative movements are much easier: Breathing and coughing are easier; getting into and out of bed and walking are easier. In all, controlling postoperative pain actually helps people heal faster with fewer complications.

Other, possibly permanent, pain problems include aching along the scar, numbness or loss of feeling around the scar, and tenderness at certain points along the scar. Internal scars left by surgery sometimes impair nerve function and cause pain. **Reflex sympathetic dystrophy** is an uncommon pain syndrome, but it can occur in people who have had lung cancer surgery. It affects blood vessels that supply blood to nerves, causing coldness of the affected arm and hand, whiteness or "blanching" when the area is pressed, and severe pain when the skin is barely touched.

The time right after surgery will be uncomfortable. Some people will be on a ventilator for a brief time, though it will be discontinued as soon as possible. The incision will hurt, and the pain will increase during the expected and necessary activities such as getting into and out of bed, walking, and doing cough and deep-breathing exercises.

There will likely be large tubes inserted into the chest to drain air and/or fluid out of the chest; they will be left in place for three to four days. Care from nurses who understand the use of chest tubes and know the signs and symptoms of problems is essential during this time.

Chemotherapy

Chemotherapy is used in treating both types of lung cancer, although surgery offers the best hope for cure in **non–small cell lung cancer.** When cure is not possible, surgery may still be used to remove as much of the tumor as possible in order to minimize symptoms.

Chemotherapy has not resulted in an increase in survival for most people with non–small cell lung cancer, though it can help to relieve such symptoms as pain and shortness of breath. The use of chemotherapy along with surgery, radiation, and immunotherapy is being studied.

Chemotherapy treatment plans for non–small cell lung cancer usually use two to four different kinds of drugs, for four to six months after the diagnosis is made. Drugs used in the management of non–small cell lung cancer include cisplatin, carboplatin, mitomycin, vinblastine, doxorubicin (Adriamycin), and cyclophosphamide (Cytoxan). Recent research provides hope that new drugs like paclitaxel (Taxol), docetaxel (Taxotere), topotecan, irinotecan, vinorelbine, and gemcitabine will be helpful in the treatment of non–small cell lung cancer.

These same drugs are commonly used to treat **small cell lung cancers** as well, though etoposide, teniposide, lomustine, and ifosfamide may be included in a small cell treatment plan. Adding radiation therapy to the treatment plan has increased the length of survival for many people, but also adds to the risk of treatment-related side effects. When two methods of treatment, such as chemotherapy and radiation, are used, a close working relationship between the medical oncologist and the radiation oncologist is essential for side effects to be minimized.

Radiation Therapy

Radiation might be used before, during, or after surgery or chemotherapy. There is continuing controversy about the use of radiation before surgery in Stage I and II non–small cell lung cancers. Other questions exist about using radiation to the brain as a way to prevent metastatic tumors from developing there. So far, the benefit of such **prophylactic brain irradiation** for people with either type of lung cancer has not been proven.

For women whose poor health rules out surgery, radiation can be used alone or along with chemotherapy. Radiation treatments are usually given on a daily basis (generally weekdays) for four to six weeks and, in some cases, for longer. Radiation used before chemotherapy can reduce the size of a tumor that is causing uncomfortable symptoms. While a chemotherapy regimen is underway, radiation might work with the drugs to increase the effectiveness of the cancer treatment. It may also be used after chemotherapy is finished if the tumor is still present or sites of metastatic spread cause problems. If this is the case, the number of radiation treatments may be fewer and will be spread over a course of one or two weeks.

Radiation therapy can be extremely effective in relieving cancer symptoms. Lung cancer often spreads to bone and causes pain, weakness, and bone fractures called **pathologic fractures**. Radiation is very useful in treating bone metastases, with people reporting pain relief within a few days of the start of treatments. Even if pain is not an issue, the potential for pathologic fracture is high when cancer has spread to the bones of the pelvis and legs. A short course of radiation directed to vulnerable boney sites can prevent fractures or speed healing when they have occurred.

To treat bone metastases, the radiation oncologist can use the standard radiation therapy machines, the linear accelerator, or cobalt equipment. A new radiation technique uses radioactive materials called **radionuclides**, radiation in liquid form that is injected into a blood vessel. The radionuclide finds its way to the places in the bone where cancer has spread, and the radioactivity is emitted just to the metastatic site. Though the radionuclide is strong enough to work on the cancer cells it comes into contact with, it is not strong enough to emit rays outside of the body—so there is no danger of accidental exposure to other people. The only necessary precaution is to flush the toilet several times when urinating or disposing of urine for seven to ten days following treatment. The doctor or nurse must provide more complete instructions.

External radiation can be useful in the management of symptoms caused by cancer blocking the airway or other major structure. Radiation effectively treats a group of symptoms known as **Pancoast's syndrome.** In this syndrome, a tumor presses on a group of nerves in the chest and neck. Symptoms include arm pain and numbness and tingling of the fingers. Left untreated, symptoms increase and pain can become quite severe. Such symptoms should be explored and treated immediately. Delays in treatment can result in permanent loss of function in the arm.

Lung cancer commonly spreads to the brain, and radiation therapy is the primary treatment for brain metastases. Lung cancer also often spreads to the backbone, or vertebrae, causing pressure on the spinal cord—**spinal-cord compression**. Signs and symptoms of spinal cord compression include back pain, numbness or tingling in the legs and feet, and changes in bowel or bladder patterns (such as constipation and inability to urinate). Spinal-cord compression is an emergency that requires immediate treatment if permanent damage is to be avoided.

Laser treatments (endobronchial laser therapy) and special application of radioactive materials directly into a tumor site (brachytherapy) are sometimes used to manage metastatic sites that block major airways.

SIDE EFFECTS Some of the side effects of radiation can occur immediately; others may not show up until one to three months after treatment. When radiation and chemotherapy are used together, side effects will be more evident.

Acute or early side effects include shortness of breath, coughing (starting with an increased amount of mucus and progressing to a dry cough), loss of appetite, fatigue, irritation of the esophagus, difficulty swallowing, and skin changes within the treatment field.

A sore throat and difficulty swallowing are usually the most troublesome side effects. It is encouraging to know that a sore throat will improve as soon as treatment is finished. In the meantime, local anesthetic preparations can be soothing. A soft, bland diet will minimize throat irritation. Liquid nutritional supplements can provide nutrients during times when swallowing is most difficult.

Shortness of breath, or **dyspnea,** may actually improve as treatment continues if the tumor blocked part of the airway. Using medications to dilate the bronchi and loosen secretions can also decrease dyspnea. Oxygen may offer some relief as well.

Fatigue is a common problem for all people with cancer, but it seems especially problematic for those with lung cancer. Rest and an appropriate activity level can help a woman manage her fatigue. Fatigue might also be a symptom of anemia; a quick examination and blood test can determine whether the woman is anemic. If so, treatment may include blood transfusions and the administration of drugs that stimulate the growth of red blood cells, or both.

Cough syrups or cough drops can help to manage coughing and to eliminate mucus. A woman might also request a consultation with a respiratory therapist.

Skin changes associated with radiation include redness and dryness in the skin included in the treatment field. More severe changes that cause the skin to break down and weep can occur in skin folds, such as in the axilla or armpit. The radiation nurse or doctor can recommend skin care products that promote healing and increase comfort.

The late effects of radiation involve changes in the healthy lung tissues. The small, delicate alveoli become thick and less elastic. Other changes occur as a result of damage to lung tissues, resulting in raw areas on the inside surface of the lungs. Prednisone is sometimes used to treat these symptoms and, to the extent possible, prevent permanent damage.

Nutritional management can reduce distressing side effects and complications and increase quality of life among women with lung cancer. Most people with lung cancer have nutritional problems, including loss of appetite and weight loss, and these result in decreased physical ability, fewer social and leisure activities, apathy, and depression. Their immune function is compromised and their wounds heal more slowly. Other symptoms relating to weight loss include shortness of breath, fatigue, infection, loss of appetite, dry mouth, difficulty or pain with swallowing, constipation, and pain. Strategies a woman might use to improve nutritional status include making deliberate attempts to eat more, adding commercial supplements to the diet, adding prescribed appetite stimulate medications, increasing exercise, and taking multivitamins. The dietician and/or nurse can offer ideas that will tailor an individualized approach for better nutritional management. The Oncology Nutrition Dietetic Practice Group of the American Dietetic Association has developed the *Handbook of Oncology Nutrition* (1999) to help guide health-care providers in solving nutritional problems. Another valuable resource is the book *Cancer and HIV Clinical*

Nutrition Pocket Guide (Jones & Bartlett Publishers, 1999) by oncology nurse practitioner Gail Wilkes.

The radiation therapy nurse and radiation oncologist should provide more complete information about how to manage side effects caused by radiation. Not all people experience all side effects—and side effects affect some people more than others. It is important to tell the radiation therapy technicians, nurses, and doctors when symptoms occur—don't assume that they know.

For more tips about coping with cancer treatment, please see Chapters 5 through 10 and scan the Resources section in the back of the book.

SUPERIOR VENA CAVA SYNDROME

In **superior vena cava syndrome**, most common in people who have small-cell lung cancer, the large blood vessel that returns blood to the heart, the **vena cava**, is compressed by a tumor around it or occluded by a clot inside it. Lymph nodes in the neck are filled with tumor cells. The enlarged nodes press on or compress the veins that carry blood away from the head, shoulders, and chest. These veins become distended, and the face and arms might appear puffy. Other symptoms include headache, cough, shortness of breath, hoarseness, difficulty swallowing, sleepiness, and blackouts after bending over or when rising from the bed or a chair. The obstruction of the blood vessels can cause swelling of the bronchi and trachea, resulting in blocked air passages. The brain can swell, and the heart's ability to pump blood is impaired.

Superior vena cava syndrome requires immediate treatment; in most situations it is considered an emergency. Treatment aims at relieving the swelling, and includes chemotherapy, radiation, or a combination of the two. Aside from treatment, elevating the head of the bed, supporting the arms on pillows, and administering oxygen can help relieve symptoms.

FOLLOW-UP AND RECURRENCE

After initial cancer treatment is finished, a woman who has had lung cancer needs to be checked often for recurrence of the known cancer and, for smokers, the appearance of new lung and other tobacco-related cancers, such as those involving the head and neck.

Follow-up will include a review of the medical history, physical exam, review of old and new chest X rays, and blood tests including the complete blood count (CBC) and possibly the carcinoembryonic antigen (CEA). This checkup should take place about every two to three months during the first two years and every four to six months thereafter. Checkups will be more frequent after small cell lung cancer. After two years, depending on general health status, exams might just be once each year.

When lung cancer recurs after initial treatment is finished, treatment options are limited. The focus will likely become the management of distressing symptoms and the maintenance of quality of life.

There is a chance that any tumor found after treatment for non–small cell lung cancer is a new cancer rather than spread of the original cancer. This "second primary" tumor may be surgically removed. If it is determined that the primary tumor has recurred, the choice of treatment depends on where the cancer has shown itself. Radiation can be used to treat symptoms caused by a new tumor that is found in only one location such as the chest, brain, or bone. Some people with recurrent cancer can get symptomatic relief from treatment with chemotherapy.

QUALITY OF LIFE, LUNG CANCER, AND WOMEN

Quality of life after a cancer diagnosis is an important issue, and a woman's quality of life after a diagnosis of lung cancer may be worse than for people who have other forms of cancer.

Women often have more distress after a lung cancer diagnosis than men; they tend to have more pain, more fatigue, more insomnia, and more problems with loss of appetite. Women are often distressed to find that their condition interferes with their ability to do household chores and other work. They also tend to worry more about the progression of their cancer and find it harder to ask others for help.

Learning new ways to cope can often help a woman regain a sense of control and competence. It can produce a greater sense of hope and well-being and help women cope better with cancer treatment.

Relaxation methods, including progressive muscle relaxation, massage, biofeedback, meditation, imagery, hypnosis, and prayer can help relieve stress. Relaxation techniques like yoga can also reduce problems with the nausea and vomiting that can occur as a result of chemotherapy, and they can decrease pain related to muscle tension and emotional distress. It might be useful to ask a nurse, doctor, social worker, physical therapist, or psychologist for help in learning how to use these techniques effectively. Many women find that audiotapes are helpful for learning and practicing various forms of relaxation. Other stress-reduction techniques that may be helpful include music therapy, exercise, nutrition therapy, humor, and interacting with pets (animal-facilitated therapy).

Shortness of breath alarms many people to the point of panic. Using diaphragmatic breathing and other relaxation techniques to manage dyspnea and anxiety can give a woman a sense of control. Focused breathing can decrease muscle tension.

Some people benefit from being part of a group. Seeing how others cope with similar problems and feeling the kinship that goes with shared experiences can be inspiring. Group processes have helped women deal with anxiety, control pain, and develop a sense of well-being and survival.

THE FUTURE

Successes in the treatment of lung cancer have been few and far between. While drugs currently being studied offer improvement in survival time and, perhaps, quality of life, it is unlikely that any of these new treatments offer new cures.

Lung cancer is one of the few cancers that, for the most part, we *do* know how to prevent. Seeking better methods to help smokers quit and more effective ways to deter young people from smoking in the first place are our greatest hope for dealing with this devastating disease.

— *Pamela Haylock*

CANCER OF THE COLON, RECTUM, AND ANUS

Cancers involving the colon and the lower part of the bowel or rectum (**colorectal cancers**) are the third most common form of cancer worldwide and the second leading cause of cancer deaths in the United States. They are also the third most common cancers affecting women—just behind breast and lung cancers. Cancers of the colon and rectum make up 12 percent of all women's cancers: Over 57,000 cases of colon cancer and over 18,200 cases of rectal cancer are diagnosed in American women each year. Every year, another 2,000 American women are diagnosed with cancers involving the anal area. More than a quarter of a million women lose their lives annually because of these cancers. This loss of life is particularly tragic: Most cancers of the colon, rectum, and anus are preventable with simple dietary measures, exercise, and use of screening tests. Found early, these cancers can be cured.

PRECANCER CONDITIONS

In most cases of colorectal cancer, there are precancerous polyps in the colon that, if found early, can be treated, which prevents a colon cancer from forming. Even though we know this, it is also true that in most cases of colorectal cancer, early signs and symptoms are ignored. More than half of all cancers of the colon and rectum are diagnosed at advanced stages, when cure is unlikely. The fact that early stage colorectal cancers are usually curable makes it urgent that we do everything we can to find precancerous polyps and have them removed. Beyond that goal, it is important to notice signs and symptoms of early stages of disease and get treatment right away.

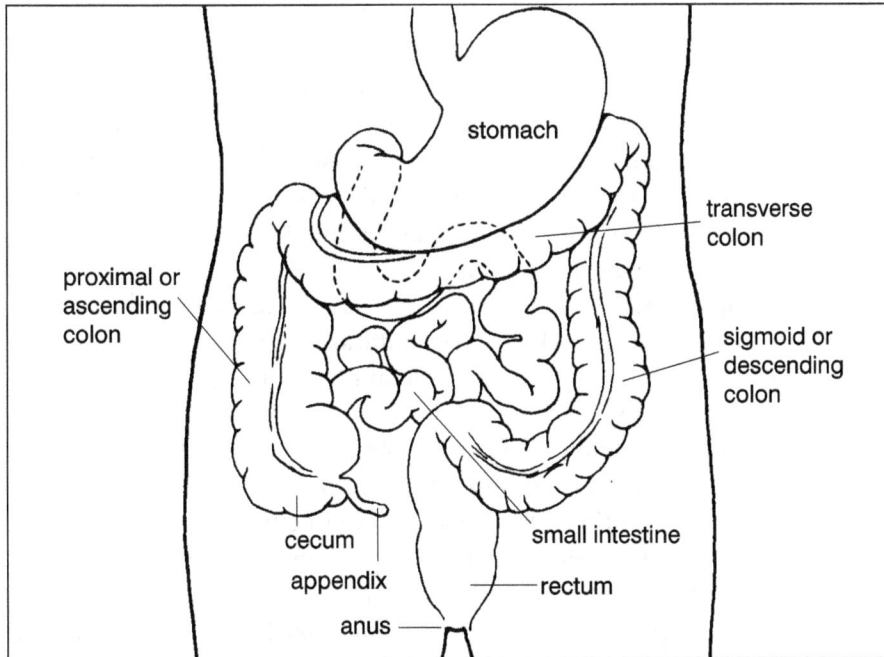

Anatomy of the colon and rectum

(reprinted courtesy of the National Cancer Institute, NIH publication Number 94-1552)

Polyps

Most (anywhere from 70 to 90 percent) colorectal cancers start from what is called an **adenomatous polyp**. One of every five persons—or 20 percent of the population—develops these benign polyps and risks the development of colorectal cancer. An adenomatous polyp starts as a tiny growth in the lining of the colon and rectum. The polyp may look like a common skin tag, except that it is on the inside of the colon or rectum. Other polyps are more flat (**flat adenomas**) and a bit harder to find using such routine tests as colonoscopy.

The cells of a polyp change into cancer cells through a slow process, which often takes as long as five to ten years. Finding and removing the polyp at any point during this stage—before it is about one-quarter inch (0.5 cm) in diameter or turns into cancer—markedly decreases the risk of developing colorectal cancer. Polyps smaller than this often disappear without treatment, though they can slowly progress to precancerous polyps. Finding polyps before they turn into cancer is the reason for regular screening using the fecal occult blood test, digital rectal exam, sigmoidoscopy, and/or colonoscopy, all of which are described in this chapter.

Cancer of the Colon, Rectum, and Anus

401

Hereditary Factors

About 25 percent of all people who develop colorectal cancer have a close family member who has had the same disease. A person with a first-degree relative (mother, father, sister, brother) with colorectal cancer is at risk for developing this cancer, especially if the relative was found to have the cancer before age forty-five. The remaining 75 percent of all people who develop colon cancer—those with *sporadic* disease, have risks that are associated with lifestyle and other factors.

Some people inherit a gene that scientists call the adenomatous polyposis coli (APC) gene. The change, or mutation, of this gene causes hundreds or even thousands of polyps to form in the colon. This gene mutation is responsible for a condition called familial adenomatous polyposis (FAP) that is passed on to children of affected parents. FAP is highly linked to the development of colorectal cancer—so much so that many people with FAP choose to have their entire colon removed even before cancer occurs. The APC gene is mutated in other inherited conditions such as Gardner's syndrome, which is similar to FAP. APC 11307K is a change in the APC gene found in about 6 percent of people of Ashkenazi Jewish descent and is linked to an increased risk of colorectal cancer.

Hereditary nonpolyposis colorectal cancer (HNPCC) is sometimes called Lynch Syndrome and Cancer Family Syndrome. It usually occurs in the right side of the colon (the proximal colon). It affects at least three people in an immediate family (for example, a mother, a sister, and a daughter), with one person being diagnosed before she reaches the age of fifty. Lynch syndrome I (named for the researcher who first described these syndromes) affects only the colon. Lynch syndrome II can affect not only the right colon, but also the uterus or endometrium, breast, bile system, and pancreas.

Inflammatory Bowel Disease

There is evidence that genetic mutations are associated with inflammatory bowel disease (IBD). IBDs such as chronic ulcerative colitis and Crohn's disease are linked to an increased risk of developing colorectal cancer. This risk is highest when the disease goes into a long-term, or chronic, active phase. People with IBD need to be watched closely—a frequent checkup schedule planned with the doctor—so that if a cancer should develop, it will be discovered and treated early.

Other Risk Factors

Several other factors may predispose a person to colorectal cancer.

AGE Colorectal cancer occurs most often in people who are over seventy years of age, followed by those in their sixties. Less than 2 percent of all colorectal cancers occur in people younger than forty years old. About one of every five cases occurs in people between the ages of forty and fifty-nine.

RACE Rates of colorectal cancer varies quite a lot by race and ethnic groups. In the United States, African Americans have a slightly higher chance of having colorectal cancer than do Caucasians, and they may develop it at a younger age. Of more importance is the death rate. Since 1950, the death rate from colorectal cancer among white women has decreased; deaths among white men from colorectal cancer have declined since 1985. The incidence—the number of new cases diagnosed and the number of deaths from colorectal cancers—is highest among African Americans. Hispanics, including those of Puerto Rican and Mexican descent, have a lower risk of colorectal cancer than non-Hispanic Caucasians. Among Native-Americans, there are tribal differences: Oklahoma tribes have the highest death rates, Alaska Natives have the second highest, while Southwestern tribes have the lowest. Racial and ethnic variations are likely linked to differences in diet and access to health care.

DIET It is estimated that at least half of all colorectal cancers are directly related to diet. Diets that are high in fat, protein, calories, and alcohol, and low in calcium and vegetable fiber, increase the risk of colorectal cancer. Colorectal cancer rates are highest among groups with high total fat intake. In Western countries where colorectal cancers are more common, fat makes up 40 to 45 percent of the total caloric intake. In populations in which fat accounts for only 10 percent of dietary calories, such as in Japan and China, colorectal cancers are less common. Some research points to red meat (beef, pork, lamb) as a culprit. Meat requires the body to produce more bile acids in the digestive process. A high concentration of bile acids may be a factor in causing normal cells to turn into cancer cells.

Heterocyclic amines (HCAs) are the cancer-causing chemicals formed when muscle meats—beef, pork, poultry, and fish—are cooked at high temperatures. Studies have linked HCAs formed in well-done, fried, or barbecued meats to stomach, pancreatic, breast, and colorectal cancers.

There is some evidence that alcohol intake relates to a slightly higher risk of colorectal cancer and strong evidence that it is related to the development of adenomas.

PHYSICAL ACTIVITY Limited physical activity has been linked to a higher risk of colorectal cancer in a few studies. Whether this factor is

Cancer of the Colon, Rectum, and Anus

important by itself, or whether limited physical activity is often part of the picture of people who also ingest a high-fat diet that increases cancer risk, has not been determined.

CIGARETTE SMOKING   Cigarette smoking has been linked to an increased risk for the development of precancerous adenomas. In addition, smokers face an increased risk that adenomas will recur after being removed.

PREVENTION

If we accept as fact the idea that at least half of all colorectal cancers relate to diet and other behaviors we can control, we have to believe that prevention is really possible. Here are some lifestyle changes every person might consider adopting to help prevent colorectal cancers.

Diet

Fiber (including wheat bran, cellulose, and dried beans) in the diet offers some protection against colorectal cancers. In one study, wheat bran at a dose of 11 grams each day reduced the recurrence of rectal polyps in people with familial adenomatous polyposis. The National Cancer Institute is conducting a trial to examine the effects of a diet low in fat and high in fiber, vegetables, and fruits on polyp recurrence in people who do not have familial polyps.

The theory of how fiber protects the colon involves the interplay of the length of time it takes digested materials to move through the colon (bowel transit time), the end products of ingested foods (especially animal fats) that seem to promote cancer, and the length of time the bowel lining is exposed to cancer-causing factors. Minimizing or completely avoiding HCAs in the diet is also important.

Calcium

Taking calcium by mouth seems to reduce the risk of colorectal cancer. It is thought that calcium attaches to bile and fatty acids and, by doing so, prevents them from attacking the inner walls of the colon. A study published in the *Journal of the National Cancer Institute* and conducted by the Harvard School of Public Health in 2002 found a risk reduction for left-side colon cancer by 40 to 50 percent with a daily dose of 700 to 800 mg of calcium.

At this time, the optimal dose is not known. In most studies, the daily calcium doses range from 1,250 to 2,000 mg. The U. S. Department of Health and Human Services' *Healthy People 2010* program recommends daily doses of between 1,000 mg (for adults nineteen to fifty years old) to 1,200 mg (for adults fifty-one and older) of calcium.

Vitamin E

A 1993 study found that women who regularly take vitamin E were slightly less likely to develop colon cancer. No real recommendations have been made based on this study. Consultation with your primary health-care provider might be useful in devising a well-thought-out prevention plan.

Folate

A daily multivitamin containing folic acid or folate may reduce the risk of colorectal cancer.

Nonsteroidal Anti-Inflammatory Drugs

The American Cancer Society conducted a study involving more than 600,000 adults and found a significant reduction in the death rates from colorectal cancers in regular aspirin users. So-called regular aspirin users were people who took aspirin at least sixteen times each month; the amount and duration of aspirin use were not reported. A study reported at the 2002 meeting of the American Association for Cancer Research reported a slight reduction in recurrence of polyps (after they were removed during colonoscopy) in people who take a daily dose of one 80 mg baby aspirin. During this meeting, experts said they are close to making a recommendation that people who have had polyps removed take a baby aspirin daily, but they are waiting for a second study to support this recommendation. Similar findings have been reported in additional studies involving aspirin and other **nonsteroidal anti-inflammatory drugs**, or NSAIDs, such as ibuprofen and indomethacin.

Although concrete recommendations based on these studies have not yet been made, some experts suggest a dose of one regular (325 mg) aspirin every other day. However, because these drugs, even if they do not require a prescription, can have serious side effects and interact with other medicines, a woman would be wise to consult with her primary care provider before taking any NSAID.

*Cancer of
the Colon,
Rectum, and
Anus*

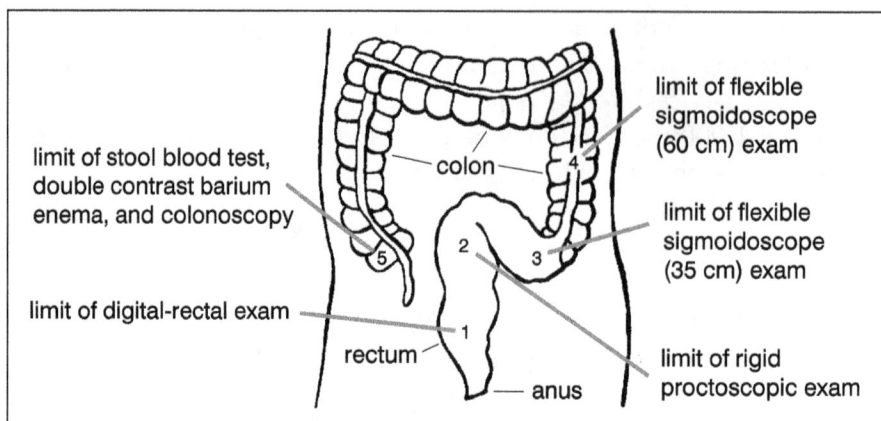

Colorectal cancer screening tests
(reprinted with permission of the American Cancer Society, Inc.)

SCREENING

Colorectal cancer is suited to using screening measures to find precancerous conditions and early stages of cancer. Using these measures, colorectal cancer can be prevented or cured. Beginning at fifty years of age, the American Cancer Society recommends that women (and men too) who have an average risk for developing colorectal cancer follow one of these five screening options:

1. yearly fecal occult blood test (FOBT) plus flexible sigmoidoscopy every five years

2. flexible sigmoidoscopy every five years

3. yearly fecal occult blood test

4. colonoscopy every ten years

5. double-contrast barium enema every five years

People at high risk should begin screening before age fifty and should undergo testing more often.

Digital Rectal Examination

The digital rectal examination (DRE) should be a routine part of every woman's regular gynecologic or medical checkup. DRE is not used alone and should be combined with screening processes such as the barium enema, sigmoidoscopy, or colonoscopy (described on the next few pages).

The doctor or nurse practitioner who performs the bimanual (two-handed) exam and Pap smear should do the DRE at the same time. In addition, many health-care plans, hospitals, and clinics request that the DRE be a routine part of all pre-admission testing regardless of diagnosis.

This simple-to-do test can locate polyps and tumors at the lowest part of the colon and rectum. There is no special preparation, other than to assure privacy and to take care to spare a woman from embarrassment to the extent possible. During DRE, the doctor or nurse inserts a gloved and lubricated finger into woman's rectum in an effort to feel any lumps or bumps that could be polyps or tumors. Any stool, or feces, removed during the exam can be tested for blood using the fecal occult blood test.

Fecal Occult Blood Test

Guidelines suggest that men and women fifty years of age and older and who are at average risk have yearly screening with fecal occult blood testing (FOBT). Finding polyps and cancers of the colon and rectum by testing for blood in the stool is based on the fact that cancers bleed more than normal tissues. Larger polyps are more likely to bleed than small polyps. People with positive fecal occult blood tests must have additional tests to rule out cancer and determine the source of the bleeding.

The most common FOBT technique is the **guaiac test**. The test cannot reveal whether a cancer is present, but it does provide a simple and inexpensive clue that further testing is needed. Substances other than blood, including red meat, bacteria, some fruits and vegetables, aspirin, and other NSAIDs can cause the test to be positive. For this reason, there are dietary restrictions that are important to follow for at least forty-eight hours before the FOBT (see table below).

Dietary and Medication Instructions to Be Followed for 48 Hours Before and During Sampling for FOBT

Include	Avoid
✦ White meats: small amounts of chicken, lamb turkey, tuna	✦ Red meats: beef, pork, veal
✦ Vegetables (cooked and raw): lettuce, corn, spinach, celery	✦ Vegetables: horseradish, turnips, broccoli, cauliflower
✦ Fruits: prunes, grapes, plums, apples	✦ Cantaloupe
✦ Cereals: bran and bran-containing	✦ Aspirin and other NSAIDs
	✦ Vitamin C and tonics that contain vitamin C

To perform the FOBT, you will be given a small test kit. Conduct the test by taking samples of stool from two different sections of a bowel movement. Using the stick from the test kit, apply a thin smear of stool onto the two windows of the testing card. Repeat this process for the next two bowel movements. Return the cards by mail, or take them to the clinic within four days. Testing will be completed in the clinic or the laboratory, and the results are known immediately.

Screening for fecal occult blood is a way that cancers are found at early and more curable stages. Still, FOBT is not proof positive that there is no cancer, nor does it prove that a cancer *is* present. It simply is one piece of a puzzle, with other pieces needed to complete the picture. If FOBT is negative, but the person has symptoms, her physician might want to repeat the test or use other tests. If FOBT is positive, the physician will require additional tests to verify the result and to pinpoint the source of blood in the feces. More complete screening will involve sigmoidoscopy, barium enema, or colonoscopy.

Sigmoidoscopy

Sigmoidoscopy can be used for screening by itself or in connection with FOBT, though sigmoidoscopy is quickly being replaced by colonoscopy. Experts recommend screening with the flexible sigmoidoscope every five years, starting at age fifty. During sigmoidoscopy, a scope is inserted into the rectum. The flexible sigmoidoscope allows the person doing the exam (the endoscopist) a view of the inside of the rectum and left (sigmoid) colon. If polyps or signs of tumor are found, a full exam of the entire colon with colonoscopy should follow, along with removal of the polyps and biopsy of possible cancers.

Sigmoidoscopy requires the patient to have a saltwater (saline) laxative enema about one to two hours before the procedure. *If removal of polyps is planned, additional and full-bowel preparation is critical.* Most people having sigmoidoscopy are not sedated. About one of every ten people who have sigmoidoscopy have discomfort. Most people find the procedure somewhat embarrassing, but good clinics that offer a quality service do everything possible to ensure privacy.

Sigmoidoscopy takes an average of eight minutes, depending on the experience and skill of the endoscopist. Doctors and nurses doing the procedure should be specially trained; experts say that skills are gained only through instruction and the experience of doing at least twenty-four to thirty exams. It is well within your rights to ask about the skill and experience of the person doing the sigmoidoscopy. In fact, every woman *should* ask.

Barium Enema

A study published in 2000 makes the point that a barium enema should be used only when colonoscopy is not available or, for whatever reason, cannot be used. If it must be used, experts suggest that a **double-contrast barium enema** should be done every five to ten years for people fifty and over.

In the double-contrast (or air-contrast) barium enema (DCBE), liquid barium is injected into the rectum through a soft tube. The barium is traced using special X rays as the patient rolls to the left and right and is tilted to a standing position; these positions allow the barium to reach every part of the colon. After most of the barium has been removed, air is injected into the rectum. Any polyps or cancer sites will be outlined by small amounts of retained barium. X rays of the colon are taken during this process.

Preparation for barium enema starts at least twenty-four hours before the exam. Preparations include eating a low-residue or liquid diet and using laxatives and enemas. Each facility, clinic, or radiology (X-ray) department will have written directions to help guide patients through the preparation. If written instructions are not offered, ask for them. Drink plenty of clear fluids to avoid becoming dehydrated during the preparation.

The exam will take about one-half hour. Some facilities give patients a drug to decrease bowel spasms, but sedatives are not part of the routine process. Patients can leave the facility right after the examination. Normally, barium will pass from the rectum for up to two days after the procedure. Barium is known to cause serious constipation, so many physicians routinely prescribe laxatives that will help patients expel the barium.

Colonoscopy

Colonoscopy is the only test that allows the entire colon to be examined, enabling detection and removal of polyps and biopsy of suspected cancers. Full colonoscopy, so far done only by doctors, should be part of the annual checkup at least once every ten years starting at fifty years of age.

During colonoscopy, the progress of the scope as it travels through the colon is photographed by a video camera attached to the scope and monitored on a video screen. Air is injected through the tube and scope to distend the bowel and offer a more complete view of its normal twists and turns. The doctor can remove polyps during this procedure.

Preparation for colonoscopy is fairly intense, requiring the use of laxatives and, usually, enemas. Most people will be given intravenous (IV) injections of enough sedatives to make the procedure as painless as possible while still allowing them to cooperate with instructions as the test is being conducted. The colonoscopy takes only fifteen to twenty minutes if an

Cancer of the Colon, Rectum, and Anus

experienced doctor does it. Most people will have some pain during and after the procedure, but can usually return home within two hours.

Older people and people with a history of heart problems need to discuss their medical history with the doctor, who may then prescribe special precautions, such as antibiotics to be taken prior to the test or special monitoring of blood pressure.

Screening for People at Increased Risk for Colorectal Cancer

Just to summarize, people considered to have higher risks for colorectal cancer are the following:

- ✦ anyone with a strong family history of colorectal cancer or polyps
- ✦ anyone whose family members have hereditary colorectal cancer syndromes
- ✦ anyone with a personal history of colorectal cancer or polyps
- ✦ anyone with a personal history of inflammatory bowel disease

Regular screening is the key to helping people with above-average risk prevent colorectal cancers from occurring or, at the very least, find and treat them when they are at their most curable stage. The American Gastroenterological Association (AGA) guidelines suggest that people with a close relative (sister, brother, parent, or child) who has had colorectal cancer or a polyp should have the same screening tests as people at average risk, but should start sooner—by age forty, if not before. A doctor or nurse who specializes in cancer risk assessment can help in developing a good screening plan.

The AGA screening guidelines for a person with a history of familial adenomatous polyposis suggest genetic counseling and genetic testing. If polyposis is found, the person might begin to think about whether and when to have the entire colon removed in a surgery called **colectomy**.

If a person has a family history of colorectal cancer in several close relatives, and especially if these cancers occurred at a young age, genetic counseling and testing for hereditary nonpolyposis colorectal cancer (HNPCC) are recommended. People with a strong family history, and particularly those who have been found to have the HNPCC genetic code, are advised to have colonoscopy every one to two years starting between twenty and thirty years of age, and every year after they are forty years old.

People who have been found to have large or several adenomatous polyps—even if the polyps have been removed—are advised to have a colonoscopy three years after polyps were first discovered. The time span between future exams depends on the type of polyps they were. This interval should be discussed with the doctor, but will be at least once every five years.

People who have actually had surgery to remove colorectal cancer are advised to have a colonoscopy within one year following the surgery. If this one-year exam is normal, a second exam should be done in three years and then, if normal, every five years.

There is an increased risk of colorectal cancer developing in people who have inflammatory bowel disease (IBD). After eight years of inflammatory bowel disease that involves the entire colon, a colonoscopy every one to two years is appropriate. For those whose IBD involves only the left side of the colon, routine or "surveillance" colonoscopy is recommended after fifteen years of active IBD.

Sometimes cost of these tests prevents people from getting them. Many insurance and HMO plans do not pay for screening tests. Fecal occult blood testing is fairly inexpensive—costing between $10 and $25, and most insurance plans (including Medicare) do cover it. Flexible sigmoidoscopy can cost between $150 and $300: Medicare, with a deductible, pays for this when it is done every four to five years. Costs of colonoscopy are considerably more—ranging from $800 to $1,600—and insurance coverage varies from one carrier to another. If cost is a problem in getting any of these tests, speak with a financial counselor, social worker, doctor or nurse at the hospital, clinic, or doctors' office: Look for ways to get this important test done.

When Is Screening No Longer Needed?

Polyps take about ten years to become cancerous, so if a person is not expected to live for another ten years, screening to find polyps may not be useful. Screening tests are more difficult for elderly people to tolerate. For these reasons, the most recent screening guidelines recommend that doctors stop screening when people are near the end of life. The age at which to cease screening varies depending on the person's general state of health and life expectancy.

SIGNS AND SYMPTOMS

The precancerous polyps do not usually cause symptoms. The signs and symptoms of actual colorectal cancer depend on the size of the tumor and where it is located in the bowel. In general, tumors in the right side of the bowel (the ascending colon) cause dull abdominal ache, black or tar-colored stool (melena), anemia, fatigue, weight loss, and indigestion. Large tumors may actually be detected during the doctor's or nurse's manual examination (palpation, or examination with the hands). Tumors located in the left side of the bowel (the descending colon) cause changes in bowel habits, cramps, gas, decrease in the size of the stool, bright red blood in the stool, and being unable to completely expel stool during bowel movements. Tumors in the rectum cause rectal bleeding and pain and cramping in the rectal area.

DIAGNOSIS AND WORKUP

When screening findings or symptoms take a person to her doctor, the workup will include an evaluation of the entire bowel. Colonoscopy allows complete examination of the bowel. The doctor may request an air-contrast barium enema too, especially if a tumor mass is blocking the colonoscope. Blood tests, including a complete blood count (CBC), CEA, and tests for liver function and liver enzymes, rectal ultrasound, CT scan, and magnetic resonance imaging (MRI) will help determine whether the cancer has spread beyond the colon or give clues to other health problems that could affect treatment choices. Endoscopic ultrasound (EUS) is used to stage rectal cancers. Colorectal cancers that are discovered at later stages are most likely to spread first to the liver, then, in descending order, to other sites in the abdomen, ovary, lung, brain, and bone.

Staging

As in other forms of cancer, the staging system defines the extent of the spread of colorectal cancer. Historically, Duke's classification system (named for the doctor who developed it) has been and is still used by many doctors. In the Duke's system, early and small tumors that have not penetrated the bowel are assigned the letter A; tumors that have penetrated the bowel and have spread to lymph nodes and other sites are assigned the letter D. Tumors that are somewhere between early and advanced are termed B and C, again depending on their size and the level of bowel penetration. The Duke's system is slowly being replaced by the TNM system, which is used for many other cancers (see the accompanying table on page 413).

Cell Types

Most colorectal cancers are adenocarcinomas, which are divided into two subclasses: **mucinous** or **colloid adenocarcinoma** and **signet-ring adeno-carcinoma**. A very small percentage of colorectal cancers are *scirrhous* and *neuroendocrine* tumors.

TREATMENT

With a few exceptions, treatment options are similar for cancers of the colon and cancers of the rectum. A woman needs to thoroughly discuss specific treatment plans with a team that includes the surgeon, the radiation oncologist, and the medical oncologist. In addition, she can include the Wound, Ostomy, and Continence Nurse (described on page 415 and also frequently called an ET nurse), the oncology clinical nurse specialist, the case manager, the nutritionist, the pharmacist, the social worker, other health-care experts, and family members and friends in the discussion of risks and benefits of all treatment options under consideration.

Comparison of Duke's and TNM Staging Systems for Colorectal Cancers

Stage	Duke's	TNM
I	A	T1 N0 M0
	B$_1$	T2 N0 M0
II	B$_2$	T3 N0 M0
III	C$_2$	T2 N1 M0
	C$_1$	T3 N1 M0

muscularis propria
serosa
lymph nodes
tumor
mucosa
submucosa

Cancer of the Colon, Rectum, and Anus

(reprinted with permission from Arnell, T.D., and Stamos, M.J. "Alternatives in therapy for low rectal cancer." Journal of Wound, Ostomy, and Continence Nursing 23(3):150–155, 1996)

Surgery

Most people with early stage colorectal cancer can be cured with surgery alone. Surgery involves removing the primary tumor and lymph nodes in the area of the primary tumor, along with the part of the colon around the tumor. Think of the colon as a garden hose: In surgery, the part of the hose where the tumor is located is sliced and cut away, and the healthy ends of the colon are sewn back together, or reconnected (resection and anastomosis).

The role of laparoscopic procedures, which are much less invasive than traditional surgical techniques, is still being assessed, but they are already being used in situations where surgery poses a high risk for the patient—such as with people who have poor lung function and other serious medical conditions. The addition of chemotherapy and radiation has increased the chances of cure for some people whose cancers have spread to the liver. Control of disease for extended periods of time is possible through chemotherapy and radiation even when cancer is found at an advanced stage.

PREOPERATIVE PLANNING   First and foremost, nutrition is key to a good, healthy healing process. Assessment for nutritional needs is an important preoperative consideration, and the woman and her family or friends—particularly if the woman might need help after surgery—should have thorough talks with the doctor or nurse to get a clear picture of what the surgery will entail and what they can expect afterwards.

Questions to Ask the Doctor or Nurse

1. Will I need a temporary colostomy?

2. Will I need a permanent colostomy?

3. Should I see the Wound, Ostomy, and Continence Nurse/ET nurse?

4. Do I need to build up my nutritional status before surgery?

5. What can I do to improve my nutritional status?

6. What can I do before surgery to decrease the chances of problems during and after surgery?

7. What can I or my family and friends do to prepare for self-care in my home after surgery?

8. Will I need home nursing services?

9. Is it likely that I will need cancer treatment such as radiation or chemotherapy before or after surgery?

10. After surgery, what symptoms (in particular, fever, wound infection, pneumonia, and blood clots) might indicate that there is a problem? When should I call the doctor and nurse?

11. What services will my insurance plan pay for?

12. What am I expected to pay for out of my own pocket?

13. Is there a social worker, case manager, or financial counselor who can help me figure out how to pay for my care?

14. How likely is it that my cancer will recur?

Before surgery, the patient will need to drink a bowel preparation fluid—a strong laxative—to clean the bowel. Oral antibiotics are prescribed for the day before surgery, and an intravenous antibiotic will be given just before and during surgery to control normal bacteria in the bowel and make infection less likely.

In years past, the presence of a medium or large tumor almost always resulted in the need for a permanent **colostomy**—the diversion of the bowel to the outside of the abdomen, which requires the use of a colostomy pouch, or bag. Modern surgical skills and techniques mean that fewer people need a permanent colostomy. Still, depending on the location of the tumor, some patients will need a temporary colostomy.

Temporary colostomy, usually lasting less than two months, allows the suture line of the resected bowel—the area where the tumor was—to heal. A colostomy diverts feces away from the fragile area. When that section of the bowel is healed, the patient has a second surgery to reconnect the bowel, and the colostomy is removed, or "taken down."

If a temporary or permanent colostomy is planned, an ET or a Wound, Ostomy, and Continence Nurse (WOCN) who is specially educated in the management of the ostomy should be called to visit the patient *before surgery* to determine the best location for the stoma. The stoma-marking procedure the WOCN uses will help the surgeon position the stoma in a place that avoids skin creases, the hip bones, body folds, and scars so that the colostomy pouch will be as easy as possible to manage. For more information about the management of a colostomy, ask to see a certified WOCN or ET nurse. The WOCN Society maintains a website (www.wocn.org) that includes a listing of certified nurses throughout the country.

The Ostomy Book (McGinn, K. Palo Alto, CA: Bull Publishing, 1992) is a terrific and easy-to-understand resource. Another helpful title is *Positive Options for Living with Your Ostomy* (White, C. Alameda, CA: Hunter House,

2002). Other information about ostomy care can be obtained from the United Ostomy Association (UOA), at 19772 MacArthur Blvd., Ste. 200, Irvine CA 92612-2405. In addition to more than 400 chapters throughout the United States and Canada, the UOA has a toll-free phone number, (800) 826-0826, and a website, www.uoa.org, that easily links to important and helpful information relating to ostomy services.

Problems linked to bowel surgery include infection, leaking from the bowel's suture line, bowel obstruction, urinary-tract infection, blood clots, and separation of the incision. Blood clots in the lungs (pulmonary embolisms) are among the most serious problems. People with a history of clotting problems, such as phlebitis, will probably be given small doses of a blood thinning or anticlotting drug like heparin. Getting out of bed and walking as soon after surgery as possible is key to preventing dangerous blood clots.

Decisions about the need for further treatment are based on the extent or stage of disease at the time of surgery.

FOLLOW-UP AFTER SURGERY In the first few weeks following surgery, the surgeon will want to verify that healing is taking place as expected. He or she will remove surgical sutures or staples within a week or ten days after the operation, depending on how well the incision has healed. If the immediate postoperative phase goes smoothly, a doctor's office visit will take place within a week or so after surgery. A woman should be sure to clarify with the doctor when the first office visit should be and what signs and symptoms indicate a need to see the doctor sooner.

A history of colorectal cancer places the person at risk for developing a new cancer. Women with a history of colorectal cancer have an increased risk of developing breast cancer and ovarian cancer. From here on out, a woman with a colorectal cancer history should have careful follow-up and screening so that new cancers can be found and treated early.

Chemotherapy

Chemotherapy is generally recommended after surgery for patients with Duke's stage B and C (or Stage II and III) colorectal cancer. The regimen most often used consists of a combination of 5-fluorouracil (5-FU) and either levamisole or leucovorin. The newer drug, Irinotecan (Camptosar or CPT-11) is often added to the treatment plan in people who have Stage III and IV disease. Other drugs that might be used include Oxaliplatin, Tomudex, and Capecitabine, especially in clinical-trial protocols.

Liver metastases denote Duke's stage D (or Stage IV) disease, which is usually not curable. If just a few metastases are found in the liver (three or fewer), surgery to remove them might actually result in cure for some patients. Other techniques used to treat liver metastases include **cryosurgery** (the combination of extreme cold and surgical methods); blocking the blood supply to the tumor sites in the liver by a process called **embolization,** in which the artery leading to the liver is blocked; and giving chemotherapy drugs directly into the major artery that supplies blood to the liver (the hepatic artery) in a procedure called **hepatic arterial perfusion**. The most common side effects of these chemotherapy agents include hair loss, skin and nail changes, sores in the mouth, nausea, diarrhea, and bone-marrow suppression. Irinotecan, like fluorouracil, causes hair loss, but its major side effects are severe diarrhea and bone-marrow suppression.

Radiation Therapy

Radiation therapy used before surgery is believed to decrease the chance of recurrence of cancer and increase chances of preserving sphincter function for patients with larger (T3 and T4) colon tumors. It might also be used after surgery for people whose cancers are probably not curable by surgery alone. In some cases, both radiation and chemotherapy are used in addition to surgery in an attempt to provide the best chance for cure. When advanced disease is present and cure is not possible, radiation often works well to control distressing symptoms.

Radiation therapy plays an important role in the treatment of rectal cancers in particular. A one-week (five consecutive days) course of radiation therapy before surgery for rectal cancer seems to increase chances for cure. After surgery, radiation can decrease the chances that the tumor will reappear. Following surgery for Duke's stage B and C (or Stage II and III) rectal cancer, radiation to the pelvic area along with chemotherapy (using 5-FU) is sometimes the treatment of choice. External beam radiation or brachytherapy techniques are used in the treatment of anal cancers.

A person getting radiation therapy directed to fields that include the rectum experiences side effects that include fatigue, bladder irritation (cystitis), diarrhea, rectal irritation (proctitis), and hemorrhoids. These side effects appear within two or three weeks of the start of therapy and can last up to twelve weeks after radiation is completed. The radiation therapy nurse, technologists, and doctor can offer guidance for the management of these symptoms.

Cancer of the Colon, Rectum, and Anus

WHEN COLORECTAL CANCER RECURS

When and if colorectal cancer recurs, the treatment options will be based on where the cancer is found. Evidence of spread to the liver is often treated in the ways described above. Chemotherapy using 5-FU alone so far appears as effective as using several drugs. Irinotecan and Tomudex seem to work well for some people in the management of advanced and recurrent colorectal cancer. Interferon has not been found to add to the overall survival rate and may actually increase the side effects of treatment.

THE FUTURE

Advances in the understanding of genetics are rapidly being translated into clinical use. A noninvasive way to detect colorectal tumors would negate the difficulties in getting people to use colonoscopy. In 2002, we saw NBC news anchor Katie Couric advocating for advances in the management of colorectal cancer—her continued interest generated by the loss of her husband to this disease. So, we were treated to watching Katie undergo what is called "virtual colonoscopy"—a computer-generated colonoscopy. This technology is predicted to be available to the general public within the next five years. Also, the *New England Journal of Medicine* published results of a research study that demonstrated the feasibility of detecting APC mutations in DNA found in feces or stool. The APC mutations were found even in people with early cancers. A genetic mutation that occurs in about 6 percent of people of Ashkenazi Jewish descent (discovered and reported in 1997) doubles the risk of colon cancer. In the not-too-distant future, blood tests should be widely available to help identify the presence of such mutations. Technologic advances and discoveries such as these will eventually help identify precancerous conditions and early cancers.

Several new chemotherapy drugs have been mentioned in this chapter as being used in state-of-the-art treatment for colorectal cancer—and surely more are on the horizon.

A related area of treatment that looks promising is the use of **biologic agents** (called **biological therapy** or **biotherapy**). These are agents made from biological sources that affect bodily systems, such as interferon, interleukin, monoclonal antibodies, and immunomodulators (biologic agents that support or increase the body's natural immune system). While they do not work well alone, they may be able to improve the effects of other drugs used to treat any number of cancers, including colorectal cancer. It is likely that the use of biologics in the treatment of colorectal cancer will increase over the next few years. Some biologic agents are already used to help manage the side effects, such as changes in the white and red blood cell counts, of other forms of cancer therapy.

The greatest hope for advances in the management of colorectal cancers lies in the knowledge of how these cancers start and grow and the ability to use this information to find precancerous polyps and remove them or to find cancers at an early, curable stage. This knowledge and the skills to apply it are available now—we just need to take advantage of what we know.

— *Pamela Haylock*

PART FIVE

LIFE AFTER CANCER

CHAPTER 23

Long-Term and Late Effects of Cancer and Cancer Treatment

There are nearly nine million Americans living today who have a history of cancer. As survival rates edge past 60 percent, the sequelae of cancer and its treatment become more apparent and of importance to a greater number of people. In addition to those people who are presumed cured, other people are living for long periods of time with cancer that is controlled, though not cured. For these people, cancer is a chronic disease.

Successes in treatment have come at the cost of ongoing and/or new health problems after treatment has ended—problems that can occur months or even years later. The survivor, her family, and her health-care providers often face the difficult task of integrating the cancer history, including its treatment, with a lifelong wellness plan that will be different for every individual. The importance of the needs of these people is evidenced by the recent creation of the Office of Cancer Survivorship within the National Cancer Institute. Its goal is to encourage research in the area of cancer survivorship.

Many survivors of the polio epidemic that swept the United States during the first half of the twentieth century are now experiencing a collection of symptoms referred to as "postpolio syndrome." Maybe it's time to consider a "postcancer syndrome"—a designation that lends credibility to the very real physical and emotional challenges of life after cancer. As more people survive cancer, we learn more about these problems and can alter treatment plans and intensities to minimize long-term and late effects.

It is important for people diagnosed with cancer today to recognize the existence of the late effects of cancer and cancer treatment. Knowing about possible late and long-term effects that are linked to a particular form of treatment—for example, a certain drug or even a certain dose of that drug or having a part of one's body exposed to a high dose of radiation—can be important information to consider when choosing from among treatment options.

In the soon-to-be-revised book from the National Coalition for Cancer Survivorship, *A Cancer Survivor's Almanac: Charting Your Journey*, Dr. Patricia Ganz, Professor of Medicine and Public Health at UCLA, differentiates long-term from late effects:

> **Long-term effects** are known or expected problems that may occur with some frequency in individuals who have received certain treatments: For example, the risk of infection after splenectomy or infertility after certain chemotherapy drugs.

> **Late effects**, in contrast, are secondary conditions that arise as a result of having received certain cancer treatments: for example, leukemia secondary to alkylating agent therapy or congestive heart failure many years after treatment with anthracycline chemotherapy.

Late Physical Effects of Cancer Treatment

Cancer treatment can alter virtually any organ system or tissue in the body. The accompanying table outlines just a few of the more common late and long-term effects: physiologic, functional, cosmetic, sensory, cognitive, or psychosocial in nature.

Change affecting the heart and its function—referred to as **cardiac toxicity**—is most often linked to the chemotherapy drugs doxorubicin and daunorubicin. Permanent damage to heart muscle caused by these drugs—**cardiomyopathy**—directly relates to the total dose: The higher the dose, the more damage. Even at lower doses, some damage is likely to occur. Heart damage increases when people who are already getting these drugs also receive radiation therapy. The heart damage may not be apparent until extra stress is placed on heart function—such as the stress imposed by a new and vigorous exercise program or a pregnancy. People who have received radiation to the chest are at risk to develop **coronary artery disease**, though newer radiation therapy techniques and equipment do minimize these problems.

Long-Term and Late Effects of Cancer and Cancer Treatment

423

Late and Long-Term Effects of Cancer and Cancer Treatment

System/Organ Affected	Mechanism of Action	Potential Effects	Possible Interventions	Wellness Planning
Cardiovascular (Heart, blood vessels)	Anthracycline-related cardio-myopathy Radiation induced cardiac changes Prolonged estrogen deprivation may increase risk of heart disease	Heart failure Coronary Artery Disease and increased risk of myocardial infarction at younger ages than the general population	There are some drugs and some radiation therapy techniques that offer protection to the heart. Ask the doctor whether these measures might work for you before beginning therapy	Include EKGs in routine medical follow-up Consult the oncologist or oncology nurse before starting an exercise program or becoming pregnant Stop smoking
Pulmonary (Lungs)	Fibrosis related to bleomycin, alkylating agents, methotrexate and nitrosureas Fibrosis related to lung tissue in radiation treatment field Anemia Malnutrition	Shortness of breath and other breathing difficulties	Learn to use "cough and deep breathing" exercises and controlled breathing, pursed lips, and use of abdominal muscles Rest Change positioning Exercise—even easy range-of-motion exercises can help Increase intake of water to help clear secretions Use a humidifier at night or when congested	Include pulmonary function tests in medical follow-up Stop smoking
Urinary Tract	Kidney damage from cisplatin, methotrexate, and nitrosoureas Bladder cancer related to long-term use of cyclophosphami de		Increase fluid intake before chemotherapy administration	Urinalysis test, urine cytology, and chemical profile blood testing as a part of medical follow-up Regularly monitor blood pressure Avoid or minimize alcohol intake Maintain a healthy diet and a healthy weight Limit salt intake Exercise moderately

Late and Long-Term Effects of Cancer and Cancer Treatment

System/Organ Affected	Mechanism of Action	Potential Effects	Possible Interventions	Wellness Planning
Nerves	Vinca alkaloids Taxol Platinol	Peripheral neuropathies (numbness and tingling in hands and feet) resulting in changes in balance, difficulty walking and performing daily activities, and mild to severe pain Hearing loss Tinnitus (ringing in the ears) Constipation Bladder problems Changes in vision Changes in muscle strength	Report symptoms to the health-care team immediately so treatment plan can be altered Assessment by neurologist may offer a useful plan of care If a painful burning sensation develops, consult a pain specialist Ask a physical or occupational therapist to advise on self-care and changes in daily living activities	Use special care when working with sharp objects (knives, needles) that may accidentally pierce the skin Monitor changes in balance, gait, bowel or bladder function, changes in vision or hearing, and report these changes to the doctor or nurse right away Get advice on self-care and protective measures from physical and occupational therapists
New Cancers	About 5% of all survivors actually develop secondary cancers. Risks are influenced by genetic tendency, lifestyle, radiation treatment, and certain chemotherapy drugs Bladder cancer secondary to chemotherapy Development of one cancer may make a person more likely to develop another	If blood tests show drops in blood counts, leukemia should be considered in medical follow-up. Monitor for potential changes in bladder function: irritation, frequent urination, blood in the urine, pain	Talk to the medical and radiation oncologists about the risks of second cancers and weigh the realistic risks against the benefits of treatment	Be aware of the potential for developing a new cancer secondary to treatment Maintain a regular schedule of follow-up and make sure any new doctor or nurse is totally aware of your complete health history Include self-care measures such as breast self-exam in a complete wellness routine Maintain a regular schedule for routine cancer screening Minimize all behavioral risks: stop smoking, limit alcohol in-take, eat a healthy diet, exercise

Late and Long-Term Effects of Cancer and Cancer Treatment

System/Organ Affected	Mechanism of Action	Potential Effects	Possible Interventions	Wellness Planning
Skeletal	Ovarian failure Use of glucocorticoids Methotrexate Cyclosporin Premenopausal use of tamoxifen	Bone loss or osteoporosis Fractures	After breast-cancer treatment, discuss use of tamoxifen to preserve bone density Discuss use of bisphosphonates to prevent loss of bone mineral density	Undergo bone density testing Discuss dietary supplements of calcium (1,000–1500 mg/day) and vitamin D (400–800 IU/day) with doctor or nurse Stop smoking Include weight-bearing exercise in an overall fitness plan
Gonadal Function	Pelvic radiation therapy Pelvic surgery Colon resection Cystectomy	Early menopause Sexual dysfunction Infertility	Increase vaginal lubrication Hormone therapy to relieve menopausal symptoms Androgen replacement Discuss possible use of medications to decrease hot flashes (Megase, Clonidine, Paroxetine, Venlafaxine, Fluoxetine)	Seek guidance for fertility concerns before starting therapy Discuss concerns with a sex education specialist or sex counselor Include partner in discussions of concerns Vitamin E and soy phytoestrogens are sometimes useful in the management of hot flashes
Immune System	Chemotherapy- and radiation therapy-related suppression of immune function Anemia	Increased risk of infection Shortness of breath	White cell growth factors might be prescribed as a precaution before white counts drop to very low levels Closely monitor for signs and symptoms of infection and report any changes to cancer care providers	Use self-care measures that protect from infection Avoid crowds and people with infections Use sharp instruments with care Wear foot coverings when walking, inside or outside Wear gloves when gardening or doing household chores

Late and Long-Term Effects of Cancer and Cancer Treatment

System/Organ Affected	Mechanism of Action	Potential Effects	Possible Interventions	Wellness Planning
Functional Changes	Lymphedema Pain Fatigue Ostomies Scarring Amputation	Alteration in body image Complicates performance of ADL Mobility alterations Chronic pain Depression	Get expert advice (from WOCN, occupational and physical therapists, doctors and nurses) before, during, and after treatment for ways to minimize damage and maximize wellness strategies	Engage in regular exercise program designed for your special needs Find a fitness instructor who has cancer-related expertise Be aware of potential problems and monitor any changes to allow for early management strategies
Cognitive Changes	Brain irradiation Chemotherapy Biologic response modifiers Side effects of antiemetics Emotional distress at diagnosis and start of treatment Fatigue Hormonal changes—especially estrogen deprivation	Loss of concentration Difficulty thinking clearly Short term memory problems Insomnia Depression Learning disabilities	Explore sleep patterns and promote adequate sleep and rest Discuss changes with a doctor, nurse, social worker, or other counselor. Clinical trials are beginning to look at cognitive changes; new and helpful interventions might be available Assessment by a neuro-psychologist can identify specific problems and devise helpful techniques	Get all important information written down: written appointment cards, letters Get printed information about all aspects of treatment Make lists of "things to do" Integrate cognitive and creative activities into daily plans Use supportive community to the extent possible for things like child-care, counseling Be open with family members Include a regular exercise plan in daily activities Engage in cognitive and social activities—a book club, crossword puzzles, word games

The lungs are prone to damage from cancer treatment. Lung—or pulmonary—toxicity in the form of decreased flexibility—**pulmonary fibrosis**—has been associated with the chemotherapy drug bleomycin, but other drugs that can cause this problem include alkylating agents, methotrexate, and nitrosurea. Radiation can also cause lung changes, with symptoms becoming more apparent as a person ages.

Kidney change—**nephrotoxicity**—is known to occur as a late effect of the drugs cisplatin, methotrexate, and nitrosurea. Usually, hydration measures can minimize kidney damage; this means oral intake and/or intravenous administration of extra fluids as the drugs are given.

Nerve damage—**neurotoxicity**—is most often thought of as occurring after use of the chemotherapy drugs cisplatin, paclitaxel, and the vinca alkaloids. Peripheral neuropathy—changes in the nervous sensations in the hands and feet—can cause various levels of discomfort, pain, and even disability. Radiation to the brain can be a cause of changes in thought processes and memory. For years, women have complained—or joked—about what they called "**chemobrain**"—changes in thought processes following treatment for breast cancer. Even though the condition has finally been recognized, and many scientists are exploring it, the cause remains a mystery.

Most changes in the blood-forming and immune systems are temporary. The blood-forming function of the bone marrow may be damaged by chemotherapy, and immune-system damage is a long-term problem for people who have been treated for Hodgkin's disease. Damage secondary radiation to the pelvis, where the large pelvic bones normally produce blood cells active in providing immunity, can create changes in immune function that last for some time. New or second cancers are also known to develop and are thought to be secondary to the altered immune function.

Radiation therapy can affect muscle, bone, and soft tissues. This is especially a problem for children and young adults in which damage to growth plates can lead to muscle wasting. Pain problems can develop as a result of scarring and loss of flexibility of soft tissues. Skin cancers can develop within radiation treatment fields.

Hormonal problems occurring as a late effect include hypothyroidism, early onset of menopause, and ovarian failure leading to infertility. Radiation therapy involving the head and neck can affect the thyroid—and thyroid function should be continually monitored. Early menopause is an effect of certain chemotherapy drugs or radiation therapy to fields that include the abdomen or pelvis. Hormone replacement therapy can be very helpful to women who experience uncomfortable and/or distressing menopausal symptoms, and can reduce the risk of osteoporosis that is often linked to estrogen deprivation. Until recently, there have been few ways to preserve fertility, but ways of preserving ova and protecting the ovaries and uterus from radiation exposure are increasingly available. A woman concerned about fertility issues should talk with fertility and/or reproductive specialists—and explore available websites—for the most current information.

SURVIVORSHIP

Mary Vachon, a nurse researcher and cancer survivor, offers the following five categories that describe approaches to survivorship:

CANCER AS A NONISSUE: Women in this category are simply able to return to their normal lives (or their newly changed lives) with little difficulty.

CANCER MINIMIZATION OR DENIAL: Denial means not believing there is a problem, and not pursuing care. Minimization acknowledges that despite the problem, one is still able to do many things. In this category, minimization is the healthier approach of the two.

CANCER AS A DEFINITION OF SELF: Some survivors are very public with their cancer experience and use it as a way to work for improving the situation for others. Programs and projects of local, regional, and national organizations such as the National Coalition for Cancer Survivorship, cancer societies, and other nongovernmental organizations offer these survivors many opportunities to advocate for changes in the way cancer is approached in our world. On the other hand, others define themselves in terms of their suffering, find secondary gain in an extended illness role, and have problems making plans for the future. There are programs and counseling available to help survivors find ways to cope most effectively with their situations.

CANCER AS A TURNING POINT: Women in this category use cancer as a chance to reflect on life, change what needs to change, and move on in new directions. In short, cancer can be a turning point in a woman's life. A woman might decide to quit a job that she really doesn't like, change or end a relationship that isn't working, or undertake other major lifestyle changes.

CANCER AS A SPIRITUALLY TRANSFORMATIVE EXPERIENCE: Spiritually transformative experiences can take any number of forms. Some descriptions that fit include experiences that connect a person with another realm, religious or psychic awakenings, and near-death experiences. However it happens, people find their lives have a more spiritual focus, and they often sense a deeper connection with a Higher Power and a stronger commitment to their own emotional healing and recovery. Being open and receptive to new thoughts—even thoughts that seem to come from nowhere—is often a first step in this personal transformation.

INTERVENTIONS: LONG-TERM WELLNESS PLANNING FOR SURVIVORS

The emotional impact of being "set free"—and some survivors instead think of it as being "cast adrift"—after active treatment ends is finally being recognized. Survivors express feelings of abandonment, fear, insecurity, and generally feel at a loss when formal cancer treatment ends (see Chapter 24). Ideally, the health-care professionals should be able to assure survivors that the "caring" continues far beyond actual treatment. Sometimes, nurses and doctors will maintain contact with their patients—an occasional and informal telephone call to say hello, or a card or note works wonders toward saying "I care" and "you are important to me." Many cancer centers that have a long history of treating children with cancer have developed "late-effects" clinics that continue to follow children through their young adulthood, assessing and suggesting strategies to deal with late effects. Although some cancer centers are starting to focus on late effects experienced by adults, the idea of an organized follow-up plan has not quite caught on yet, even though so many adults now live for decades after cancer treatment. The ways to manage the long-term and late effects of treatment are subjects that each woman will need to consider, and often, take charge of herself.

Survivor's Owner's Manual

Throughout the cancer treatment period, but especially as a course of therapy concludes, women can keep things organized by compiling a complete and accurate history of their illness and treatment. A three-ring binder with page dividers for different aspects of the cancer journey works well. I call this "the cancer survivor's owner's manual," and compare it to the owner's manuals we get with a new car: a guide that tells us when to do important maintenance tasks and serves as a convenient place to keep all of the receipts that record how well we've taken care of this car. The record is valuable when we take the car in for repairs or wish to know its trade-in value.

The survivor's owner's manual, likewise, documents how well we take care of ourselves. One section can be set aside for the names and current contact information of all health-care professionals who have been involved in our care. A section might contain reports from laboratories, clinics, and X-ray departments. Another section might document the course of treatment, treatment-related side effects, and descriptions of measures that were helpful or of no use in managing these problems. A section might be devoted to describing other physical and emotional problems that relate to the cancer. A section might address life beyond cancer and describe plans for establishing a lifelong wellness plan, including such things as hints for dietary changes, smoking cessation ideas, and exercise strategies. A special section can be used to keep track of follow-up appointments and any pertinent information to review with the doctor or nurse at follow-up—such as a new health issue, a change that is of concern, or (and health-care professionals love this) the positive changes that have occurred in your life. This notebook can be a virtual lifesaver whenever a woman relocates throughout her life and must establish relationships with a whole new set of doctors and nurses.

As treatment ends, a woman can ask for a sort of "exit interview" with the oncologist or the oncology nurse. This "exit interview" could be similar to the interviews conducted when an employee leaves a job. What went right? What could be done better? What still needs attention? Cancer centers are increasingly making the exit interview a formal part of their services and recommending that each patient get, in writing, an outline of her cancer experience: the diagnosis, stage, treatment regimen, including doses, schedules, initial and final test results, side effects that were experienced, and plans for follow-up. However this conversation takes place, it does set the stage for what comes next, and can include plans for wellness. The doctor, nurse, social worker, dietician, physical therapist, and any other member of the health team can offer guidance about wellness-oriented interventions such as smoking cessation, diet, follow-up, complementary and supportive care, learning self-advocacy skills, and community resources that might be tapped to enhance quality of life.

— *Pamela Haylock*

CHAPTER 24

FEELINGS AFTER TREATMENT ENDS

I swallowed my final three chemo pills with three glasses of water. Pills 250, 251, and 252. (I counted!) For months I had mentally checked off each injection and pill and wondered if this day would *ever* come.

An hour later, my husband and I packed up my cold cap and the empty pill container and headed for the county dump. There we ritually crushed the container (driving back and forth over it several times) and tossed the cold cap into the deepest garbage pit. An exhilarating moment....

So why did I feel more terrified than exhilarated? Why this jolt of anxiety? What in the world was the matter with me?

Nothing. I had just learned the hard way that the after-treatment road is not all rainbows and bluebirds, although there are plenty of those.

At any point after she finishes cancer treatment, a woman may struggle with

- ✦ her feelings, including fear, anger, sadness, and guilt

- ✦ her self-image and body image

- ✦ her relationships

- ✦ her goals

Some of these may be more of the same old problems that came up during treatment. Others may be new, or may be more pressing now.

Ending cancer treatment is a predictable emotional pothole on the cancer survivorship journey. Many people feel anxious, vulnerable, uncertain, ambivalent. It is common, normal—and temporary.

In sharing stories of life after treatment, cancer survivors have discovered that almost everyone goes through certain emotional bad patches along the way.

The timing of some is predictable: However many years or decades it may be after treatment, no breast cancer patient ever undergoes mammography again without trembling a little inside.

The timing of others is less predictable, but just about everyone with cancer eventually experiences a painful range of feelings about the disease: fear that cancer will return, grief at the losses she has had, uncertainties about her self-image.

One woman may grieve most intensely right after diagnosis or during treatment. (Of course, one never tidily "finishes" a feeling and then puts it behind forever.) Another woman, conserving all her emotional energy just to get through treatment, may not face that first excruciating blast of sorrow until after treatment ends.

What has been postponed, however, cannot be put off indefinitely. Thus, when treatment ends, some women find themselves struggling not only with the common after-treatment feelings but also with the postponed or "holdover" ones. They may doubt their ability to survive, let alone thrive. They feel wobbly and unsure, both physically and emotionally; the journey ahead looks like one rock, rut, and jolt after another.

But it gets better—and knowing what to expect and when makes it easier to get through. Techniques that other cancer survivors have found helpful may prove useful. But, whether it is the day therapy ends or decades later, simply getting through the rough spots as easily as possible is part of the challenge of living well after cancer treatment.

But not the only part.

Like other major crises, cancer provides a window of opportunity for change and growth. Eventually, many women—no matter how much they hate the disease—become aware of positive changes in themselves that would not have happened without cancer. Whether or not they feel "transformed," they may become conscious of a new sense of clarity, of fresh eyes for the world and the people around them. Many just enjoy and appreciate life more. Some gain a better idea of who they really are and what they truly want out of life.

Sometimes women have learned through cancer to be kinder to themselves, or have been astonished at their own strength and resilience. Whatever the good changes are, many women want to hold on to them, build on them.

As time passes, however, and the immediacy of the cancer experience fades, it is all too easy to slip back into old ways. If a woman wants to live better than ever after cancer treatment, her second challenge is to keep alive all the positive changes that have happened because of her response to cancer.

GENERAL STRATEGIES

The general strategies for coping with feelings after treatment are similar to those that can be used during treatment. Whatever the difficult feeling, acknowledging and naming it take away some of its power.

A woman can examine what she is feeling by herself, in a group, or with a mentor, therapist, or close friend. Like women at earlier stages of the cancer journey, some women make the unspoken spoken by keeping journals or diaries. A woman can also draw her feelings, sculpt them, dance them, or write poetry about them, using the creative process not only to express her emotions but to begin "resolving" them. Many women find it useful and safe to read about feelings.

For the woman who belongs to a cancer support group, the immediate posttreatment period is not the time to leave. Some localities offer after-treatment groups (often listed with the local American Cancer Society unit). Any mentor should be a woman who has navigated the posttreatment period successfully. The breast cancer patient who had a helpful Reach to Recovery volunteer earlier might contact her again. If necessary, a mentorship can be by long-distance telephone, letter, e-mail, or Internet chat room. Y-ME (breast cancer), DES Action, and the National Coalition for Cancer Survivorship are possible resources (see Resources). The Cancer Survivors Network link on www.cancer.org brings multiple possibilities for connecting with other survivors.

A psychotherapist or counselor may be able to help a woman integrate what she has experienced with cancer into the rest of her life. Many women look to a special friend who does not have cancer or to a noncancer-related group for techniques and support in identifying and coping with strong emotions: Cancer patients have no monopoly on feelings of anger or vulnerability. Such groups include general women's support groups, twelve-step groups, and informal gatherings of women friends talking about what bothers them.

After some time passes, many women begin serving as mentors for other women or as cancer volunteers and discover that they are helped as much as they help. As she works with the cancer "novice," the woman reexamines her own feelings, but in a new context. Being a mentor or a cancer volunteer does not require that a woman know all the answers. It simply means that she has passed this way before and is willing to listen and share her experiences.

Many women invest some of their feelings and energy in cancer political action groups or the national survivorship movement. In fact, in 1996, the National Cancer Institute established an Office of Cancer Survivorship to provide an official home for research and activities related to the "physical, psychological, and economic well-being of individuals following cancer treatment" (www.survivorship.cancer.gov). On the other hand, the woman who finds she is spending every waking moment on cancer-related activities may need to create more balance in her life.

AFTER-TREATMENT FEARS

The "what ifs"—what if cancer comes back? what if I need more treatment? what if I die?—bedevil most cancer survivors at least once in a while. Most admit they never completely get over the fear that cancer will return. Living with a cancer diagnosis means living with a certain degree of uncertainty forever. For most of us, however, the fear eventually recedes into the background of our everyday lives. The fear and uncertainty are just there, rather like emotional background music.

But there are the "high-decibel" times. One, as unexpected as it is unwelcome, often comes at the completion of basic cancer treatment (surgery, chemotherapy, radiation).

A woman expects to feel jubilant, relieved. Instead, what she experiences is so at odds with what she thought she would feel, thought she *should* feel, that it staggers her.

"I just can't believe how terrified I feel—and how weird it is," confided one woman right after she finished chemotherapy:

> For months, I've been trying to reach this day, cheering myself on. At the doctor's office, the nurses even gave me flowers and a big certificate to congratulate me on finishing treatment. My family and friends are all geared up to celebrate with me at this big party I was planning.
>
> Instead, here I am, so scared I can barely function. I haven't been this frightened since I got my diagnosis. What if it comes back? How do the doctors know I'm okay? Sometimes I even feel like asking the doctor if I can have more chemo. I hated it—but it was my powerful weapon, keeping me safe. Is it always going to be like this?

Her panic is common, and it doesn't seem to matter whether treatment involves a single surgery or months of treatment. At the end, many a cancer survivor feels "as if I've been thrown out of the nest and don't know if I even have wings."

Some women on long-term hormonal therapy for cancer, such as tamoxifen for breast cancer, continue to feel "protected"; others do not. The end of hormonal therapy can also be an anxious time.

As treatment ends, a woman may be physically weak, severely fatigued, hard pressed to believe that she will ever feel healthy again. Whatever cancer therapy she has undergone, it takes weeks, months, or even longer for the body to recover fully—and it is difficult to wait with patience and confidence.

In addition, as a woman's treatment ends, much of her support may vanish. During treatment a woman yearns for the day when she can measure her life by something other than doctors' appointments, but right after therapy finishes, she may ache for that reassuring surveillance. And family and friends may be less "there" for her after therapy ends. They have been grappling (often with little help) with their own feelings of helplessness, anger, and sadness. Like her, they've been focusing on that magical end-of-treatment day. Now they may be so ready to get back to "normal" that they do not want to listen to her fears. No matter how much they care, they just can't take any more.

Dealing with "What Ifs"

We fear what *might* happen in the future. But, as oncologist William M. Buchholz, M.D., writes in the newsletter *Surviving* (July/August 1989), "You become tense in anticipation of being powerless some time from now.... The antidote for fear is returning to the present."

When I am pondering what ifs, I keep reminding myself that, *whatever* happens to me, I will never, *ever,* have to face more than one day at a time. While the prospect of *"The Future"* may sometimes overwhelm me, I can manage twenty-four hours.

Sometimes I turn and face my fear, remembering the Bene Gesserit creed from Frank Herbert's science fiction adventure *Dune:* "I will face my fear. I will permit it to pass over me and through me. And when it has gone past I will turn the inner eye to see its path. Where the fear has gone there will be nothing. Only I will remain."

If we feel overwhelmed by the what ifs, relaxation techniques can bring us back to the moment and serve as first aid for fear. Slow breathing makes us pay attention to what is happening *now*. In progressive relaxation, we experience each part of the body as it tenses and then releases. We can soften the belly or *feel* our feet solidly connected to the ground.

Taking concrete action lets a woman feel more in control. She might draft a will or fashion a fallback plan for the care of her children, for instance; this practical planning (appropriate for everyone, with or without cancer) is prudent rather than morbid and allows her to relax and get on with life.

Sometimes we have to remind ourselves that the body's own strong immune system is still the state-of-the-art mechanism for destroying cancer cells. After a cancer diagnosis, we forget how long and well the body's defenses have protected us. We may blame our bodies for betraying us; we have to relearn to trust them.

After treatment ends, energy returns in bits and spurts. Many of us tend to overdo one day, suffer for it the next, and then wonder if we will ever feel really healthy again. But if we give them a fair chance, our bodies work diligently to get healthy again—and then to stay healthy.

Some women swear by improved nutrition: "I've really decreased the amount of fat in my diet. When I cook a delicious low-fat, high-fiber meal for myself and my family, I know I am doing something special for all of us. It gives me back a sense of control, too, in a situation in which I felt little control. I can do something to make me healthier."

Other women start an exercise program, perhaps a postmastectomy class. Our bodies, made to fight or flee anything that causes distress, crave physical activity. Taking it slowly at first is better. Rushing into vigorous exercise with a not-so-vigorous body invites discouragement as well as sore muscles.

Some women meditate, stop smoking, sip special herbal teas, or listen to relaxation tapes. Some just try to be kinder to themselves, becoming readier to say "yes" to themselves and "no" to others. One way of being kinder involves setting realistic health expectations, ones that allow for the occasional chocolate bar or missed exercise class.

Many women, having put together a "healing package" for themselves during treatment (perhaps a combination of chemotherapy, walking, visualization exercises, and herbal teas), continue everything but the medical therapy, and maybe add other techniques that make them feel healthier, stronger, and more at peace. It helps many women to think of their cancer diagnosis and treatment as a kind of "midcourse correction" in life's journey, an opportunity to see what is wrong and make it better.

Yes, it is important to celebrate the end of treatment and to mark closure of a difficult phase. A woman *deserves* to congratulate herself and to bask in the love and good wishes of others. But she also needs to know that fear and ambivalence commonly appear as unwelcome guests at the celebration—and to realize that she has some effective strategies for throwing them out.

Fear that Comes from Nowhere

Sometimes a woman experiences sudden, fierce anxieties, seemingly from nowhere. I use these as an emotional barometer: What have I been ignoring?

I may find that the painful feelings have little to do with cancer per se, more to do with vulnerability, or fear of making a choice, or something else. Once I know what I am really dealing with and begin to take some action, the fear passes.

Some women, often those who "sailed through" treatment and the immediate posttreatment period, encounter an unexpected and totally unsettling period of acute anxiety several months (or even years) later. This often comes at just about the time the woman is congratulating herself on how well she has coped with the whole experience. This happens to be her individual timetable for integrating cancer into her life, and the techniques she can use to deal with it are the same: acknowledging and naming the fear, shedding some tears, talking about it, and so on.

With most cancer-related fear, the common remedies are sufficient. If fear hangs on, causes severe and continuing distress, or immobilizes a woman, it is definitely time for professional help. This might include psychotherapy (often brief) or the short-term use of antianxiety medication.

OTHER PREDICTABLE DIFFICULT TIMES

As time passes, we recover more confidence in our ability to survive and thrive. But there are other predictable scary moments.

Any symptom, whether a twinge, a cough, or a phone number we cannot recall, can trip our internal alarm system. It doesn't take much, especially at first. (One of my doctors called this the "cancer of the hangnail" syndrome.) Most symptoms have nothing to do with cancer, of course, and go away on their own, but sometimes it is hard to believe that.

It makes sense to get information from the doctor about follow-up care, prognosis, common symptoms that don't mean anything, and problems that need to be reported. Knowing what is important and what can be safely ignored lets a woman adjust her emotional alarm system. However, if a woman is seriously concerned about *any* symptom, it is reasonable to check with the doctor.

Are there skills she needs to know in order to monitor her continuing health? One woman reports that she felt much better after breast-cancer treatment when she visited a hospital-based breast-health center and learned the most effective way to examine her own breasts.

Routine checkups and tests, even when there are no symptoms, can be times of predictable anxiety. Many women felt perfectly healthy when their cancers were diagnosed. Taken by surprise once, they worry that feeling fine now is no guarantee of health.

"Before my regular mammograms, I still can't sleep," admits a woman treated for breast cancer several years ago. "I thought that after a year or two, I would face checkups with total calm and equanimity, but I don't. I don't get *quite* as worked up now though!"

People who survive cancer sometimes experience the post-traumatic stress syndrome (complete with sudden distressing flashbacks) common to soldiers after a war. For instance, on a cancer-related anniversary, a woman may find herself reliving the scene in the doctor's office, struggling with the excruciating fear she felt then.

It is also a common experience to develop symptoms right before a checkup or test. Many women have learned from experience that symptoms that develop right before checkups have more to do with anxiety than with any physical problem. Relaxation techniques, talks with a support group sister, and positive "self-talk" can all help. Sometimes I "fast forward" myself a few days mentally so that I am looking *back* at the event, savoring my relief. I hunt for distractions and promise myself that I will not do this again—until the next time. Mentally reframing checkups and anniversaries into reassuring milestones helps many women. Focusing on the champagne afterward makes the temporary anxiety more tolerable. It is cause for celebration to check off another test, another year!

Other predictable occasions of anxiety include hearing about the death of a woman from a similar cancer. In the case of a personal friend, the fear is overshadowed by grief but still exists. The death of a public figure can also feel almost like the loss of a friend. Many women reported finding the autobiographies of Gilda Radner or Jill Ireland, for instance, painful and anxiety-raising—but also cleansing and cathartic. News stories or obituaries may make us pause and worry; movies, TV dramas, or novels may tap into an undercurrent of anxiety.

ANGER AND SADNESS

Cancer wounds us with visible and invisible scars. We grieve and feel angry—and that is how it should be.

Aside from any "holdover" feelings of sadness that she may have postponed until after treatment, a woman may face specific posttherapy losses. What appeared to be a temporary loss, for instance, may prove permanent. A woman may suffer what turns out to be permanent major damage from chemotherapy, radiation, or surgery. A woman in her thirties who underwent chemotherapy for breast cancer may discover, perhaps, that her periods do not return and that she cannot give birth to the baby she longs for.

*Feelings
after
Treatment
Ends*

439

Or she may mourn an accumulation of "little" physical losses: a scar that has healed well according to the surgeon, but is still there; a continuing numbness under her arm that always feels strange when she shaves; lessened vaginal lubrication during intercourse. Almost everyone treated for a women's cancer faces a few long-term reminders that she has had cancer. Admitting that these sometimes bother her in no way means that she is ungrateful to be alive.

As treatment ends, a woman may *know* intellectually that she no longer needs the close attention from her doctors that she was getting, but that may not keep her from *feeling* a sense of loss. Women, far more than men, tend to see a relationship with the doctor as a personal one and to want to be liked by their health professionals. Especially when therapy has been protracted, it is not uncommon for a woman to have a sense of being rejected and abandoned when she is sent on her way after treatment ends.

If she stifled any anger or resentment toward her doctor during treatment in order to be a good or lovable patient, a woman still has those feelings simmering within. In addition, many patients feel angry that their health professionals did not prepare them for the difficult transition after treatment.

There are other kinds of scars. The process of renegotiating relationships may be painful. The friends who could not tolerate any part of cancer and dropped from view during the woman's treatment may be gone forever. Other people may continue to treat her differently than they once did. If a support group sister dies of cancer, a woman grieves the loss. Uninsured medical bills may come due, imperiling a woman's financial security.

Guilt enters the scene when what she thinks or does or feels does not match her expectations, usually internalized from her culture. Some of this is a holdover from the period right after diagnosis when the woman was trying to make sense of why she got cancer. That the cause is not knowable in most cases, with the current state of medical information, does not deter her from blaming herself: "I didn't eat right. I didn't manage stress right."

After treatment, she can feel even more culpable. Now she knows better—and still may not eat right or do her relaxation exercises! Or, expecting a transformation in herself because of cancer—and seeing few changes—she wonders where she has gone wrong. It is usually the expectation at fault, not the woman.

Many women are hard on themselves at the best of times. They struggle to meet the expectations of a society that keeps changing what it wants of them. Cancer can give a woman the opportunity to look at what she expects of herself and those around her. Changing the expectations to something more realistic reduces the guilt.

Although, amazingly enough, women cancer survivors do not appear to be *more* at risk for severe depression (and other acute psychiatric ills) than the general populace, they are not immune. The woman who feels immobilized by sadness for more than two weeks (major sleeping or eating problems; persistent severe "empty," guilty, hopeless feelings; a "slowed down" or very restless feeling; continuing thoughts of suicide) urgently needs professional help and perhaps antidepressant medication.

HOW WE FEEL ABOUT OURSELVES

All through her life, a woman's internal computer keeps adding to her mental picture of herself, her self-image (including her body image). Words women use to describe themselves during and after treatment include victim, ugly, weak, stupid, dependent—and strong, survivor, sensitive, magnificent, focused.

Crises in self-image can occur any time during the cancer experience. Reentering "normal" life after treatment ends can make a woman question again just who and what she is. Body-image concerns, however, often reach critical mass about the time treatment ends. No matter that she is an ardent feminist, no matter that she is truly convinced that what's inside is far more important than what's on the surface, a woman may still be shaken by what she sees. In fact, many of these changes improve rapidly after their low point as treatment ends. Scars fade over time, though this depends on the individual woman's body. Hair regrows, often thick, lustrous, and curly, after chemotherapy ends. Her complexion gradually returns to normal.

A woman recovering from breast cancer may choose breast reconstruction to replace a missing breast, use a secure prosthesis, or simply enjoy her Amazon-woman chest (the ancient Amazons removed a breast so they could shoot their arrows better). I love the striking poster that shows a woman named Deena Metzger, her arms stretched wide as she embraces life, with a delicate tracing of leaves tattooed over her mastectomy scar.

Many women find that the hardest body-image change they have to cope with is weight gain during chemotherapy. Weight losses may reverse relatively quickly as a woman feels healthy again, but the extra pounds common after breast cancer chemo hang on tenaciously. If she wants to lose weight, a slow, steady pace of about one to two pounds a month through healthful eating and exercise seems to work best.

Women who have undergone radical colorectal or pelvic surgeries may now have one or more openings on the abdomen, new exit(s) for the digestive tract and/or urinary tract. A plastic pouch is worn over the ostomy (opening) to collect stool and/or urine. Specially trained health profession-als called *enterostomal therapy nurses* (known as ET nurses or WOCNs) can help the woman with both the practical and psychological adjustments to these changes.

RELATIONSHIPS

During treatment many relationships enter a holding pattern. Nobody wants to rock the boat much, and the woman undergoing therapy may lack the energy and will to make changes.

As treatment ends, exhausted family and friends may crave an emo-tional break from the intensity of diagnosis and treatment. Although this is usually temporary, it conflicts with the woman's need for support during this difficult transition. Everyone is upset and resentful and no one quite understands why. Information and direct communication are key: If the woman, her family, and her friends all know that this is normally a trying time and that it passes, they can relax more and help each other while pro-tecting themselves.

A woman may feel angry at family and friends who want to "get back to normal" and expect her to do the same. She knows intuitively that she is not physically or emotionally ready for normal yet.

Or she may realize, consciously or not, that normal as defined by other people is not where she wants to be. During cancer treatment, many women begin paying attention to their own legitimate needs and desires, often for the first time. Reluctant to return to the precancer status quo, a woman may seek new rules for her relationships. But making these kinds of changes (and then making them stick) takes more emotional energy than she is likely to have now; the attempt may leave her feeling angry, frus-trated, and powerless. Time, returning energy, and some negotiating skills can bring about a more successful outcome later.

At the same time, the other person in each of these relationships has also been changing. Thus the relationships must be renegotiated gradually between two individuals who are in some ways new and different from what they were.

Partners

Some cancer doctors recommend that, if a woman has a partner, they plan an official getaway by themselves for a few days about a month or so after treatment ends, a sort of second honeymoon. This is one way to mark the end of one phase of their lives and start on a new life together. It is only a start, however, since this is an ongoing process.

It helps if neither the woman nor her partner expects too much yet: The physical and emotional wounds of cancer and its therapies are still relatively fresh and unhealed. Recognizing that this can be a difficult period is half the battle. But if they can talk about their separate and mutual uncertainties and hopes, they can use these to forge new and stronger connections.

Psychotherapist Diane W. Scott, R.N., Ph.D., in her work with women with cancer, says that in a close relationship there is not only the woman's ego and the partner's ego, but a separate something that she calls the *couple ego*. As they struggle together through the crisis of cancer, the process may strengthen not only each one of the pair, but also their shared sense of what they have together. The woman may feel grateful for what her partner has done to make life easier during treatment; many a woman finds wonderful and unexpected depths in her mate. The partner may experience with awe the courage and lovability of the woman. Knowing that they could lose each other lends a sweet and urgent edge to their journey of mutual discovery.

But, with or without cancer, most relationships do not run like Swiss watches all the time. Cancer may make some good relationships idyllic, but it may also show clearly that some are poisonous and unsalvageable. Like most people, however, most relationships are neither perfect nor dreadful; they repay the time and effort spent making them better.

It is a temptation for some women to want to change their lives drastically after cancer or to hold a flawed relationship accountable for causing the disease. Often, it makes sense to consider the first months after treatment a "sit back and take a deep breath" time. This gives both partners a chance to heal and the relationship space to settle a bit before a woman makes any radical decisions.

It is not uncommon for one or both partners to blame the cancer for all their problems. Sometimes that is an excuse, a camouflage for bigger but unacknowledged problems and feelings. Only after admitting they have these feelings can partners begin to accept them, communicate them, and begin working together to resolve them.

If the situation does not improve after some time and effort, both partners have to decide whether their relationship is worth saving. Counseling may be able to help them sort out tangled feelings and perhaps learn better ways of being together.

What if a woman does her part to build the relationship and the other person still rejects her, giving cancer as the reason? Obviously, this can be devastating. As hard as it is to keep the situation in perspective, the woman must remind herself over and over again of all the wonderful things she is and can do. Cancer has changed her, perhaps, but it has not diminished her.

It is the partner's loss. Some people, because of their own fears and conflicts, cannot tolerate the reality of cancer in someone close to them. This is not in any way the woman's fault, but that does not mean that she will not feel outraged and shed many tears before beginning a new phase of her life.

Other Family Members

What about her children? How children respond depends on the individual child, the age, and the situation. Young children can be told that Mom's treatment is finished and (if appropriate) that she will start feeling better again. Again, children need to know clearly that *they are in no way to blame* for the illness and that there will always be someone to care for them.

Older children (including teenagers) who may have taken on more family responsibility during the treatment phase may keep some of it, or may happily or very reluctantly relinquish it. Getting back to "being a kid" can be a tricky transition, another relationship change to renegotiate. As always, talking openly means that children can get their questions answered and their fears resolved. Teenagers and parents sometimes benefit from using a "buffer" adult to help with communication, perhaps a school counselor or a trusted family friend.

Just being older doesn't save adult children from their own terrors when a mother has cancer, and they need to be included in the communication loop. When family history increases the risk of this cancer, the end of treatment period is a natural time to open the issue of how a daughter can protect herself.

This can be a difficult subject to broach. The woman may feel guilty for handing down a vulnerability to the cancer to her child, or may not know how to raise the subject. Some daughters react by denying the danger, others by becoming panicky about their risk. If the woman can admit her feelings to herself and perhaps rehearse what to say—by herself or with a mentor or support group—it is easier to begin. Then, of course, she needs accurate information to pass along. A caring doctor, a medical geneticist, or a women's health center may be able to guide the daughter to take appropriate measures to protect herself.

If the woman's parents and siblings have been part of her support team during cancer treatment, this relationship too may need to be renegotiated when treatment is over. Sometimes a woman does not know what she wants now (being "babied" may have been rather pleasant) and may feel like a touchy, ambivalent adolescent all over again.

Friends and Others

Each woman decides how open she wants to be about the cancer with friends, acquaintances, and coworkers. There is no one right solution, but many women handle the subject after treatment more or less the way they handled it earlier.

After treatment, however, the changes made because of cancer are less obvious. The wig is gone, and the lunch date does not have to be postponed because of the radiation therapy appointment. As cancer comes less often to mind, it is natural to speak of it less frequently. If the woman finds herself sharing her cancer experiences nonstop with everyone long after treatment ends, she may need to remind herself that there are plenty of other fascinating topics of conversation.

It is a woman's decision what to do about friends who drifted away after the diagnosis because they couldn't handle it. If they drift back and she is interested in being friends again, she may overlook the earlier defection and consider their behavior now a reaffirmation of her current healthiness.

What about a new friendship after treatment ends? Does this person need to know about the cancer? If the relationship is becoming a close one (certainly if the person is a potential "significant other"), it is not fair to either party to withhold the information.

SETTING GOALS

"Enjoy the moment. Live for today!" Yes—and no.

As she is going through cancer treatment, a woman's goal often is just getting through it. After treatment, she may want simply to get back to normal. Many women, however, feel a need to make something fresh and special of their lives, perhaps to set out in a new direction entirely. They feel a sense of rebirth, of having a second chance. They do not want to spin their wheels going nowhere. But, physically and emotionally drained, they do not know where to begin.

On the other hand, a woman may be scared to set goals for fear that cancer will disrupt them again; she has been through that once already. Sometimes there may be a deep-down feeling of not tempting fate: Could planning far beyond today *trigger* a return of the cancer? Knowing this is superstition may not protect her from this common feeling.

Many women alternate between the two, one moment eager to brave new worlds and the next moment fearing to stick a toe in the water. They do not feel transformed, but sense some changes in themselves and wonder where they will all lead.

The will to set goals usually requires some physical energy, and that comes in time as the woman's body recovers. During this time she takes baby steps: What can she do to make her life better in the next week? This means setting a reachable, concrete goal for the near future ("I will walk half a mile tomorrow and increase the distance a little bit every day until I am walking three-quarters of a mile a day one week from tomorrow").

The more concrete the goals are, the more achievable they are. "I will get in shape" is less helpful than "I will take this ballet class three times a week." Simply concentrating on one or two goals at a time seems to be more effective than reaching out in all directions at once. The woman also needs to include some intermittent monitoring: Is this, in fact, a helpful goal for her?

Many women set goals for themselves, fail to meet them, and then not only give up on the goals completely but feel bad about themselves. It helps if the woman rehearses in her mind beforehand what she will do if she stumbles. This gives her a plan so that she can pick up where she left off, rather than becoming bogged down in self-loathing.

When she becomes more comfortable with short-term goals, the woman can set goals that are a little bigger and a little longer term... eventually....

— *Kerry McGinn*

CHAPTER 25

AFTER TREATMENT ENDS: THE OTHER ISSUES

In black moments, I sometimes think, "You mean I went through everything I went through and now there's this too? That's the *last straw!*"

Indeed, after treatment ends, a woman may discover that cancer and its therapy have affected many areas of her life besides her feelings, raising questions about

+ sexuality

+ pregnancy

+ lymphedema

+ early menopause

+ employment and insurance

Sometimes I get downright furious. It's not fair, and there is no way to pretend it is. I keep trying to remember the Serenity Prayer—although I do not always get serene.

The fact is, some things cannot be changed, and a woman simply exhausts herself trying to make them go away. But other things are challenges, opportunities to make life better—or at least more interesting. By looking at a problem squarely, getting information about it, talking about it, and finding out strategies other people have used to deal with it, a woman learns what reasonable action she can take. Who knows? She may be able to take that "last straw" and weave it into something beautiful.

SEXUALITY

No cancer makes it impossible for a woman to give and receive pleasure from touching. If this is important to her, there is always a way.

However, some women's cancers and their treatment put hurdles in the path of a woman's sexuality. She and her partner may need to keep open minds about ways to feel sexual pleasure. Changing techniques and expectations can broaden lovemaking horizons.

During treatment, women may find that they have less interest in sex, simply because mind and body are so involved in getting through this phase. Then treatment ends and the woman and her partner wonder, "What now?" She may fear possible rejection at the same time her partner is concerned about appearing overeager and insensitive.

What happens now depends on what is happening in the woman's mind, in her body, and in the relationship. Whatever happens, it is likely to take some time for recovery and renegotiation. The woman and her partner need to remind themselves of this before immediately worrying that things are not back to normal.

It helps to realize that the first experiences with lovemaking after surgery, or after a period without much sexual touching, are sometimes awkward and disappointing. The woman tries to protect new scars and her partner worries about hurting her. This situation can improve dramatically as the woman continues her recovery and they both relax.

The Mind

The most important female sex organ is not the clitoris or the vagina, but the brain. Many sexual difficulties start there—and that is also where they can be solved.

How a woman thinks of herself and her body (self-image, including body image) plays a crucial role in how she responds sexually. She needs to like herself, to think she is "worth it," desirable, and deserving of sexual pleasure. In addition, she has to be sufficiently free from fear and other overpowering negative emotions to muster the energy for lovemaking. Depression is one of the major inhibitors of sexual response: It tamps down all the feelings and vanquishes joy, spontaneity, and pleasure.

Since the period immediately after treatment ends is often full of negative feelings and fears about pain, it is a tricky one for lovemaking. If a woman engages in intercourse before she is emotionally ready, her body may not respond—and she may feel worse about herself and resentful toward her partner. The more tense she gets, the more painful it is. That means her body is even less likely to respond the next time. This can become a vicious cycle.

On the other hand, satisfying lovemaking helps both mind and body to recover. Aside from the pleasure, it makes a woman feel good about herself and feel that she is no less a woman because of what she has gone through. It can distract her from fear and draw her back to "normal" again. It can bond partners tightly at a time when they may especially need closeness.

Satisfying lovemaking depends less on bedroom acrobatics than on *communication*. If a woman and her partner can say to each other directly, "That feels good," or "I'm scared that touching that spot will hurt," and can trust that the other will listen, then both can relax. Expecting a partner to be able to read one's mind simply does not work.

Thinking of lovemaking itself as a special communication, as a way to give and receive pleasure in many ways, takes the pressure off and lets both partners enjoy the journey. They can caress, stroke, touch, laugh, and cuddle to their hearts' content. The woman who masturbates can explore her body, listening to its old and new messages of what feels right.

The Body

Many women feel violated, both physically and emotionally, by the treatments for women's cancers. To get through therapy, they begin considering their body a *thing* unrelated to them, and it takes time to move back into their altered bodies.

Possible physical changes include scars, missing organs or parts of organs, different sensations in sensitive areas, and altered hormonal balance. Obvious scars ordinarily fade in time; as long as they are healing normally they do not need any special physical consideration during lovemaking—just some tender loving emotional care for these badges of courage.

With no uterus after a hysterectomy, a woman can continue to have orgasms but they may feel a little different because the spasm no longer includes the uterus contracting; on the other hand, she may be more free to respond because she no longer experiences bleeding or fear of pregnancy.

If the vagina is all or partially removed, it may be rebuilt with reconstructive surgery. To keep the vaginal channel open the woman can use either a vaginal dilator or have regular intercourse.

The woman who has lost her clitoris in surgery for cancer of the vulva may have the most difficult sexual road to travel, because the clitoris is where the most intense sexual sensations occur. For her, recovering or retaining her sexuality means becoming sensitive to the pleasures available from the rest of her body (breasts, thighs, and so on).

Many women experience altered sensations, such as numbness, a pins-and-needles feeling, or increased sensitivity. Some are shocked by bizarre sensations in the armpit and along the arm after a breast-conserving surgery and lymph-node surgery; they thought that only women who had mastectomies felt those sensations. While many women are tempted to avoid these areas, consistent touching and stroking during lovemaking and at other times may actually reeducate the nerve endings and reduce the negative sensations.

When both ovaries are removed with surgery or are made nonfunctional with treatment, the premenopausal woman catapults into menopause. If she cannot (or does not) take hormone replacement therapy, she will experience physical changes in the vagina (see "Menopause—Without Hormone Therapy," in this chapter).

Even in the best of relationships and with a healthy vagina, some women experience very decreased sexual desire or difficulty with arousal because of hormonal changes from chemotherapy and/or tamoxifen. These women can ask their doctors for a blood test to measure their testosterone level. Testosterone, a hormone associated with sexual desire, is considered a male hormone but it normally occurs in smaller amounts in women too. If the testosterone level is very low, some women are choosing to replace the deficiency with pills or injections of the hormone. The one concern that a few doctors have raised is whether the body could convert the testosterone into another hormone capable of nourishing some tumors; this is a possible but unproven risk.

Any major physical change requires adjustments in lovemaking: more comfortable positions, lubricating jelly, more attention to other sensitive areas, use of fantasy, and so on. In many cases, including vaginal surgery and menopausal changes in the vagina, fairly frequent intercourse helps keeps the vagina in good condition—a clear case of use it or lose it.

The woman needs clear information from her doctor, a nurse, a sex therapist, or a good reference book about the changes that occur. This is a legitimate part of cancer therapy for women *of any age* who are interested in continuing or beginning a sexual relationship. But many women feel reluctant to ask—and too many health professionals, raised in the same atmosphere of sex being a thing we do not talk about, either do not know the answers or feel uncomfortable telling women what they need to know.

The booklet *Sexuality and Cancer: For the Woman Who Has Cancer, and Her Partner,* available on request from the local American Cancer Society unit, contains information about both the physical and emotional aspects of sexuality after a cancer diagnosis. Also, many a woman finds, in talking with friends or opening up in a support group, that she is not alone—that her questions and problems are all too common. Participation does not mean she has to tell other people every detail of her sex life, of course. She might ask a simple question, such as, "Is anyone having trouble getting interested in sex?"

The Relationship

Anyone eavesdropping on Cinderella and her Prince Charming a few years after "happily ever after" would doubtless hear a few spats and misunderstandings. Even the most long-term relationships experience some sexual difficulties at one time or another. These go with the territory when two imperfect human beings try to communicate (including sexually) over time.

Because people can use a sexual relationship to express many different aspects of themselves, sexual problems may mask all sorts of personal or relationship difficulties, big and small. Sometimes the partners themselves can disentangle the threads and work to make the situation better, but it may take a counselor to step in and take an impartial look.

After cancer diagnosis and treatment, some women in a reasonably good, established relationship feel a need for a new relationship—perhaps an affair—to affirm that they are still desirable. The thinking may go, "Of course, my regular partner will act as if I'm desirable, but that does not *prove* that I really am." It makes sense to think long and hard before acting on this kind of impulse.

Beginning a New Relationship

When a woman and her partner have been together for some time before her cancer diagnosis, they have a shared history, good or bad. A woman interested in beginning a new close relationship does not have that—but she does have a clean slate.

At the best of times, however, it can be scary to reach out for a new friendship. A woman may feel vulnerable, unsure of herself and of how much she can trust the partner. Cancer and the changes it has brought may make her question her desirability as a partner: Who would want someone with one breast or a missing uterus or a cancer diagnosis?

She focuses so much on the negative changes that have occurred that she cannot remember the exciting positive changes, as well as the wonderful things about herself that have not changed. Cancer scars can become a convenient cover for more basic feelings of inadequacy: a reason not to reach for the relationship at all or a scapegoat if she is rejected.

Cynthia, for instance, was a most attractive single woman who underwent mastectomy surgery with reconstruction using a breast implant. The tissue around the implant hardened somewhat, and she became acutely self-conscious about it. She began seeing herself (as she admitted later) as a horrible rock-like breast which just happened to have a walking, talking person attached. She was convinced that everyone else was just as aware of her breast as she was. If she ever went on a date, she spent the whole time protecting herself from "discovery," maneuvering herself away from even a hug. No date had a chance to discover the warm, intelligent, funny Cynthia underneath—and no date ever came back.

It took some months of therapy before Cynthia realized how much she had been using her "different" breast as a scapegoat for all the doubts she'd had about herself long before surgery. When she began liking herself more, she no longer had to spend all her energy protecting herself. Now she had more interesting tasks: listening to her date, talking, having fun. She learned that a woman who sincerely likes herself is profoundly desirable.

To her astonishment, she found that when she did engage in sexual relations, her partner barely noticed the scars or the "different" breast, just as she did not pay much attention to the reddened appendectomy scar that made her partner self-conscious. Each had the same reaction to the other's "disfigurement": "Is that all? What's the problem?"

After cancer, there is another possible scenario: the woman who collects sexual "scalps" in order to prove she is still desirable. Aside from the dangers in a time of deadly sexually transmitted diseases, this woman is not coming any closer to liking herself as a real person.

How and when does a woman tell a prospective partner? Neither Miss Manners nor Emily Post has offered guidelines about this. Some people tell casual dates; some do not. But before committing to a long-term relationship, certainly a potential lifetime partner has the right to know of a previous cancer diagnosis. And some people feel so much more at ease after they tell that they explain fairly early in any possibly serious relationship.

Explanations can be simple, honest—and honestly optimistic: "A few years ago I was diagnosed with cancer of the uterus. I had a hysterectomy and, as you can see, I'm doing very well!" (She can also enlist her doctor's help to talk to a potential mate.)

One of my favorite strategies was the one used by a friend who took her date to a Survivors' Day picnic sponsored by the National Coalition for Cancer Survivorship. Surrounded by other obviously healthy, thriving people who had been through a cancer diagnosis, she felt comfortable broaching the subject.

Occasionally, a partner cannot deal with the cancer—or gives that as an excuse to discontinue the relationship. This is not easy to handle, but it is still better to discover the problem before wasting too much time on a fruitless relationship.

PREGNANCY

Saving the woman's life is the first priority in treating any cancer. Considerations of becoming and staying pregnant take second place. Some cancers and their treatments make pregnancy afterward impossible, highly unlikely, or inadvisable.

However, some women do become pregnant and deliver healthy babies after treatment for a women's cancer. These are among the women who cheered when actress Ann Jillian gave birth to a beautiful, healthy boy a few years after a double mastectomy and chemotherapy for breast cancer.

Childbearing is an individual question, and it makes sense for the woman who truly wants to have a baby after treatment to ask questions beforehand. Occasionally, there are two equally effective treatment options and the doctor and the woman can choose the one less likely to hurt her chances of having a baby.

After treatment, a woman should consider any limiting physical factors. Have any parts of her reproductive tract been removed or severely damaged? This could be from surgery, such as removal of both ovaries so that the woman can no longer provide the ova (eggs) necessary for a pregnancy. Radiation can cause similar local damage. Or a woman could have such heavy scarring after conization of the cervix that she has difficulty carrying a pregnancy to term. It is worth consulting a gynecologist who specializes in fertility issues.

During chemotherapy for breast cancer, especially with the drug cyclophosphamide (Cytoxan), many premenopausal women stop menstruating. The younger the woman is, the more likely it is that her ovarian function will resume after she finishes treatment; however, the woman over forty or so may be close enough to normal menopause that this tips the balance permanently.

Tamoxifen (Nolvadex), a common long-term treatment after a breast cancer diagnosis, blocks the hormone estrogen in the breast but actually acts as a weak estrogen elsewhere in the body. It does not make a woman infertile, but it can cause severe damage to the fetus in the uterus. Thus a premenopausal woman who uses the drug needs to use effective birth control at the same time. Removing both ovaries or destroying them with radiation so that they do not produce hormones to "feed" a breast cancer used to be more common. Now, tamoxifen usually does the job.

Even if she remains physically capable of becoming pregnant, a woman wants to know whether she can have a healthy baby and whether pregnancy poses any special risk to her continuing health. For several reasons, many doctors advise the woman to wait two years or so after treatment ends before trying to become pregnant. The first two years are the most common time for cancer to reappear. This waiting period also allows the woman time to recover her health and energy before coping with pregnancy and the challenges of new motherhood. It is especially important after chemotherapy to protect the baby from residual effects of the powerful

*After
Treatment
Ends:
The Other
Issues*

453

drugs, and that means taking time for them to leave the body (although some women have become pregnant only a few months after chemotherapy and have given birth to healthy babies). Of course, this also means that if there is any chance a woman could be fertile, she needs to use an effective method of contraception during this time. Not having menstrual periods is no guarantee of infertility.

There are many questions and few answers about pregnancy as a risk to a woman's continued health. Especially after diagnosis of a hormone-nourished cancer, both doctors and women worry that any stray cancer cells lingering in the body will thrive on all those pregnancy hormones. However, while the studies and literature are scant, they seem to show that women who become pregnant after cancer treatment tend to live as long (or even longer) than women who do not become pregnant. These studies have tried to eliminate the factor that women with a good cancer prognosis may be more likely to attempt pregnancy.

More research is long overdue. Many women argue that for them the benefits of having a baby outweigh the risks from cancer cells that may or may not be there. Still, it makes sense for any woman contemplating pregnancy to sit down with her cancer doctor first so that she can make her decision based on both head and heart. Adoption may be a good option if a woman has a positive bill of health from her doctor but cannot or does not want to become pregnant.

One of the unspoken questions for many cancer survivors is, "What are my chances of living to bring up this baby?" It needs to be spoken. In a sense, it is an appropriate question for *any* woman who wants to become pregnant or adopt, but the woman with a cancer diagnosis is more intimately acquainted than most with uncertainty and her own mortality. Each woman's answer must be her own, but it is prudent (for every woman) to consider who will raise her child if she cannot.

LYMPHEDEMA

After cancer treatment, many women are at risk for **lymphedema:** edema, or swelling, of an arm or leg that occurs from the buildup of lymph fluid that cannot drain freely. This can happen because a tumor is pressing on the lymph nodes in the armpit or the groin. More often, it occurs as a complication of cancer treatment: The lymph nodes have been removed to check for the presence of cancer or have been purposely destroyed with radiation therapy to the area. Lymphedema does not mean that the treatment itself was unsuccessful or poorly done.

Lymph is a sticky, protein-rich fluid. If it cannot drain normally, it builds up like water before a dam. If it pools long enough, it begins to stick to the linings of the lymph channels in the arm or leg, forming protein plaques that harden and make the channels even narrower and less elastic; this makes the drainage even worse and means that less oxygen reaches the tissues. In addition, since bacteria thrive in any quiet pool of protein-rich fluid, the arm or leg with lymphedema is prone to infection, which can further damage the lymph vessels.

Right after surgery, many women develop some temporary tissue swelling in an arm or leg. This goes away by itself and usually does not indicate the chronic high-protein swelling of lymphedema, which tends to develop later.

Lymphedema is unsightly, and finding attractive clothing to fit over a grossly swollen limb may be next to impossible. It can also be very difficult to use a swollen arm or leg. The limb may be quite uncomfortable and heavy, although, surprisingly, pain is rare unless there is infection or another problem.

Prevention

Preventing lymphedema is the first goal. A lymph system damaged by surgery or radiation may still be able to function well unless an infection or other "insult" tips the delicate balance into lymphedema. That is the idea behind the common sense do's and don'ts after surgery or radiation to either armpit or groin.

A woman avoids infection by keeping the arm or leg clean and taking reasonable care to prevent any break in the skin: wearing gloves for household or garden work after breast cancer surgery, for instance, and not allowing the arm to be used for injections or blood drawing (unless there is no other option, and then the site needs to be very carefully prepared with antiseptic). To prevent nicks, she shaves with an electric razor rather than a safety razor and does not cut her cuticles. She cleans and cares for any tiny cut or injury thoroughly and seeks medical help at the first sign of infection.

The woman avoids constriction of the limb or pressure on any lymph nodes in the area because that makes it harder for the lymph to circulate normally. This means no tight bands or jewelry and no blood pressure readings in the arm after breast surgery. She protects the lymph nodes along the collarbone by not wearing over-the-shoulder handbags on that side or a very heavy breast prosthesis.

She also uses gravity to help keep the lymph from pooling in the limb. If the arm is at risk, for instance, she does not carry things with a straight arm hanging at her side, and periodically she raises the arm so that the

*After
Treatment
Ends:
The Other
Issues*

455

hand is above her heart. She exercises the limb. This maintains or increases the muscle tone to help move lymph fluid out of the arm or leg.

These precautions mean being reasonably careful. They do not mean that a woman should become so petrified at the possibility of lymphedema that she wraps herself in lambswool and refuses to budge. Most women never develop lymphedema.

Treatment

If the arm or leg does become swollen, a woman needs to seek help as soon as possible. Expert care from a health professional who specializes in lymphedema care can make the difference between a condition that is a mild nuisance and one that makes a woman chronically miserable. A lymphedema clinic, a physical therapist who treats the condition frequently, or a cancer center are possible resources.

Early mild lymphedema is usually relatively easy to treat. First, any threatening factor is removed (an infection is cured with antibiotics, for instance). Swelling can be reduced by elevating the limb; after the swelling is gone, the woman may use compression sleeves or stockings (like heavy-duty support hose) to help lymph fluid leave the area before it can build up protein plaques along the lymph channels. These compression garments may encourage the body to form new "collateral" lymph drainage channels.

Treatment for more severe or advanced lymphedema includes use of pressure pumps, lymph-drainage massage, a low-salt diet, and special bandaging techniques. The specialist also teaches the woman how to prevent more injury and prescribes antibiotics at the first hint of possible infection. Some surgeons, primarily in Europe, are working on microsurgery techniques to increase lymph drainage. Drugs to reduce the development of the protein plaques that often occur with lymphedema and to control the amount of protein in the lymph are also being studied; diuretics (water pills) do not work with lymphedema because the lymph fluid is too "thick."

The pressure pump blows air into an inflatable "sleeve" that fits over the whole limb. Effective pumps use a sequential pattern of inflation. The sleeve is divided into several channels circling the limb, which inflate and deflate in turn to provide deep massage, increase circulation, and push the lymphedema fluid out of the arm or leg. The safest pumps use a system of gradient pressures, which means they compress most firmly at the wrist or ankle (a high grade of pressure), less firmly as they move up the arm or leg.

Manual lymph drainage massage helps open existing lymph channels. The gentle, circular motions focus on the connective tissue rather than the muscles. Physical or massage therapists with training in these special techniques can often reduce lymphedema symptoms dramatically.

Bandaging techniques developed especially for lymphedema, standard compression sleeves and stockings, or one of the newer compression devices with Velcro closures may help keep the limb compressed after use of a pressure pump or manual lymph drainage—or may be all the woman needs. A woman may be able to learn and use manual lymph drainage and bandaging techniques herself at home; sequential gradient pumps are often available for rent or sale.

Unfortunately, many doctors are not yet aware of new advances in lymphedema treatment. Many believe lymphedema occurs so rarely in their patients that it is not their problem, often because it happens years after surgery or radiation when they no longer routinely see the patient. And some ignore or undertreat lymphedema because of their personal—and very human—difficulty coping with the fact that the therapy they gave is partially responsible for a difficult problem. The National Lymphedema Network—(800) 542-3259 or (510) 208-3200, website: www.lymphnet.org —provides information, support, a newletter for people with lymphedema and their health-care providers, and a conference every other year to spread news of advances in treatment. Another helpful resource is Jeannie Burt and Gwen White's book *Lymphedema* (Alameda, CA: Hunter House Publishers, 1999).

MENOPAUSE—WITHOUT HORMONE THERAPY

Menopause occurs when the ovaries dramatically decrease their production of the sex hormones estrogen and progesterone. The major physical concerns are immediate problems such as hot flashes, night sweats, and vaginal changes, and potential long-range problems such as osteoporosis ("thinning" bones) and heart disease.

Normally, menopause is a gradual process, occurring over several years as the body adjusts to these natural changes. Some kinds of cancer therapy, however, can send a woman into an abrupt, all-at-once menopause. This usually happens when her ovaries are removed surgically or become nonfunctional after radiation or certain kinds of chemotherapy.

Many women in the United States now rely on **hormone replacement therapy** (HRT) to counter the effects of naturally decreased hormones after menopause, although enthusiasm has dimmed somewhat with the findings in the Women's Health Initiative study (see Chapter 11: "Hormonal Events and Taking Hormones"). This therapy is an option for many women with a cancer history, but most doctors currently consider it too risky to use when the woman has been treated for a cancer that can "feed" on hormones. If there are stray cancer cells anywhere in the body, the doctors want to starve them, not nourish them. On the other hand, many women do not have stray cancer cells around after treatment, many stray cells that do exist would not be nourished by hormones, and many women successfully undergo pregnancy—with its major hormonal upheaval—after cancer treatment. Clinical trials are under way now to see if some groups of breast cancer patients can take HRT with relative safety for severe menopausal symptoms. One trial in Britain hopes to enroll three thousand women; early results of the small "pilot" study of one hundred women have been surprisingly positive.

From another point of view, some women are alarmed that a normal human event like menopause has been "medicalized" and that hormones with some known risks (and possibly some unknown ones) are being prescribed so widely to prevent possible problems.

Plus, alternative strategies exist for dealing with menopausal changes. Not many years ago, all women went through menopause without replacement hormones—and billions of them survived and even thrived! (Of course, women do tend to live longer now, with many more post-menopausal years.)

With an abrupt menopause, a woman's symptoms might come on more dramatically than those of other women. However, menopause is an absolutely individual experience; some women experience minimal symptoms while others suffer significantly. Any woman with concerns deserves to get clear, factual information and help with symptom relief from her doctor.

No one knows yet exactly how the drop in hormones triggers the sudden expansions and contractions in the blood vessels that can leave a woman suddenly dripping with sweat. Simple strategies for warding off hot flashes and night sweats include dressing lightly so that she does not get too hot, layering clothing, and keeping a paper fan handy.

"Keeping cool" emotionally can help but is not usually a cure. Yoga or slow, deep breathing works for some. Some women find symptom relief through such complementary health therapies as herbal medicine and acupuncture or acupressure. Also, engaging in stimulating activity can distract a woman from hot flashes and may actually make them occur less often.

My friend Marilyn took another tack, changing her diet dramatically to decrease fats and sugars and increase soy products, and found her hot flashes vanishing. A bonus: Her weight dropped and she just felt all-around healthier and more energetic. (While soy products have been touted for their possible effects on menopausal symptoms because of their natural estrogen effect, some critics caution that they may not be safe in large amounts simply because of this estrogen effect. Too, clinical trials have come up with conflicting results about whether soy products help the symptoms more than a placebo does. More questions to answer!)

Specific drugs from the selective serotonin uptake inhibitor (SSRI) class of antidepressants have proved quite effective in clinical trials to relieve hot flashes and other symptoms. Paroxetine (Paxil), venlafaxine (Effexor) and fluoxetine (Prozac) are the three SSRIs most studied so far for menopausal discomforts. Since nobody knows exactly why hot flashes happen, it is not clear just how these drugs work to relieve them, but it appears to be more than simply lifting depression.

Other possibilities for hot flashes include a pill or patch of clonidine (Catapres) or propanolol (Inderal), usually used as blood pressure medications and both with their share of side effects. The Food and Drug Administration has approved Bellergal, a combination drug, for severe menopausal symptoms, but it contains small amounts of two drugs, belladonna and phenobarbital, that could be addictive. Diphenhydramine (Benadryl, found in several over-the-counter sleep medicines), an antihistamine that also makes people drowsy, is a mild sleeping aid that lets some women sleep through the night. More potent sleep medications tend to lose their effectiveness and cause drug dependence if they are taken for more than a few days.

Dryness and thinning of the vaginal walls can make sexual penetration uncomfortable. It can also make the woman more prone to infections, because of tiny breaks in the vaginal lining. Drug stores offer several over-the-counter, water-based lubricants that can be applied to the vagina or penis during intercourse. (Vaseline works poorly, does not clean off well, and is a haven for the organisms that cause yeast infections.) Some doctors recommend a vaginal moisture-replenishing product such as Replens to use routinely a few times a week, unrelated to intercourse, to keep the vagina more comfortable. Other doctors are convinced that, even if the estrogen pills are too risky after breast cancer, a small amount of an estrogen cream can relieve the local changes to the vagina with minimal effect on the rest of the body.

Some women find that tamoxifen, used as anti-estrogen therapy for breast cancer, makes hot flashes and night sweats worse but acts as a mild estrogen in the reproductive tract and may relieve vaginal thinning slightly. Other women have not found it effective for vaginal changes and some complain that it causes increased vaginal discharge which can be a problem. Regular sexual activity, including masturbation, helps keep the vagina open and healthy.

For the woman experiencing problems with menopause, there may be a specific menopause group in her area, since this is a problem for many women with no cancer history. Several books on menopause offer hints on dealing with both physical and emotional concerns. The woman who has been advised not to use hormone therapy needs to choose a book that does not focus entirely on the benefits and joys of replacement therapy. *Dr. Susan Love's Hormone Book* presents a relatively balanced picture. The menopause section on the website www.breastcancer.org contains all sorts of valuable information, updated constantly; http://project-aware.org and www.power-surge.com are other Internet possibilities. Pamphlets published by drug companies naturally tend to stress the hormone medications from which they make their profits.

Women begin to lose bone mass during young adulthood, but the process accelerates dramatically when estrogen decreases at menopause. If the bones become too porous, in a condition called **osteoporosis,** they break easily. Estrogen protects a woman's bones somewhat, and post-menopausal women who do not take estrogen need other strategies to maintain as much bone density as possible—including regular exercise, especially weight-bearing exercises such as walking, jogging, jumping, and dancing, which build bone in legs, hips, and spine.

A well-balanced diet can help prevent osteoporosis. It should include generous servings of foods rich in calcium and vitamin D, which the body needs to absorb calcium. There are many calcium-rich foods besides the obvious dairy products, but women who like and can digest dairy products can make tasty blender drinks from nonfat (or low-fat) milk and yogurt, one or more kinds of fruit, and perhaps a bit of sweetener; these give plenty of calcium but few calories and minimal fat. Calcium from pills can supplement calcium from food. In fact, it is the rare woman who can get the 1,500 mg of calcium she needs each day after menopause from food alone (an eight ounce glass of milk provides about 250 mg of calcium), so most women need to supplement with calcium pills.

Yo-yo dieting, in which a woman frequently loses weight and then regains it, changes the body's metabolism and draws calcium out of the bones. Smoking, too, decreases the effectiveness with which the body processes calcium.

One class of drugs, the bisphosphonates, slows down bone loss, which may help women maintain bone density. If a bone density study shows that a woman's bones are more porous than they should be, her doctor may prescribe the very effective bisphosphonate drug alendronate sodium (Fosamax), currently available in pill form with either daily or weekly dosing. The woman taking Fosamax swallows her pill with a full glass of water first thing in the morning; she does not eat or drink anything else for at least half an hour to increase pill absorption and she stays upright during that period to avoid heartburn or other problems with the esophagus (the tube for food passage from throat to stomach). Tamoxifen and raloxifene both appear to have some protective effects against osteoporosis, although their effects are probably not as strong as those from estrogen or Fosamax

The possibility of preventing some heart disease has long been a big selling point for estrogen therapy, although recent studies have raised some doubts. Tamoxifen, as a weakened estrogen, may have some effects on the heart, but researchers need to learn more about this. Although we do not have a great deal of data yet on how lifestyle factors such as diet, no smoking, and exercise affect women's hearts, we know they make a huge difference for men—and they may well make the same kind of difference for women.

So all those osteoporosis strategies probably work to keep the heart healthy as well. Many researchers believe that diets low in saturated fats build up less "sludge" in the body's blood vessels so that the blood moves freely; that means less work for the heart and less chance of a clot forming in the heart. Other researchers are convinced that a diet low in all fats decreases the risk for breast cancer and some other cancers.

Menopause is a normal, natural process. But because menopause means that a woman can no longer bear a child, she may equate this stage of life with growing old or with losing her femininity and worth. A cancer diagnosis can make those feelings more acute.

Many women, however, happily bid adieu to menstrual periods. Because she no longer has monthly blood loss, a woman may feel more energetic than she has felt for years. *Postmenopausal zest,* a phrase coined by anthropologist Margaret Mead, says it accurately for many women. Freed from the possibility of pregnancy, they are eager to dream new dreams, step out in new directions.

EMPLOYMENT AND INSURANCE

Some women with a job never break step after a cancer diagnosis. They may take sick leave for treatment, but they have secure jobs they like and can continue to perform, and they never face an employment problem.

For others, employment after cancer is a major concern. Some have lost jobs during a period of disability, or for another reason, and fear their health history will make it more difficult to find a new job. Some women can no longer meet the physical demands of a particular job, such as heavy lifting, or find that the job makes them feel so stressed and unhappy that it is probably not healthy for them. And some women just want to spread their wings and do something new.

Whenever a woman looks for a new job, there are some basic tips she can follow that are appropriate for all job seekers, such as arriving on time, dressing appropriately for interviews, and applying for only those jobs for which she is qualified. The woman who can no longer perform her former job because of cancer or its treatment may be able to get the state department of rehabilitation to finance job retraining.

Liking oneself and communicating that good self-image to a potential employer make a difference. The woman can give herself positive "self-talk" and possibly role-play with a mentor or support group. It helps to practice answering questions beforehand that the personnel department might ask so that she can appear confident rather than defensive. The library or bookstore, state department of employment, and private employment agencies all offer information about basic job-seeking skills.

Specific tips include downplaying any cancer-related gaps in employment history by organizing a résumé by skills and achievements rather than chronological dates of employment. In any job application or interview, the woman must answer honestly any direct questions about her health history (although employers are legally limited in the questions they can ask), but is not obliged or advised to volunteer any information. She can make honest positive statements about her health. If her health history comes into question, her doctor can write a letter to the employer.

In the United States, the employment rights of the person with a cancer history are protected somewhat by the Rehabilitation Act of 1973 and the Americans with Disabilities Act of 1990. Many U.S. employers can no longer base hiring decisions on what are perceived to be disabilities. State laws may also apply. Federal and state agencies give information about these laws and enforce them.

The National Coalition for Cancer Survivorship offers packets of current information about both employment and insurance issues—and fights to make the situation better. *Facing Forward: A Guide for Cancer Survivors,* a pamphlet that is a joint venture of the National Coalition for Cancer Survivorship and the National Cancer Institute, is available free from NCI's Cancer Information Service, and gives tips about these practical problems as well as about emotional and physical survival. Another free booklet, *Cancer: Your Job, Insurance, and the Law* is available from the American Cancer Society Hotline at (800) ACS-2345. Local units of the American Cancer Society can provide information about current laws and how to fight apparent discrimination.

Insurance

To remain profitable, most health insurance companies prefer to insure people who will not cost them much money. This often means that the people who need health insurance most have the most trouble getting and keeping it. After treatment, a cancer patient may cost no more than anyone else—in fact, she may cost less because she takes better care of her health—but insurance companies look at actuarial tables of statistical averages rather than at individuals.

If a woman is insured through work, she may cling to a job she does not like in order to keep her health insurance ("job lock") or may have trouble finding a new job that covers her. Since insurance companies may pass on their potential future costs to employers or a group of employees, an employer could be leery of hiring a woman who might cost more. Other potential problems include obtaining new insurance that covers her preexisting condition, getting the insurance company to pay for procedures, especially ones it sees as experimental, and affording premiums and copayments.

These are not concerns in countries with national health insurance, such as Canada. In the United States, federal or state governments offer basic health care for some groups of people: most people sixty-five or older and the permanently disabled (Medicare), armed service veterans (VA), and some people in low-income brackets (Medicaid, or Medi-Cal in California). Any kind of large-group insurance plan in which the risks and costs are spread out among many people is generally easier to obtain and pay for than individual or small-group policies. Besides a regular company plan for the employed woman with a cancer history, options include dependent coverage under a spouse's insurance plan, a health maintenance organization (HMO) with an open enrollment period in which a person must be accepted regardless of health history, and group insurance through a professional or other organization to which the woman belongs.

The woman who is insured under a group health plan through an employer and leaves her work for any reason can continue the same coverage for eighteen months under the federally mandated COBRA program (Consolidated Omnibus Budget Reconciliation Act of 1985). She pays the full cost of the policy, including what her employer used to pay, but because it is a group-rate policy, the cost is much less than for individual coverage. After eighteen months, she may be able to convert to an individual policy with the same company, which will cost more and often cover less but will insure her despite her preexisting condition.

The Health Insurance Portability and Accountability Act (HIPAA, or Kassenbaum-Kennedy Bill), signed into law in 1996 and slowly being put into effect, is a first step toward protecting people with preexisting conditions from losing insurance if they change jobs. While it does not cover employees in very small businesses, it does make insurance coverage portable from job to job for many people, which means they do not have to cope with "job lock." It also forbids some kinds of discrimination against people with preexisting conditions. Whether this will make a real difference remains to be seen. For more information, see the HIPAA area on the website www.hcfa.gov.

Some states offer high-risk health insurance pools for people who cannot get insurance any other way. Blue Cross and Blue Shield have open enrollment periods in some states. A phone call to the National Coalition for Cancer Survivorship will bring information. Some independent insurance brokers can match a woman with some kind of insurance, although the coverage may have high premiums and deductibles and limited coverage.

Occasionally, legal action about insurance becomes appropriate, especially in cases in which the insurance company refuses to pay for a procedure it considers experimental but that the medical community contends is state-of-the-art. Currently, however, the federal Employee Retirement Income Security Act (ERISA) provisions mean that most cases involving insurance through an employer must be tried in federal court. Since federal courts do not allow damages for emotional distress or punitive damages, this reduces incentives both for attorneys to take on the woman's case and for insurance companies to settle (since it costs them little to stall).

More and more people consider health insurance in the United States an expensive scandal, but it does not look as if the country is going to adopt a unified health system any time soon. The current trend is toward hospital and insurance company mergers, with enormous growth of for-profit health maintenance organizations and a substantial portion of the health-care dollar going to investors and insurance corporations. The few recent attempts to regulate the insurance industry have been modest baby steps.

One of the greatest changes in health insurance, with huge effects on cancer care, has been the major switch from traditional "fee for service" to systems of "prospective payment." Under fee for service, the more the doctors or hospitals did, the more money they received. According to the insurance companies, this led to runaway health costs because the doctors and hospitals had no incentive to keep services and prices reasonable and tended to supply *more* services than patients really needed.

Prospective payment turns the fee-for-service system on its head. It works in two ways. Using "diagnosis-related groups," Medicare and some other insurance companies reimburse hospitals and some specialists a set amount based on the patient's diagnosis. Thus, the hospital receives the same amount for a woman undergoing mastectomy surgery whether she stays twenty-three hours or six days—and loses money if the woman requires more services than the average mastectomy patient.

With "capitation," the insurance company pays the doctor (often the primary care doctor, such as the internist or family doctor) a set amount each month for each patient in the doctor's panel who is insured by the company, regardless of how much or little service the patient receives. Thus, with capitation, if the doctor receives twenty dollars a month per patient and never sees the patient, the doctor pockets twenty dollars. However, if the patient needs multiple services, as the typical patient with cancer does, the doctor loses money on that patient, a strong motivation to limit services. In theory, however, the doctor has enough patients so that those who do not need services balance out those who need many services.

The plus side of moving from fee for service to capitation is that it provides new incentives for doctors to focus on preventing diseases, since they save money over the long term if their patients stay healthy. However, the key question with both of the prospective payment systems—diagnosis-related groups and capitation—is whether patients are now getting *fewer* services than they need and are suffering because of that.

◆

Creating the best possible health-care system—which we definitely do not have yet in the United States—means asking how limited health dollars should be allocated to best serve both individuals and society. Balancing the needs of the individual woman for health insurance, of all insured people for coverage at reasonable rates, and of the insurance company and/or the employer to remain profitable enough to stay in business, can call for the wisdom of Solomon—and probably the charity of Mother Teresa.

— *Kerry McGinn*

CHAPTER 26

CANCER IS STILL
A POLITICAL ISSUE

In 1992, when we wrote the first edition of *Women's Cancers,* friends and colleagues were shocked that we said "cancer is a political issue." In the second edition, this information was presented in the chapter titled "Cancer Is (More Than Ever) a Political Issue." As nice as it would be to say that politics plays no role in who gets cancer, who gets treated, and who survives, that just isn't true. Cancer—and health care in general—are *still* very political issues. Health care assumes a prominent place in local and national political campaigns, and certain issues are very hot topics.

The major advances that have taken place in medical science offer hope for the future for many people with cancer, and they also create social, economic, and political dilemmas for individuals, groups, communities, states, the country, and indeed, the world. Politics can and does affect access to doctors and nurses who know about and understand cancer and the latest and best therapies. Politics affects how much each of us is expected to pay for the care and services we use. Political processes determine how much money is allocated to cancer research and what sorts of treatment are approved and available to the general public. Politics affects support for education for the next generation of cancer doctors, nurses, researchers, and the entire spectrum of professionals that it takes to provide good cancer care. If you really think about it, politics affects just about every aspect of cancer care, and it is important to understand how many political decisions can affect the kind of cancer care that is available.

There are a growing number of political issues to be considered and they cannot all be included in this brief chapter. Even so, I hope this chapter will capture your interest and spur your involvement in some level of cancer-related advocacy. There are many levels of political involvement open to every person—and if everyone contributes what she can, important and valuable changes will take place.

WHO PAYS? WHO PROFITS?

Like it or not, the U.S. health-care system—and some health-care systems in European countries too—are shaped by market forces and by the myriad governmental and business entities that are involved in one or another aspect of health care. These entities—the two parties of the American political system for example—are often characterized by philosophical differences. Republicans traditionally favor minimal government involvement and support measures that reflect individual responsibility. Democrats tend to consider the government as a protector. You can see these differences in their health-care proposals. Historically, the Democrats have been in favor of a government-sponsored "universal" health-care program: a basic level of care to which every American citizen would have equal access. Republicans have favored the free market approach to health care and lean toward allowing charitable organizations and public teaching hospitals to assume the role of "safety net" for people who cannot otherwise get care. Obviously this is oversimplifying, but nevertheless, the most important policy and political issues affecting cancer care now relate to the question of "Who pays?" Interestingly, related and important questions are "Who profits" and "How much profit is permitted?"

The pharmaceutical industry gets a lot of bad press. Whether you think this is deserved or not depends on where you stand on the "who profits and how much" issue. But other types of businesses are involved in the business of health care too, and for the most part they seem to escape the criticism showered on the pharmaceutical industry. Every piece of medical equipment or material used today is designed by someone who expects to profit from his or her invention or design. The companies that produce the equipment and supplies—ranging from X-ray machines, hospital beds, needles, syringes, IV tubing, and waste supply bags to shoes, uniforms, and laboratory coats, sheets, pillows, and blankets—all operate on a for-profit basis and must answer to their boards of directors when profits are not high enough. And, while we tend to think doctors make a lot of money, it is also true that they have invested heavily in their education and training, put in long hours, and assume very high expenses to set up and maintain their medical practice. Nurses usually don't have high income levels (and, in fact, rank with teachers in being among the most underpaid professionals), but they still must be paid by their employers. And, of course, no one expects to operate a business at a loss or to work without pay.

Reducing the cost of health care is a congressional priority, and cancer care is a big target. The National Institutes of Health estimates that cancer-related costs in the United States now top $180 billion a year, and the federal government pays for more cancer-related expenses than all other

Cancer Is
Still a
Political
Issue

467

public or private entities. Most people who have needed cancer treatment know that the costs of chemotherapy and radiation therapy are shockingly high. Politicians think the costs are high too, and keep looking for ways to limit the federal government's health-care spending. Almost every presidential administration gets accused of spending too much for health care in the face of proposed tax cuts and efforts to rein in all forms governmental spending. Once again, political questions about money and health care collide.

Medicare and Medicaid

Medicare and Medicaid are among the most expensive programs in the federal budget. Medicare is the federal government-sponsored insurance program that primarily covers health-care costs for people aged sixty-five and older. Medicaid (and in California, MediCal), funded and governed jointly by the federal government and each state, provides help for people who meet low-income requirements. As the population of America (and all Western societies) ages, Medicare costs are expected to soar. Because Medicare is such a big budget item, it is a highly visible and attractive target for policymakers looking for ways to cut costs. At the same time, the people who qualify for and use these government-sponsored insurance plans want expanded, not less, coverage, such as payment for prescription drugs and for some of the more popular complementary therapies. Medicare is the largest payer for cancer care, which is to be expected, since most people diagnosed with cancer are sixty-five and over and qualify for Medicare. And since Medicare handles so much cancer care, other private insurance companies often follow its lead in determining what it will pay for and what it will not.

States try very hard to control Medicaid spending and are focusing on the costs of prescription drugs used by Medicaid recipients. Some states are increasing the copayments for prescriptions (the amount that patients are expected to pay themselves). Some states limit the number of prescriptions covered for each patient and also determine which of many similar drugs will be included in their "formulary"—the list of drugs they cover. The result is that a growing number—one report says 26 percent—of Medicaid beneficiaries cannot afford to get all their prescriptions filled. Eight percent of the elderly covered by Medicare and a growing number of people covered by employer-sponsored health care also say they cannot afford to buy all of their needed medicines. Nearly 30 percent of people who are totally uninsured cannot afford prescription drugs.

The issue of Medicare payment for chemotherapy drugs has consumed the energies of many advocates in the cancer community over the past several years and exemplifies the many forces in play in policymaking decisions. All the settings where patients can receive chemotherapy—hospitals, clinics, doctors' offices—keep a substantial supply of the most commonly used drugs on hand. That way, when it is decided that a patient should get a certain drug, it is readily available. These settings (the hospitals, clinics, and doctors' offices) have to buy these drugs. Then, the drugs have to be properly stored, handled, and when the time comes, prepared or mixed for use by someone who knows how to do this correctly and safely. Cancer care settings that treat a large number of patients buy a large quantity of drugs and are often given a discounted price based on volume. Medicare currently reimburses the care facility for the costs of drugs using a complicated formula. The reimbursement formula that Medicare has traditionally used does not take into consideration the storage, handling, preparation, and administration costs that accompany the safe use of chemotherapy drugs. The formula has allowed practice settings to receive a small percentage over and above the cost of the drugs. This "profit margin" has been used to cover expenses such as the costs of hiring qualified nurses and social workers and other common expenses of a modern cancer care facility.

Recently, Medicare officials have tried to decrease reimbursement, and cancer care providers contend that eliminating that profit margin would also eliminate their ability to continue to provide the safe and expert levels of care that should be the cancer patient's right. And nurses have asked that the Medicare formula formally recognize the nursing component of cancer care—removing it from its hiding place among charges for drugs and supplies. Medicare has issued several proposals over the past several years, but so fa, not one has met with the approval of cancer care providers and the grass roots cancer advocates.

Another idea proposed by Medicare officials and congressional representatives who oversee the Medicare budget involves cutting reimbursement for any drug that could possibly be self-administered—even if the patient who needs the drug is incapable of taking it or administering it to herself. Although this idea is not specific to cancer-related medications, it does have special ramifications for people affected by cancer. On one hand, the idea has some logic. Many of the newer drugs used in cancer care, such as the drugs that can be taken orally, could be self-administered. Growth factors, for example, the drugs that help the body form new white and red blood cells, can be self-administered. Many of the medications used to treat pain and other distressing symptoms can be self-administered too. Growth factors are among the most costly medications on the market, but anti-nausea medications and some forms of pain medicines are also quite expensive. Eliminating Medicare payment for these expensive drugs would definitely cut the government's health-care costs, but from a humane and ethical perspective, is this the right thing to do? The fact that a drug can be self-administered doesn't mean that it should be self-administered, nor are self-administered drugs free from potentially harmful side effects. Many people battling cancer are older and are experiencing other health problems aside from their cancers that can cause them to be frail. Manual dexterity is a problem for many people in this population as well. Add in the fatigue, weakness, stress, and confusion so common among cancer patients and you see the increased potential for problems if this policy were to be put into practice. Regardless of who administers the drug, whether it's the nurse or the patient or a caregiver, administration necessitates instruction and careful monitoring. For example, chemotherapy drugs can still cause the common side effects of nausea, vomiting, and suppression of the immune system—side effects that require patients and caregivers to learn potentially life-saving self-care strategies and close monitoring by the cancer care team.

Radiation therapy is another target for those looking to save Medicare dollars. Cutbacks in payments to radiation therapy facilities and radiation therapy doctors have resulted in the closure of some facilities and reduced services in others. This is especially problematic in rural settings that offer therapy to patients coming from great distances, who would otherwise need to travel even further to treatment centers in larger urban settings. The payment offered by Medicare for this form of treatment is often *less* than it costs these centers to provide safe, state-of-the art therapy and to complete the required documentation of their care services. What is the incentive to continue to offer these therapies when it actually costs providers to stay in business?

One last but especially compelling issue regarding Medicare is the lack of its coverage for drugs used outside of the physician's office or the hospital. Hospital costs are paid under Medicare Part A. Costs incurred in the physician's office are paid by Medicare Part B. But, if the physician writes a prescription for a pain medicine or an anti-nausea medicine that the patient is expected to take on an ongoing basis after discharge from the hospital, the cost of the prescription is not paid for by either Medicare Parts A or B. Patients are expected to pay these costs out of their own pockets (hence the term, "out-of-pocket expenses"). So, even though effective symptom management is possible with a fairly simple plan using oral medicines, many cancer patients won't be able to afford them.

All these scenarios represent a great deal of misunderstanding on the part of Medicare policymakers. Bad policy is usually made, not by mean-spirited people, but by people who simply do not understand the realities their policy imposes. Our politicians usually employ a number of young, bright, recent college graduates who have little or no "life experience."

These aides are expected to produce information and plans to address a whole host of issues, including cancer, but also such diverse topics as railroad use, highway expenditures, and defense spending. What is needed is the perspective of "people who know"—cancer survivors, caregivers, and cancer care professionals. This is the best hope for new policies that will truly work for everyone, policies that ensure access to safe, humane, necessary care, and the most cost-effective use of what we all know are limited financial resources.

Haves and Have-Nots: Insurance

Almost fifty thousand Americans do not qualify for either Medicare or Medicaid and have no other form of health-care insurance. Another ten to twenty million Americans lack insurance at some time during any calendar year. Lack of insurance relates directly to access to care. It is well-known that people without insurance are more likely to have their cancers found at later, less curable stages. Public hospitals and clinics that would generally assume the care for uninsured people are reducing services, closing, or being sold to for-profit companies.

The Unequal Burden of Cancer

The government report issued by the Institute of Medicine (IOM), *The Unequal Burden of Cancer: The Assessment of NIH Research and Programs for Ethnic Minorities and the Medically Underserved* (1999), finally verifies what many people have suspected for some time: U.S. citizens are not uniformly benefiting from the advances in prevention, early detection, treatment, and supportive care that have been described throughout this book. Congress has mandated that programs to study health disparities be established, and there is much work to be done.

People of all ethnic backgrounds who are poor, and who lack insurance and access to high-quality cancer care, get cancer more often, experience more pain and other distressing symptoms, and die from cancer more quickly than do people who are not poor. African Americans and Hispanics or Latinos are less likely to benefit from sophisticated diagnostic tests and treatment than other Americans. After the Breast and Cervical Cancer Prevention and Treatment Act was signed into law in late 2000, allowing underserved women to receive breast and cervical cancer detection and treatment services under Medicaid, it took an additional two years for public law to be signed making Native American women eligible for the same care. This, despite the fact that Native American women have a higher incidence of these cancers than other groups of American women. Native

American women and women native to Alaska have a 52 percent greater cervical cancer death rate than all other races in the United States. And, even now, there are provisions of Medicaid that exclude some Native American women.

There are troubling reports that pharmacies in poor neighborhoods are less likely to stock the medicines most commonly prescribed to manage symptoms such as pain, nausea, and vomiting. Maybe even more troubling are the studies that find that poor people are also less likely than their more affluent counterparts to have these medicines prescribed by doctors. Dr. Lovell Jones, Professor of Gynecologic Oncology at the University of Texas M.D. Anderson Cancer Center and Director of its Center for Research on Minority Health says (in an editorial in the *Houston Chronicle* from 31 March 2003) that the "odds for beating most cancers are so different for minorities, especially black Americans." He goes on to note that policymakers and medical providers are aware of these problems, but many are unconcerned about finding effective methods to deal with this health crisis. And, of course, the poor are the least likely to have a strong political voice.

TECHNOLOGY AND POLICY

Scientific advances in technology have outpaced the making of policy that relates to how and when we use these advances, and again, how we pay for them. Some of the most visible issues involve advances in genetics, electronic technology, and the many questions swirling around the stem cells.

GENETIC RESEARCH is paying off. The blueprint of the DNA sequence of the human genome that was revealed in 2001 brings social, ethical, and legal questions about how the information is used, how it is interpreted, and how it will be merged into everyday health care and public and professional education.

We have new knowledge about how genes cause cancer. Gene mutations have been indicated in several kinds of cancers, including those of the breast, colon, ovary, and lung. This information will help identify high-risk women and result in better programs for screening, early detection, and treatment. But, who pays for expensive genetic testing? Should insurance cover it? What sort of counseling should accompany genetic testing? Who is qualified to offer this counseling? After the results are known, what actions should be next? And inevitably the question, who pays for that?

Genetic information also threatens our right to privacy. Who should have access to our genetic information? If you have some sort of genetic testing, will the results be added to your medical record? Will your insurance company have access to this information? And if your insurance company has access to the information, and your employer pays for your insurance, should your employer have access too? Is it possible that your genetic information could be held against you—or your daughters and sons? If your genetic information reveals that you are at risk for cancer or some other genetic disease, will you be able to get that new job? or to obtain health insurance? How do you talk about these genetic risks with your children?

STEM CELL use in cancer care has given rise to some new policy questions, and, remarkably, new business and marketing opportunities. Placental or umbilical cord blood is a would-be source of blood-forming stem cells. The potential value of this placental blood is the basis for the new business of placental blood banking. The ethical, legal, and social policy issues regarding ownership, consent, privacy, and profit have yet to be addressed.

ELECTRONIC AND COMPUTER-BASED TECHNOLOGIES offer exciting health-related applications. Telehealth—the blending of telephone and satellite communications with computer imaging technologies—can bring sophisticated health-care technology and a variety of cancer care specialists to remote, rural settings. What communities get this access? What companies get the contract to bring in the technology? These can be very politically charged decisions that need to be made by local, state, regional, federal, and international policymakers.

The privacy of medical records is an issue linked to electronic technology and the ease with which information is shared among facilities and agencies. Complete medical records can be transferred to several different agencies, doctors' offices, and insurance plans in a matter of seconds via computer-based messaging—and the rules for this sharing of information have yet to be decided. Privacy rules were established during President Clinton's last few months in office and took effect under President Bush in April 2001. In March 2002, President Bush announced plans to repeal requirements that health-care providers get patients' written consent before using or disclosing medical information. Proponents of these changes, which were favored by the health-care industry, claimed that excessive privacy requirements could delay care. Opponents, including consumer-advocate and patients'-rights groups, viewed the changes as a major threat to privacy. The public was allowed several weeks for public comment, and a final rule was issued in August, 2002, with the force of law.

Final modifications to the standards for privacy of health information covered marketing, consent and notice, uses, and disclosures regarding Food and Drug Administration-regulated products. In practice, patients will be asked to acknowledge in writing that they have been notified of their rights and providers' disclosure policies, but will not have to provide written permission. Implementation of these rules affects every doctor, patient, hospital, pharmacy and health plan in the United States, but how they will actually work has yet to be seen. There are endless questions and not many answers. For additional information, see the U.S. Department of Health and Human Services' website page devoted to "The Privacy Rule" (www.hhs.gov).

TOBACCO

Tobacco use places a huge financial burden on individuals, communities, and nations. According to a study released in 2002 by the U.S. Centers for Disease Control and Prevention (CDC), total costs of smoking in the United States are close to $4,000 per smoker, or $157.7 billion. These figures factor in medical costs (at $3.45 per pack) and lost job productivity ($3.73 per pack) for a total of $7.18 for every pack of cigarettes sold in the United States. The conclusion is that the current level of cigarette tax does not cover the costs of health problems caused by smoking.

The issue of tobacco taxation does make for interesting public debate. Take, for example, the perspective that city and state taxes on cigarettes are sometimes used to replenish dwindling public funds. The Mayor of New York, Michael Bloomberg, has suggested raising his city's cigarette tax from $.08 to $1.50 per pack. Politicians in other states have made similar proposals. Critics say that raising cigarette taxes hurts the poor and middle class who spend a greater portion of their income on cigarettes than do wealthier people. Economists at the Massachusetts Institute of Technology say that smoking is a "price-sensitive" habit: A 10-percent price increase produces about a 5-percent drop in smoking. They conclude that taxes can push people to stop smoking.

Globally, tobacco products kill millions—and tobacco company stock values are higher than ever. Tobacco industry executives grow rich, and the tobacco industry makes huge profits. As an increasing percentage of Americans become concerned about the health effects of tobacco and nicotine, the tobacco industry simply shifts its focus to developing countries. The Republic of Georgia, a former member of the Soviet Union that is burdened by years of civil war, has the world's largest per person consumption of cigarettes and yet cannot afford to rebuild roads, bridges, and buildings. The giant tobacco company Philip Morris funded a study in the Czech Republic. The final report called the cost savings from Czech smokers' early deaths one of the "positive effects" of cigarette smoking. A summary of the study and its conclusions was published in *The Wall Street Journal* in July

2001, causing a public relations crisis at the tobacco company. Columnist Ellen Goodman wrote that "tobacco companies used to deny that cigarettes killed people. Now they brag about it." Children in Europe, China, and other Asian countries are taking up smoking at an alarming rate. Experts predict that a deadly lung cancer epidemic will start in twenty to thirty years in these countries.

CANCER RESEARCH

In the "war on cancer," there are victories and defeats. Efforts to understand cancer have greatly increased since 1971, when President Nixon signed the National Cancer Act. Provisions of this act created the National Cancer Institute, which directly influences the way cancer care is provided today.

In spite of all these advances, over fifteen hundred Americans die every day from cancer. This is equivalent to the total passenger loads of at least three Boeing 747 jets crashing, killing all aboard, every day of the year. Three out of every four of the research grants that are approved by the National Institutes of Health go unfunded. And for every ten dollars you and I pay in taxes, just one penny goes to fund cancer research. At the same time, cancer costs exceed a billion dollars every year, and only 2 percent of these costs are actually invested back into research to find effective prevention, treatment, and cures for cancers. Without research, there will be no advancement in the way cancer is managed. Many cancer experts believe that the "war on cancer" has never been mounted at all—that there have been only minor skirmishes. Still, the number of cancer deaths each year exceeds all U.S. combat deaths in all the wars of the twentieth century. Growing numbers of grass roots cancer advocacy groups work to increase the political will on Capitol Hill to fund cancer research. Some groups are composed of people with very specific interests, for example, various groups support pediatric cancer research, breast cancer research, ovarian cancer research, and prostate cancer research. Other advocacy groups are interested in employment issues or the long-term effects of cancer treatment. There's a place among these advocacy group efforts for anyone with the desire to be part of the political side of fighting cancer.

The National Cancer Institute is responsible for the direction of cancer research in the United States. The federal government, through the NCI, determines cancer research priorities. Through its research grant processes, the NCI decides which projects and which researchers receive funding. The U.S. Congress determines how much money the NCI has available to offer researchers, but the NCI budget competes with all other federal budget items, from Medicare to the military.

The federal government and the NCI have historically funded almost all cancer research. The NCI still funds and directs most cancer research in the United States, but drug companies and other privately owned companies are increasingly using their own resources to fund such research.

The Feinstein-Smith Cancer Bill, drawn up by the National Cancer Legislation Advisory Committee and named for California's Senator Dianne Feinstein and Oregon's Senator Gordon Smith, has thirteen provisions covering research, translation (moving from research to clinical, or from "bench to bedside"), cancer care access, quality of care, and cancer prevention activities. The bill would increase the NCI budget by 10 percent every year after 2003, eventually allowing NCI to fund 40 percent of the fundable research grants—up from the current rate of less than 25 percent. It would increase clinical trials; require insurers to pay routine medical care costs of clinical trials; provide incentives for manufacturers to produce drugs to treat rare cancers; and attract and train health-care professionals including the full range of nurses committed to providing cancer care, giving preference to people who make a commitment to working in underserved communities. Under preventive provisions in this bill, insurers would be required to pay for cancer screening tests, smoking cessation programs, genetic testing, and nutritional counseling. The bill's authors propose paying for costs associated with these plans with federal excise taxes on all tobacco products. A provision of the bill would give the U.S. Food and Drug Administration the authority to regulate tobacco—a provision that is sure to be heavily contested by tobacco interests and one that some experts think could "kill" the entire bill. The future of this particular piece of legislation is at present unknown, but pass or fail, it is clear that some legislators are looking for creative ways to address the cancer problems this country faces.

CANCER POLICY

In addition to setting the course for cancer research, the NCI, its various advisory panels, and the National Institutes of Health guide the development of policies and regulations that determine how and what health care is provided in this country. Policy is a reflection of the values of a country—or, at least, the values of the decision makers. At the National Cancer Institute, policy decisions guide what the government is prepared to support and pay for.

A controversy over the effectiveness of mammography screening among women under the age of fifty took center stage in 1997. Even though a panel of experts would not deny the value of mammography for women under age fifty, panel members could not confirm the cost-effectiveness of mammography for the total population of American women under fifty. Since offering mammography screening to all women under fifty would ultimately affect millions of women and cost millions of dollars for a screening test that would detect a relatively small number of cancers, the panel chose not to endorse mammography screening for women under fifty.

Another emerging mammography issue is that involving even younger women—premenopausal women. It is acknowledged that use of mammography in premenopausal women is less than perfect: Breast tissue in these women is more dense and mammography images can be difficult to read. But there is some speculation that biopsy or breast surgery on the basis of these hazy images may not only be unnecessary, but might also possibly be harmful. A few scientists propose a theory that the wounds from biopsy or surgery in combination with menstrual cycle hormonal changes may cause an existing tumor to grow and spread more rapidly. While it is too early for application of these findings to public policy, they do give some credibility to a long-standing suggestion that the scheduling of biopsy and surgery should take into consideration each woman's menstrual cycle.

A new controversy over mammography screening policy emerged in 2002 when two Danish scientists published a report in the medical journal *Lancet* that questions the overall value of mammography. This report, called a "meta-analysis," is an attempt by the authors to summarize all the studies that have been done on mammography to date and come up with a concise finding reflecting all of the compiled data. The analysis includes studies that go back to the early days of mammography—and judges the old studies by today's much higher standards. With the old and new data combined, the Danish researchers concluded that there was no lifesaving benefit from routine mammography. Needless to say, this report created headlines throughout the media, including a cover story in *Time* magazine. Editorials from health and cancer experts appeared in major newspapers and as lead stories on television news reports.

So, what's the real story? Basically, most cancer professionals acknowledge that mammograms, as they are today, are not perfect: Even the best miss 10 percent of all breast cancers. Abnormal mammographic findings alone do not predict what the abnormality is and certainly do not predict the woman's future. There is a high rate of false positives—readings that seem to indicate a problem when, in fact, there is none—resulting in unnecessary anxiety for these women. But, finally and most importantly, at this point in time mammograms find more breast tumors at earlier, more manageable stages than any other available breast cancer screening test.

MANAGED CARE

There are many concerns about the rapid growth of managed care in the United States. Since the introduction of employer-sponsored health insurance after WWII, most Americans have come to rely on their employers for access to care. Governmental agencies have been charged with guaranteeing the quality of care received in hospitals and other health-care institutions. But so far, there has been minimal monitoring and regulation of managed care systems or of the office-based physician practices where most cancer care is provided.

The news about managed care is not all bad. Since the idea behind HMOs is to "maintain health," it follows that they should promote prevention measures that are important to women, and to some degree this appears to be true. Pap smears, mammograms, and other screening tests are offered more often by HMOs than by doctors who see women in the old fee-for-service plans.

The bad news is that some HMOs encourage doctors *not* to order important tests or refer women (and men and children) to specialists. Among managed care executives, there is debate about whether an oncologist can be a primary care doctor—or whether a woman with a history of cancer must always go through a generalist who then refers her to an oncologist.

Legislators have begun to address the shortfalls of managed care. The Newborns and Mothers Health Protection Act requires health plans to allow new mothers at least forty-eight hours in the hospital. Legislation in some states bans outpatient mastectomy. A Connecticut law established an appeals process through which consumers can file complaints about decisions to deny care, and other states are considering similar measures.

The Health-Care Nonsystem

Health care in the United States is not a "system" at all, since the word *system* indicates some master plan or organization. Many people say what we have is a "nonsystem." Health care in the United States is a fragmented patchwork of programs and plans with many cracks—and many of our citizens fall through these cracks. While universal access to care or a single-payor system would solve many of these problems, the American public and the U.S. Congress have been unwilling to support this kind of system.

The only thing that is certain is that more piecemeal regulation will be put in place in response to gaps in the present system.

It is vital that every woman knows and understands her health-care needs. With this knowledge, a woman can advocate for services that are important for her health and that of her family and her community.

NO MONEY? NO MISSION!

It might be cynical to voice the opinion that "money makes the world go 'round," but as most people involved in political advocacy know, the "no money—no mission" chant holds true. It takes money to educate people to become doctors, nurses, social workers, and other experts in cancer care. It takes money to set up and staff prevention and screening programs. It takes money to build and maintain health-care facilities and to pay people to work in those facilities. It takes money to support good cancer research.

Money by itself is not the answer. It will require a coordinated plan in which everyone knows her or his job, there is no duplication of effort, and people work together instead of competing with each other. The decision to fund basic cancer research, cancer nursing research, and clinical trials of new treatment methods are all choices—choices of consumers, choices of constituents, and choices of policymakers and legislators. We have the power to influence the choices legislators make, and we must use that power. The National Coalition for Cancer Survivorship is a leader in cancer policy advocacy efforts. Its website (www.canceradvocacy.org) offers information about how to get involved in cancer advocacy and also provides up-to-date information about the most compelling current policy issues.

Consumers of Health Care?

Sue Berkman, author of *Surviving Your H.M.O.* (Villard, 1997), says, "patients might have to redefine the role they play in their care." She encourages women to have a more aggressive attitude when dealing with the health-care system. In the new millenium, her words are still good advice: If the health-care industry thinks of us as clients or customers, we can act that way. Consumers have *choices*.

Every woman, man, or child who uses a health service is a consumer. Be a choosy buyer—as when you shop for the best deal on a car, select a meal in a restaurant, or purchase furniture. You can bargain for the options and price you want when you buy into a health plan, just as you would when buying a car. Being a good health-care consumer means knowing what you want and expect from a service. If an employer offers a plan, make sure the

Oncology Nursing Society
Position Paper* on Quality Cancer Care

(approved by the ONS Board of Directors, April 1997)

The ONS uses the Institute of Medicine's definition of quality of care: "the degree to which health services for individuals and populations increase the likelihood of desired outcomes and are consistent with current professional knowledge." A quality cancer care program takes into account each part of life that cancer could affect, from prevention and early detection, to treatment and cure, and at the end of life. A team of healthcare professionals who specialize in cancer care, including registered nurses, doctors, pharmacists, social workers, physical and occupational therapists, and dietitians, work with patients and families in planning and giving care. These elements form a quality cancer care program.

Prevention: Quality cancer care programs create and support ways to teach the public about cancer risks and lifestyle changes that decrease cancer risk, using teaching methods that reach various cultural and ethnic groups.

Early detection: Screening programs for colon, cervix, testicle, and breast cancers are part of a quality cancer care program. Insurance companies, HMOs, Medicare, and Medicaid will pay for screening methods that help find cancers when they are most curable.

Treatment: There is quick and easy access to treatment proven to work best for the specific cancer. Available treatments include surgery, radiation, chemotherapy, bone marrow or peripheral blood stem cell transplant, hormonal/biological therapies, complementary therapies, and rehabilitation services.

Supportive care: Cancer treatment, the control of cancer symptoms, and the control of side effects of treatment are equally available. Patients and family members learn to care for themselves to the extent possible, and community and home care resources are routinely used.

Long-term follow-up: Rehabilitation services help people learn to live with cancer as well as the physical and emotional aftereffects of cancer. Follow-up by oncology specialists focuses on health, prevention, early detection, and treating the physical and emotional aftereffects of cancer and its treatment.

End-of-life care: Patients and families have quick, easy access to humane and dignified care at the end of life.

(Adapted from the original paper and reprinted with permission of the Oncology Nursing Society)

employer keeps your needs in mind. A group of employees can pressure employers to make good health plans available. This type of negotiation is politics in action.

The National Commission on Quality Assurance (NCQA) accredits HMOs. So far, accreditation is voluntary—HMOs choose whether they want to go through the NCQA accreditation process—so not all HMOs are evaluated. There is no national "report card" that grades HMOs or helps us determine whether all HMOs provide quality care. The American Nurses Credentialing Center recognizes the "best" hospitals in America through its Magnet Nursing Services Recognition Program. These "magnets" are recognized as hospitals that create environments in which excellent nursing care is provided. Magnet hospitals have lower mortality rates and higher levels of patient satisfaction. Since excellent nursing care is critical in the safe and competent delivery of cancer care services, it makes sense to seek care in designated "magnet" facilities. There is no "magnet"-like credential for community-based treatment centers—at least not yet—but this idea is catching on and is likely to be evident in all sorts of health-care facilities in the not-too-distant future.

Several cancer-related professional organizations have offered definitions of quality cancer care. The synopsis on page 480 of the Oncology Nursing Society's *Position on Quality Cancer Care* outlines the important elements of a quality cancer care program. A copy of the original position paper is available from the Oncology Nursing Society (ONS) by calling (412) 921-7373 or visiting the ONS website at www.ons.org.

WHAT YOU CAN DO

Politics is more than people who work on Capitol Hill or in offices in state capitols. Politics means finding ways to meet the needs of a community health center or a prevention and screening clinic. It can be letting elected officials know what you think about issues. Letters to these people have meaning. Legislators and city council members respond to constituents. But they are not mind readers—and they interpret silence as approval.

Our ability to influence our health-care system on the local, state, or national level begins long before we call or write a city council member or senator. The most important step in the process is to influence who is nominated and elected. Women can participate in campaigns to help elect officials who are sensitive to their views. Political party activity provides a way to develop relationships with elected officials. Simple things like helping on a telephone bank or volunteering time in an elected official's office give a woman an "inside track" in the political process.

There is power in numbers. Working with groups that reflect your views is important. For example, it helps support my opinion to say that thirty thousand other cancer nurses in this country share it, or that my idea is endorsed by a particular professional organization. The power of numbers is an important reason for organizations like the National Coalition for

*Cancer Is
Still a
Political
Issue*

Cancer Survivorship and Y-ME to exist. I have become a "pen pal" to my elected officials. I write to them about legislation I think might curb the tobacco industry's efforts to addict more people (like selling cigarettes in foreign countries). I write to express objections to the gag rules that prevent doctors and nurses from discussing all relevant treatment options. I write or call when pending legislation might affect women's health—particularly when the issues involve cancer prevention, early detection, and care. And I write about funding for nursing education and nursing research.

Let elected officials know who you are, what you think, and what you would like to see them do. The addresses and telephone numbers of all officials are in the phone book. If you are not sure who to contact, call the local League of Women Voters for information. Internet sites also provide this information. Western Union offers a public opinion message service; call them at (800) 325-6000. Ask to send a public opinion message to the representative you need to reach. It doesn't matter how you do it. A handwritten letter is usually more likely to get attention; it is obvious this letter is not mass-produced and that the writer went to some trouble to write it.

Tips on writing to an elected official:

+ Be concise, informed, and polite

+ Stick to one typewritten or handwritten page; if writing longhand, write legibly

+ If you are writing about a bill, cite it by name and number

+ Be factual, and support your position with factual information about how the bill might affect you

+ If you believe that legislation or a proposal is wrong, say so; state the likely adverse effects and suggest a better approach

+ Ask for the official's views, but do not demand support

+ Be sure your name and return address are legible

Most important, be visible. Express your opinions and ideas. After all, elected officials will not know your opinion unless you tell them. The people in charge of writing new policy—those recent college graduates—are unlikely to have your cancer expertise and experience. If good policy is to be written and enacted, these people need to know what *you* know.

Politics goes beyond what we think of as the traditional political arena. The media, for example, is a powerful political tool. Women can write letters to the editors of newspapers and magazines to present pertinent ideas or respond to issues of the day. Television and radio offer public service announcements and other free public opinion forums. Boycotts of products (including magazines and television shows) accompanied by written and publicized messages of protest can send a potent message. Silence is approval. Visibility creates reality.

In *1 in 3: Women with Cancer Confront an Epidemic,* Judith Brady summarizes the need for women in cancer-related politics:

> Our ultimate salvation from the ravages of cancer lies neither in the doctor's office nor the pharmaceutical laboratory, but in the political arena.

— *Pamela Haylock*

AFTERWORD

I can check them off on my fingers, my "sisters" from the Monday night cancer support group alumnae:

Margaret is enjoying her husband and her handsome and lively seventeen-year-old son, her challenging job, and the completion of the extensive home remodeling project which none of us thought would ever end.

Jenny quit the job she detested, pulled up stakes, and happily worked as a park ranger in national parks all over the United States before retiring last year to hone her impressive creative writing skills.

Ellen continues running her own tax accounting business and spends as many hours as possible gardening during the less "taxing" seasons.

Elizabeth is now taking a well-deserved break after putting her amazing organizational skills into the breast cancer foundation she started. (She was a force behind breast cancer survivors' ascents of such mountains as Mount Aconcagua in Argentina and Mount Fiji in Japan.) We all find it almost impossible to believe that her daughter, whom we met as an impish six-year-old, is now in college.

And Linda... Linda died of her cancer. We will never forget Linda, with her keen artistic eye, her spunk, and that crazy sense of humor. She was the one who coined the term "CRS syndrome" ("can't remember shit") for the memory glitches we all complained about during chemotherapy. We honor her memory and will always mourn her loss.

But then there's Marty....

That's what cancer is. Both sadness and joy. Both dreams put on hold— and bright new beginnings.

And that is why I treasure, and wear with pride, the bold yellow button given to me by one of my "sisters": *Enjoy life. This is not a dress rehearsal.*

— *Kerry McGinn*

GLOSSARY

adenocarcinoma—a tumor originating in a glandular structure

adjuvant chemotherapy—anticancer drugs used after all the known cancer has been removed with surgery/radiation and when there is a high risk of hidden cancer cells in the body

alopecia—partial or complete hair loss

aneuploid—cancer cells that do not contain the standard number of chromosomes

angiogenesis—the process by which cancerous tumors are able to induce the production of new blood vessels

anti-oncogenes—normal genes that suppress cell division

atypia—cells that look abnormal under the microscope

aromatase inhibitors—a class of hormone drugs used for breast cancer that affect the adrenal glands

autologous bone marrow transplant—the planned infusion of a patient's own tissue, previously withdrawn from the body and stored, as a rescue after very high-dose chemotherapy has destroyed the bone marrow in the body

axilla—armpit

axillary lymph nodes—the lymph nodes (bean-shaped filters) in the armpit

axillary-node dissection—removal of the lymph nodes from the armpit during breast cancer surgery

barium enema—special X ray of the colon and rectum after liquid barium has been given in an enema

benign—not cancerous

benign breast changes—collective term for any breast lump, lumpiness, nipple discharge, or pain that is not caused by cancer

bimanual pelvic examination—examination of the internal reproductive organs using both hands, two fingers of one hand in the vagina and the other hand on the abdomen

biological-response modifier—a naturally occurring substance, often grown in the laboratory, that changes the body's defenses

biological therapy—use of biological response modifiers to fight cancer

biopsy—removal of a piece of body tissue so that it can be examined under a microscope

bisphosphonates—a class of drugs used to stop or slow bone loss, used for osteoporosis and hypercalcemia

bone marrow—the place in the center of most bones where blood cells are made

brachytherapy—radiation therapy given from a sealed radioactive source placed in the body

BRCA1 and BRCA2—mutated genes associated with increased breast and ovarian cancer risk

breast reconstruction—surgery to restore the breast mound (and sometimes areola and nipple) after a mastectomy

bronchoscopy—passage of a long tube through the mouth into the bronchi (upper lung passages); biopsies can be taken

BSE (breast self-examination)—inspection and palpation of the breast tissue by the woman herself

CA 15-3—a breast cancer tumor marker measured with a specific laboratory blood test

CA 27-29—a specific substance found in the blood, increased in breast cancer

CA 125—an ovarian cancer tumor marker measured with a specific laboratory blood test

calcifications—see microcalcifications

cancer—a condition in which highly abnormal cells, with the capacity to invade nearby body tissues and spread to other organs in the body, are growing abnormally

cancer-risk counseling—advice given by medical geneticist or other health professional based on an individual's family history and other risk factors for cancer

capsular contracture—the formation of a fibrous shell around a breast implant

carcinogens—substances that can cause cell changes leading to cancer

carcinoma—cancer that develops in the covering or lining tissues of body organs

carcinoma in situ—presence of highly abnormal cells confined within a local area, without evidence of any invasion of nearby tissues. Some people consider this the earliest stage of cancer while others believe it may be the most abnormal form of benign breast changes

cardiac toxicity—changes affecting the heart and its function that is most often linked to the chemotherapy drugs doxorubicin and daunorubicin.

cardiomyopathy—permanent damage to heart muscle caused by the chemotherapy drugs doxorubicin and daunorubicin and direct radiation exposure to the heart

CEA (carcinoembryonic antigen)—a tumor marker in some breast cancers and other kinds of cancers, measured with a specific laboratory blood test

"chemobrain"—a term that many women use to describe the changes in their thought processes following treatment for breast cancer

chemoprevention—preventive medicines for people thought to be at high risk for cancer

chemotherapy—treatment of cancer with drugs to kill cancer cells

CIN (cervical intraepithelial neoplasia)—premalignant changes in the cervical cells

clinical trial—a study that tests the safety and effectiveness of a new treatment in humans

colonoscopy—passage of a flexible, lighted tube from the anus through the entire large intestine to inspect the colon and remove biopsy specimens if needed

colony stimulating factor (G-CSF or GM-CSF)—a substance that increases the blood cell production of the bone marrow

colposcopy—inspection of the cervix, vagina, and vulva through special lighted "binoculars" on a stand with wheels

Community Clinical Oncology Program (CCOP)—one of the local community programs that participates in clinical trials under the direction of the National Cancer Institute

complementary therapy—a treatment from a source other than traditional Western medicine that a patient uses along with traditional therapy

complete remission—disappearance of all signs of a cancer

Comprehensive Cancer Center—a specialized cancer hospital/research center that meets criteria set by the National Cancer Institute

computerized thermal imaging—a way of picturing the breasts using a sensitive infrared camera, with findings analyzed by computer

cone biopsy (conization)—removal of a cone of tissue around the opening of the cervix to check for the presence of cancer cells

cone view—a mammography technique in which a small part of the breast is compressed to give a clearer image of a suspicious area than can be seen on routine views

consent form—a piece of paper a patient signs before surgery or other procedures to indicate that she or he has been informed about the procedure and agrees to it

core biopsy—withdrawal of a core of tissue from a suspicious area through a special, wide-bore needle

counterconditioning—*see* systematic desensitization

CT scan (CAT scan, computerized tomography)—a special X-ray study that gives cross-sectional views of the body organs

culdoscopy—inspection of the area behind the uterus and between the uterus and the rectum through a tube inserted through a tiny incision in the vagina

cyst—a benign fluid-filled sac

cystoscopy—inspection of the bladder (and removal of tissue specimens as needed) through a lighted tube inserted through the bladder opening

cytology—examination of cells under a microscope for the presence of cancer (as with a Pap smear)

D&C (dilatation and curettage)—a gynecological procedure in which the cervix is enlarged (dilated) with a special instrument and the lining of the uterus in scraped out for diagnosis and/or treatment

DES (diethylstibesterol)—a synthetic estrogen given at one time to prevent miscarriages, now known to initiate rare gynecologic cancers in offspring; still used as treatment for some metastatic cancers

DNA (deoxyribonucleic acid)—genetic material in cells that determines inherited cell characteristics

detection—finding a body change that could be either benign or malignant *diagnosis*—the process (or the doctor's conclusion) when the pathologist examines body tissues under the microscope to discover what a change means

digital mammography—a variation on breast X rays using a detector that "reads" breast tissue for a computer screen

diploid—cells having the normal number of chromosomes (46)

disease-free interval—the period of time after initial cancer therapy during which the person has no signs or symptoms of cancer

distant metastasis—spread of cancer cells through the blood or lymph system to a body organ away from the site where it started

dominant breast lump—in breast examination, a three-dimensional lump that stands out from the surrounding tissue

Doppler study—a technique that images the blood vessels by transmitting sound waves through them

doubling time—the time it takes for a group of cells to double

duct carcinoma in situ (DCIS, intraductal carcinoma, noninvasive carcinoma, non infiltrating carcinoma)—highly abnormal cells confined within the ducts of the breast

dysplasia—abnormal cells; often used to refer to atypical cells of the surface layer of the cervix

early detection—finding cancerous changes during their silent period or soon after, before they cause symptoms

endometrial biopsy—removal of a small piece of tissue from the lining of the uterus for examination by a pathologist

endometrium—inner layer of tissue in the uterus

endoscopy—examination of a hollow organ or body cavity with a tubular instrument

estrogen—the female hormone that acts on the reproductive tract and the breasts

estrogen receptor—protein on some cells that attaches to the female hormone estrogen. A cancer tumor that is estrogen-receptor positive has this protein on its cells and responds to the hormone

excisional biopsy—removal of the entire lump during an open surgical biopsy

external radiation—radiation therapy delivered from a machine outside the body

false negative—an imaging study or biopsy that does not show cancer although cancer is present

false positive—an imaging study that shows suspicious changes that do not prove to be cancer

fibroadenoma—a kind of benign solid breast lump

"fibrocystic breast disease"—inaccurate and outdated term used for any breast change that is not cancer

flow cytometry—a test that analyzes the DNA content of a cancer to see if the cells have the normal number of chromosomes

FNA (fine needle aspiration)—withdrawal of fluid or a few cells from a breast lump through a needle into a syringe for diagnosis

frozen section—the freezing and slicing of biopsy tissue to make a slide for immediate diagnosis

grading—a way of judging how aggressive a cancer is likely to be by its appearance under a microscope

Health Insurance Portability and Affordability Act (HIPAA)—a law passed by U.S. Congress that allows many persons to carry their health insurance to a new job

hematoma—a "pocket" of blood, usually as a complication of surgery

HER-2/neu oncogene—a specific rapid-growth gene found in about 30 percent of breast cancers

hormone receptor assay—test to check whether breast cancer cells contain specific proteins sensitive to the female hormones estrogen and/or progesterone

hormone replacement therapy (HRT)—the use of hormone drugs, usually estrogen and often progesterone, for menopausal symptoms and to prevent bone thinning

hormone therapy—use of female or male hormones or antihormones to influence cancer growth

HPV—human papillomavirus, or genital warts

HRT—hormone replacement therapy

HSV—herpes simplex virus type II, or genital herpes

hypercalcemia—a dangerous increase in calcium in the blood, often caused by cancer metastasis to the bone

hyperplasia—too much cell growth

hysterectomy—surgical removal of the uterus

hysteroscope—lighted tube that can be inserted through the cervix to see inside the uterus

imaging technique—any one of several techniques to picture the inside of the body without direct visualization (e.g., X rays)

incisional biopsy—removal of a piece of a suspicious lump during an open surgical biopsy

infiltrating cancer—*see* invasive cancer

informed consent—a legal standard of minimum information a patient must receive before agreeing to surgery or other invasive procedure

initiators—substances or factors that cause direct cell damage leading to cancer

internal radiation—radiation therapy using a source of radiation inside the body, such as ovoids

interventional radiologist—a person skilled in performing procedures using radiologic (X-ray) imaging guidance

intra-arterial chemotherapy—a way to deliver chemotherapy agents directly to a body organ by infusing them into the artery leading to that organ

intraperitoneal chemotherapy—delivery of chemotherapy through a special catheter into the space around the abdominal organs to "bathe" the tissues there

intravenous pyelogram—a special X ray of the urinary tract after a contrast fluid has been injected into the patient's vein

invasive cancer—cancer cells that have penetrated and taken over surrounding normal tissue

Kaufman axillary treatment scale—a tool being investigated to classify breast cancers by how much axillary node surgery is needed

Ki-67—a test done on a small amount of a breast cancer tumor to estimate the percentage of dividing cells, a clue to how fast the tumor is growing

laparoscopy—use of a narrow, lighted tube inserted through a small skin incision to see inside the body

LATS flap (latissimus dorsi flap)—a breast reconstruction procedure in which skin and a piece of muscle from below the shoulder blade area are tunneled under the skin to help form a new breast covering

linear accelerator—a type of machine that delivers external radiation therapy

locally advanced breast cancer—stage III breast cancer with a large tumor or certain other specific changes but no evidence of distant metastasis

local therapy—a treatment for cancer in the organ where it originated

lumpectomy (tylectomy, quandrantectomy, wide excision, partial mastectomy)—removal of a cancerous breast lump with a margin of normal tissue as treatment (with radiation) of some breast cancers

lymphatic system—the system of lymph vessels and lymph nodes

lymphedema—swelling of an arm or leg because of blocked drainage of lymph fluid in the armpit or groin

lymph nodes—bean-size filters along the lymph system that contain special white blood cells and that sometimes trap cancer cells

magnification views—special mammogram views that show breast tissue in more detail

malignant—cancerous

malignant transformation—the process by which a healthy cell becomes a cancer cell

mammograms—X rays of the breasts

margin—the strip of apparently normal surrounding tissue removed with a cancer or a biopsy specimen

mastalgia—breast pain

mastectomy—surgical removal of the breast

metastasis—the spread of a cancer from one organ to another via the bloodstream or lymph system

microcalcification (calcification)—tiny calcified specks seen on a mammogram that can be associated with either benign or cancerous breast changes

microscopic nodal invasion—spread of cancer cells to nearby lymph nodes in numbers that can be seen only with a microscope

microsurgical free flap procedure—a breast reconstruction surgery technique in which a piece of tissue is removed completely (perhaps from the abdomen) and then moved to the breast area where the blood vessels are reattached to blood vessels in the new location

mitosis—the process of cell division

modified radical mastectomy—removal of an island of breast skin with nipple and areola, all the breast tissue, and some or all of the armpit lymph nodes, but no chest muscle

MRI (magnetic resonance imaging)—method of imaging the body by using magnetic field and radiowaves

multiple hits—a theory that an individual cancer requires several changes, or "hits," to the normal cell

mutagen—anything that can cause a cell to change (mutate)

mutation—the process by which a cell changes

nadir—after a chemotherapy drug is given, the point at which the white blood cells and platelets reach their lowest count

needle-localization biopsy (wire-localization biopsy)—special technique for surgical biopsy of the breast when the abnormality appears only on mammogram. The radiologist marks the area first with one or more needles (or wires) and often dye, and then the surgeon cuts out the marked area

neo-adjuvant therapy—giving chemotherapy to shrink a tumor before surgery

neoplasia—abnormal new growth that can be either benign or malignant

nephrotoxicity—kidney change that is known to occur as a late effect of the drugs cisplatin, methotrexate, and nitrosurea

neurotoxicity—nerve damage most often thought of as occurring after use of the chemotherapy drugs cisplatin, paclitaxel, and the vinca alkaloids

neutropenia—the condition of having too few of the white blood cells that protect against infection

noninfiltrating carcinoma—*see* carcinoma in situ

noninvasive carcinoma—*see* carcinoma in situ

nonproliferative change—a benign increase in body cells because the old cells are not being disposed of as fast as they should be

nuclear grade—a way of estimating the aggressiveness of a cancer by its appearance under the microscope

nuclear scan (bone scan, brain scan, etc.)—an imaging study done after an injection of a small amount of radioactive tracer into the vein

oncogenes—specific pieces of DNA in the cell that can be activated and cause uncontrolled cell division

oncologist (medical oncologist, radiation oncologist)—a doctor who specializes in cancer treatment

oophorectomy—surgical removal of the ovaries

open biopsy—surgery to obtain a specimen of tissue that can be examined under the microscope

osteoporosis—low bone mass and deterioration of bone tissue that results in fragile bones and increased risk for bone fractures

ostomy (colostomy, urostomy, etc.)—rerouting the healthy end of the digestive or urinary tract to a new opening on the abdomen

Paget's disease—a rare condition in which a rash signals highly abnormal or cancerous cells

palliation—the giving of treatment to relieve symptoms

palpation—examination of body tissue by feeling with the fingers

Pap smear—process of scraping a few cells from the cervix, placing them on a slide, staining them, and examining the slide under a microscope for presence of abnormal cells. Similar experimental process for fluid suctioned from nipple of breast

partial remission—decrease in size of tumor by at least 50 percent

pathologist—doctor who specializes in examining tissue under a microscope for diagnosis

PCA (patient-controlled analgesia)—use of a preprogrammed intravenous pump that delivers a set dose of pain medicine when the patient pushes a button

PDQ (Physician Data Query)—computer information service run by the National Cancer Institute to make current cancer treatment information available, primarily to physicians

peripheral neuropathy—numbness, burning, tingling in feet or hands, a side effect of certain chemotherapy drugs

permanent section—lengthy process by which the pathologist slices and prepares biopsy tissue for definitive diagnosis

poorly differentiated—cancer cells that look very different from normal cells in the same organ, associated with poorer prognosis

positive lymph node—a lymph node with cancer cells in it

proctosigmoidoscope (sigmoidoscope)—a lighted instrument inserted through the anus to look directly at the last 12 inches of the large intestine and take biopsy specimens if needed

p.r.n.—"as needed or requested," usually referring to when medication is given

progesterone—female hormone associated with producing breast milk and female reproductive functions

progesterone receptors—proteins that some cells have that are sensitive to the female hormone progesterone

prognosis—the statistically likely outcome of a disease

proliferative change with atypia—benign buildup of cells because abnormal cells are dividing more often than normal

proliferative change without atypia—benign buildup of cells that appear normal themselves but are dividing more often a normal

promoters—factors that encourage the development of cancer, but do not initiate the process

prophylactic mastectomy—surgical removal of a breast where there is no known cancer as a preventive measure

proto-oncogenes—normal genes that stimulate cell division

psychoneuroimmunology—the study of the influence of the brain on the immune system and the development of disease

pulmonary fibrosis—lung (pulmonary) toxicity in the form of decreased flexibility that has been associated with the chemotherapy drug bleomycin, alkylating agents, methotrexate, and nitrosurea

radiation oncologist (radiation therapist)—doctor who specializes in treating cancer with radiation

radiation therapy (radiation oncology)—treatment of cancer with energy from atoms in transition

radiologist—doctor who specializes in imaging studies such as X rays and CT scans

Reach to Recovery—American Cancer Society volunteer organization that pairs a woman undergoing breast-cancer treatment with another woman who is a veteran of that treatment

recurrence—return of cancer after a period when it was thought to be gone (used by some people to mean only the return of cancer in the same organ)

regional extension—spread of cancer cells directly to an adjoining organ (not through bloodstream or lymph system)

RNA (ribonucleic acid)—material associated with the control of cell level chemical activities and DNA replication

s-phase—the time in the life of a cell when it is preparing to divide; checking what proportion of cancer cells are in s-phase gives information about how fast-growing the cancer is

sarcoma—a cancer that begins in the connective or supporting tissue of the body (bones, muscle, etc.)

scintimammography (Sestamibi nuclear medicine breast imaging)—a way of picturing the breasts after injection of a tiny amount of radioactive material into the woman's vein, with the image shown on computer monitor

sclerosing adenosis—a benign breast change, sometimes marked by microcalcifications on mammograms

screening tests—physical examinations, imaging studies, and/or laboratory tests used to check for the presence of disease in apparently healthy people

second opinion—therapy recommendation from a doctor other than the treating physician

selective estrogen receptor modulators (SERM)—a class of hormone drugs that act as "weakened" estrogens in the body; they are used for breast-cancer treatment and are being investigated as a possible way of preventing or postponing cancer; tamoxifen and raloxifene are the best known SERMS

sentinel lymph node sampling—a surgical technique to mark the axillary lymph node(s) directly in line with a breast cancer (with dye and radiation) so that the surgeon removes only one or a very few nodes; the node is checked for cancer and, if positive, more nodes are removed

seroma—a collection of tissue fluid under the skin, usually after surgery

silent period—the time between when a cancer begins growing and when it begins causing signs or symptoms

simulation—a "mockup" of radiation therapy from machine, done before the treatment begins

sonography (ultrasound)—an imaging study that records the echoes of sound waves passing through the body

specimen radiography—a technique for examining by X ray a biopsy specimen of a breast change that cannot be palpated but shows on mammograms

squamous—of or relating to the epithelial or skinlike tissue

staging—a process for classifying a cancer by how extensive it is

STAR trial—a clinical study looking at the hormone drugs tamoxifen and raloxifene to see if they can prevent or postpone breast cancer in high-risk women

stem cells—immature white blood cells usually found in the bone marrow

stem-cell transplants—the collection and storage of "baby" blood cells from a woman so that they can be given back to her after high doses of chemotherapy to "rescue" her white blood cells

stereotactic guided needle biopsy—a procedure for using a needle placed by computer to obtain a biopsy specimen of a breast change that shows only on mammography

stomatitis—inflammation of the lining of the mouth, often as a side effect of chemotherapy

systemic desensitization—a way to prevent anticipatory nausea or vomiting that involves gradually exposing the woman to the stimulus of the chemo experience until she no longer automatically reacts to the prospect of having chemo by becoming nauseous

systemic therapy—cancer therapy that treats the whole body

T-scan imaging—a way of picturing the breasts by passing tiny amounts of low-level electrical current through them, with the information displayed on a computer monitor

tamoxifen—a hormone medication commonly used in breast-cancer treatment

thermography—a breast imaging technique that measures body heat at skin level to identify hot spots due to inflammation or cancer

thrombocytopenia—the condition of having a serious deficiency of platelets in the blood

tissue expander—a kind of breast implant used in breast reconstruction, consisting of an expandable chamber connected to a port; the chamber is slowly expanded with weekly injections of salt water through the skin into the port

TNM classification—a system to classify cancers by the size of the tumor (T), lymph-node involvement (N), and distant metastasis (M)

TRAM flap (transverse rectus abdominus myocutaneous flap)—a technique for reconstructing the breast by tunneling abdominal muscle, skin, and fat under the skin to make a new breast mound

transvaginal sonography—an imaging technique for the ovaries that measures the echoes of sound waves transmitted by a probe placed in the vagina

tumor—a swelling or lump that can be either benign or malignant

tumor board—a group of cancer doctors from different specialties who meet periodically to pool their expertise and recommend therapy for individual cancer patients

tumor marker—a physical change that is not itself cancer but often occurs in connection with a cancer (e.g., elevated CEA or CA-125 in blood tests)

tylectomy—*see* lumpectomy

ultrasound—*see* sonography

upper GI series—X rays taken of the upper digestive tract after the patient swallows barium

VAIN (vaginal intraepithelial neoplasia)—carcinoma in situ of the vaginal canal

Van Nuys Prognostic Index (VPNI)—a way of classifying ductal carcinoma in situ of the breast by certain characteristics to decide what kind of treatment should be done

VIN (vulvar intraepithelial neoplasia)—carcinoma in situ of the vulva

well differentiated—cancer cells that still look somewhat similar to normal cells from the same organ, usually associated with a less aggressive cancer

wide excision—*see* lumpectomy

wire localization biopsy—*see* needle localization biopsy

BIBLIOGRAPHY

In this third edition, we have discovered that we are getting a major amount of information from reputable Internet sites rather than from print journal articles. This means a shorter bibliography.

Chapter 1: Cancer Basics

Ruoslahti, E. "How Cancer Spreads." *Scientific American*. 275(3):72–77, 1996.

Scanlon, E. F., and Murthy, S. "The Process of Metastasis." *CA: A Cancer Journal for Clinicians*. 41(5):301–305, 1991.

Weinberg, R. A. "How Cancer Arises." *Scientific American*. 275(3):62–70, 1996.

Chapter 2: Cause and Prevention

American Cancer Society. *Cancer Facts and Figures—2002*. Atlanta, GA: American Cancer Society, 2002.

American Cancer Society. *Cancer Facts and Figures for African Americans, 2000–2001*. Atlanta, GA: American Cancer Society, 2000.

Frank-Stromberg, M., and Cohen, R. F. "Assessment and Interventions for Cancer Detection." In Yarbro, C. H., et al. (eds.) *Cancer Nursing Principles and Practice*, Fifth Edition. Boston, MA: Jones and Bartlett, 2000, 150–188.

Hay, L. L. *Heal Your Body*. Carson, CA: Hay House, 1988.

Jemal, A., Thomas, A., Murray, T., and Thun, M. "Cancer Statistics, 2002." *CA: A Cancer Journal for Clinicians*. 52(1):23–47, 2002.

Johnson, E. Y., and Lookingbill, D. P. "Sunscreen Use and Sun Exposure: Trends in a White Population." *Archives of Dermatology*. 120:727–731, 1984.

LeShan, L. "An Emotional Life-history Pattern Associated with Neoplastic Disease." *Annals of the New York Academy of Sciences*. 125:780–793, 1966.

Moulder, J. E., et al. "Cell phones and Cancer: What Is the Evidence for a Connection?" *Radiation Research*. 151(5), 513–531, 1999.

Rowe, W. "Identification of Risk." In P. Oftedal and A. Brogger (eds.) *Risk and Reasons: Risk Assessment in Relation to Environmental Mutagens and Carcinogens*. New York: Alan R. Liss, 1986, 3–22.

Samet, J. M., and Nero, A. V. "Indoor Radon and Lung Cancer." *New England Journal of Medicine*. 320(9):591–593, 1989.

Selye, H. *The Stress of Life*. New York: McGraw-Hill, 1956.

Siegel, B. S. *Love, Medicine, and Miracles*. New York: Harper and Row, 1986.

United States Department of Health and Human Services, Public Health Service. *Healthy People 2000: National Health Promotion and Disease Prevention Objectives*. Publication 017-001-00474-0, 1990.

United States Department of Health and Human Services, Public Health Services. *Healthy People 2010*. www.dhhs.gov.

Chapter 3: Detecting a Change

Miettinen, O. S., Henschke, C. I., Pasmantier, M. W., et al. "Mammographic Screening: No Reliable Supporting Evidence?" *Lancet.* 359:404–406, 2002.

Olsen, O., and Gotzsche, P. "Cochrane Review on Screening for Breast Cancer with Mammography." *Lancet.* 358: 1340–1342, 2001.

Smith, R., Cokkinides, V., von Eschenbach, A., et al. "American Cancer Society Guidelines for the Early Detection of Cancer." *CA: A Cancer Journal for Clinicians.* 52 (1): 8–22, 2002.

Chapter 4: Diagnosis and Beyond

Benedict, S., Williams, R. D., and Baron P. L. "Recalled Anxiety: From Discovery to Diagnosis of a Benign Breast Mass." *Oncology Nursing Forum.* 21(10):1723-1727, 1994.

Chapter 5: A Woman and Her Doctors

"Cancer Survival Toolbox." Audiotape set. Available from National Coalition for Cancer Survivorship; see Resources.

Chapter 6: The Rest of the Team

Spiegel, D. "Health Caring: Psychosocial Support for Patients with Cancer." *Cancer.* 74(4, Supplement):1453–1457, 1994.

Spiegel, D. "Mind Matters—Group Therapy and Survival in Breast Cancer." *New England Journal of Medicine.* 345 (24):1767–1768, 2001.

Chapter 7: Local Treatments for Cancer

Sitton, E. "Early and Late Radiation-Induced Skin Alterations. Part I: Mechanisms of Skin Changes." *Oncology Nursing Forum.* 19(5):801–807, 1992.

Sitton, E. "Early and Late Radiation-Induced Skin Alterations. Part II: Nursing Care of Irradiated Skin." *Oncology Nursing Forum.* 19(6):907–912, 1992.

Chapter 8: Systemic Treatments for Cancer

Groenwald, S. L., Frogge, M. H., Goodman, M., and Yarbro, C. H. *Cancer Symptom Management.* Sudbury, MA: Jones and Bartlett, 1996.

Mock, V. "Fatigue Management." *Cancer.* 92(6, Supplement):1699–1707, 2001.

Preston, F. A., and Cunningham, R. S. *Clinical Guidelines for Symptom Management in Oncology.* New York, Clinical Insights Press, Inc., 1998.

Winningham, M. L. "Strategies for Managing Cancer-Related Fatigue Syndrome: A Rehabilitation Approach." *Cancer.* 92(4, Supplement):988–997, 2001.

Chapter 9: Complementary and Alternative Therapies for Cancer

Achterberg, J. *Woman as Healer.* Boston: Shambala, 1991.

American College of Sports Medicine Preventive and Rehabilitative Exercise Committee. *Guidelines for Exercise Testing and Prescription*, Fourth Edition. Philadelphia, PA: Lea and Febiger, 1991, 178–180.

Bach, M., and Schleck, L. *ShapeWalking: Six Easy Steps to Your Best Body.* Alameda, CA: Hunter House, 2003.

Burton Goldberg Group. *Alternative Medicine: The Definitive Guide.* Puyallup, WA: Future Medicine Publishing, 1994.

Carlson, R., and Shield, B. *Healers on Healing.* Los Angeles, CA: Jeremy P. Tarcher, 1989.

Cassileth, B. "Alternative and Complementary Therapies." *Cancer.* 77(6), 1996.

Collinge, W. *The American Holistic Health Association Complete Guide to Alternative Medicine.* New York: Warner Books, 1996.

Cousins, N. *Head First: The Biology of Hope.* New York: E. P. Dutton, 1989.

Decker, G. M. (ed.). *An Introduction to Complementary and Alternative Therapies.* Pittsburgh, PA: Oncology Nursing Press, 1999.

Decker, G. M. and Myers, J. "Commonly Used Herbs: Implications for Clinical Practice." *Clinical Journal of Oncology Nursing,* 5(2), pullout insert, 2001.

Dehart, O. W. "Quackery: The Modern Highwayman." Editorial. *Southern Medical Journal.* 85(8):793–794, 1992.

Eisenberg, D. M., et al. "Trends in Alternative Medicine Use in the United States, 1990–1997." *Journal of the American Medical Association,* 280(18):1569–1575, 1998.

Federation of State Medical Boards. "New Model Guidelines for the Use of Complementary and Alternative Therapies in Medical Practice." *Alternative Therapies,* 8(4):44–47, 2002.

Frankl, V. E. *Man's Search for Meaning.* Boston, MA: Beacon Press, 1992.

Geffen, J. R. *The Journey Through Cancer.* New York: Crown Publishers, 2000.

Gordon, J. S., and Curtin, S. *Comprehensive Cancer Care: Integrating Alternative, Complementary, and Conventional Therapies.* Cambridge, MA: Perseus Publishing, 2000.

Harner, M. "The Hidden Universe of the Healer." In R. Carlson and B. Shield (eds.) *Healers on Healing.* Los Angeles: Jeremy P. Tarcher, 1989.

Healy, B. *A New Prescription for Women's Health.* New York: Penguin Books, 1995.

Henig, R. M. "Medicine's New Age." *Civilization.* 4(2):42–49, 1997.

Jacobsen, J. S., and Verret, W. J. "Complementary and Alternative Therapy for Breast Cancer: The Evidence So Far." *Cancer Practice,* 9(6):307–310, 2001.

Kabat-Zinn, J. *Full Catastrophe Living: Using the Wisdom of Your Body and Mind to Face Stress, Pain, and Illness.* New York: Dell, 1990.

Khalsa, D. S., and Stauth, C. *Meditation as Medicine.* New York: Pocket Books, 2001.

Krieger, D. "The Timeless Concept of Healing." In R. Carlson and B. Shield (eds.) *Healers on Healing.* Los Angeles, CA: Jeremy P. Tarcher, 1989.

Labriola, D. *Complementary Cancer Therapies.* Roseville, CA: Prima Health, 2000.

Lane, D. "Music Therapy: A Gift Beyond Measure." *Oncology Nursing Forum.* 19(6):863–867, 1992.

Lane, I. W., and Comac, L. *Sharks Don't Get Cancer.* Garden City, NJ: Avery Books, 1992.

Lane, I. W., and Comac, L. *Sharks Still Don't Get Cancer.* Garden City, NJ: Avery Books, 1996.

Lerman, C., Rimer, B., Blumberg, B., Cristinzio, S., et al. "Effects of Coping Style and Relaxation on Cancer Chemotherapy Side Effects and Emotional Responses." *Cancer Nursing.* 13(5):308–315, 1990.

Lerner, M. *Choices in Healing: Integrating the Best of Conventional and Complementary Approaches to Cancer.* Cambridge, MA: MIT Press, 1996.

Moore, K., and Schmais, L. *Living Well* with *Cancer: A Nurse Tells You Everything You Need to Know About Managing the Side Effects of Your Treatment.* New York: G.P. Putnam's Sons, 2001.

Nessim, S., and Smith, D. S. (eds.). *A Dialogue with Cancer.* Los Angeles, CA: Cancervive, 1996.

O'Connor, A. P., Wicker, C. A., and Germino, B. B. "Understanding the Cancer Patient's Search for Meaning." *Cancer Nursing.* 13(3):167–175, 1990.

Pasquali, E. A. "Learning to Laugh: Humor as Therapy." *Journal of Psychosocial Nursing and Mental Health Services.* 28:31–5, 1990.

Payer, L. *Medicine and Culture: Varieties in Treatment in the United States, England, West Germany, France.* New York: Holt, 1988.

Pert, C. B., Dreher, H. E., and Ruff, M. R. "The Psychosomatic Network: Foundations of Mind-Body Medicine." *Alternative Therapies,* 4(4):30–41, 1998.

Pert, C. B. *Molecules of Emotion: The Science Behind Mond-Body Medicine.* New York: Touchstone, 1997.

Radziewicz, R. M., and Schneider, S. M. "Using Diversional Activity to Enhance Coping." *Cancer Nursing.* 15(4):293–298, 1992.

Sagar, S. M. *Restored Harmony: An Evidence Based Approach for Integrating Traditional Chinese Medicine into Complementary Cancer Care.* Hamilton, Ontario: Dreaming DragonFly Communications, 2001.

Siegel, B. S. *Love, Medicine, and Miracles.* New York: Harper and Row, 1986.

Siegel, B. S. *Peace, Love, and Healing.* New York: Harper and Row, 1989.

Simonton, O., Simonton, S. M., and Creighton, J. *Getting Well Again.* Los Angeles, CA: Jeremy P. Tarcher, 1978.

Vines, S. W. "The Therapeutics of Guided Imagery." *Holistic Nursing Practice.* 2(3):34–44, 1988.

Waitzkin, H. "Information-Giving in Medical Care." *Journal of Health Social Behaviors.* 26:81–101, 1985.

White, J. A. "Touching with Intent: Therapeutic Massage." *Holistic Nursing Practice.* 2(3):63–67, 1988.

Winningham, M. L., and Barton-Burke, M. *Fatigue in Cancer: A Multidimensional Approach.* Boston, MA: Jones and Bartlett Publishers, 2000.

Winningham, M. L. "Walking Program for People with Cancer: Getting Started." *Cancer Nursing.* 14(5):270–276, 1991.

Winningham, M. L., and MacVicar, M. G. "The Effect of Aerobic Exercise on Patient Reports of Nausea." *Oncology Nursing Forum.* 15(4):447–450, 1988.

Chapter 10: Feelings

Glover, J., Dibble, S. L., Dodd, M. J., and Miaskowski, C. "Mood States of Oncology Outpatients: Does Pain Make a Difference?" *Journal of Pain and Symptom Management.* 10(2):120–128, 1995.

Holland, J. C., and Rowland, J. H. (eds.) *Handbook of Psychoncology: Psychological Care of the Patient with Cancer.* New York: Oxford University Press, 1989.

Payne, D. K., Sullivan, M. D., and Massie, M. J. "Women's Psychological Reactions to Breast Cancer." *Seminars in Oncology.* 23(1, Supplement 2):89–97, 1996.

Price, M., Tennant, C., Smith, R., et al. "The Role of Psychosocial Factors in the Development of Breast Carcinoma; Part I: The Cancer Prone Personality." *Cancer.* 91(4):679–685, 2001.

Price, M., Tennant, C., Butow, P., et al. "The Role of Psychosocial Factors in the Development of Breast Carcinoma; Part II: Life Event Stressors, Social Support, Defense Style, and Emotional Control and Their Interactions." *Cancer.* 91(4):686–697, 2001.

Chapter 11: Questions about Breasts

Hoskins, K. F., Stopfer, J. E., Calzone, K. A., Merajver, S. D., Rebbeck, T. R., Garber, J. E., and Weber, B.L. "Assessment and Counseling for Women with a Family History of Breast Cancer: A Guide for Clinicians." *JAMA.* 273(7): 577–85, 1995.

Johnson-Thompson, M. C., and Guthrie, J. "Ongoing Research to Identify Environmental Risk Factors in Breast Carcinoma." *Cancer.* 88(5):1224–1229, 2000.

McGinn, K. A. *The Informed Woman's Guide to Breast Health*, Third Edition. Palo Alto, CA: Bull Publishing, 2001.

Melbye, M., Wohlfahrt, J., Olsen, J., Frisch, M., et al. "Induced Abortion and the Risk of Breast Cancer." *New England Journal of Medicine.* 336(2):81–85, 9 January 1997.

Weiss, S. E., Tartter, P. I., Ahmed, S., et al. "Ethnic Differences in Risk and Prognostic Factors for Breast Cancer." *Cancer.* 76(2):268–274, 1995.

Chapter 12: Detecting and Diagnosing Breast Changes

Neuschatz, A., DiPetrillo, T., Steinhoff, M., et al. "The Value of Breast Lumpectomy Margin Assessment as a Predictor of Residual Tumor Burden in Ductal Carcinoma of the Breast." *Cancer.* 94(7):1917–1924, 2002.

Silverstein, M. J., Lagios, M. D., Craig, P. H., et al. "A Prognostic Index for Ductal Carcinoma in Situ of the Breast." *Cancer.* 77(11):2267–2274, 1996.

Wood, W. C. "Management of Lobular Carcinoma in Situ and Ductal Carcinoma in Situ of the Breast." *Seminars in Oncology.* 23(4):446–452, 1996.

Chapter 13: Treating Invasive Breast Cancer

Antonelli, N. M., Dotters, D. J., Katz, V. L., and Kuller, J. A. "Cancer in Pregnancy: A Review of the Literature. Part 1." *Obstetrical and Gynecological Survey.* 51(2):125–134, 1996.

Baron, R. H. "Dispelling the Myths of Pregnancy-Associated Breast Cancer." *Oncology Nursing Forum.* 21(3):507–512, 1994.

Booser, D. J., and Hortobagyi, G. N. "Treatment of Locally Advanced Breast Cancer." *Seminars in Oncology.* 19(3):278–285, 1992.

Buzdar, A. U., Singletary, S. E., Booser, D. J., Frye, D. K., et al. "Combined Modality Treatment of Stage III and Inflammatory Breast Cancer: M. D.

Anderson Cancer Center Experience." *Surgical Oncology Clinics of North America.* 4(4):715–734, 1995.

Ingle, J. N. "Aromatase Inhibition and Antiestrogen Therapy in Early Breast Cancer Treatment and Chemoprevention." *Oncology.* 15 (5, Supplement 7):28–34, 2001.

Moore, M. P., and Kinne, D. W. "The Surgical Management of Primary Invasive Breast Cancer." *CA: A Cancer Journal for Clinicians.* 45(5):279–288, 1995.

Muss, H. B. "Breast Cancer in Older Women." *Seminars in Oncology.* 23 (1, Supplement 2):82–88, 1996.

NIH Consensus Conference. "Treatment of Early-Stage Breast Cancer." *JAMA.* 263(3):391–395, 1991.

Nixon, A. J., Troyan, S. L., and Harris, J. R. "Options in the Local Management of Invasive Breast Cancer." *Seminars in Oncology.* 23(4):453–463, 1996.

Perez, C. A., Fields, J. N., Fracasso, P. M., Philpott, G., et al. "Management of Locally Advanced Carcinoma of the Breast: II. Inflammatory Carcinoma." *Cancer.* 74(1, Supplement):466–476, 1994.

Perez, C. A., Graham, M. L., Taylor, M. E., Levy, J. F., et al. "Management of Locally Advanced Carcinoma of the Breast: I. Noninflammatory." *Cancer.* 74 (1, Supplement):453–465, 1994.

Petrek, J. A. "Breast Cancer During Pregnancy." *Cancer.* 74(1, Supplement): 518–527, 1994.

Schain, W. S., and Fetting, J. H. "Modified Radical Mastectomy Versus Breast Conservation: Psychosocial Considerations." *Seminars in Oncology.* 19(3): 239–243, 1992.

Schwartz, G., Giulano, A., Veronese, U., et al. "Proceedings of the Consensus Conference on the Role of Sentinal Lymph Node Biopsy in Carcinoma of the Breast, April 19–22, 2001, Philadelphia, Pennsylvania." *Cancer.* 94(10):2542–2551, 2002.

Sledge Jr., G. W. "Implications of the New Biology for Therapy in Breast Cancer." *Seminars in Oncology.* 23(1, Supplement 2):76–81, 1996.

Smith, G., and Henderson, I. C. "New Treatments for Breast Cancer." Seminars in Oncology. 23(4):506–528, 1996.

Stevens, P. E., Dibble, S. L., and Miaskowski, C. "Prevalence, Characteristics, and Impact of Postmastectomy Pain Syndrome: An Investigation of Women's Experiences." *Pain.* 61(1):61–68, 1995.

Chapter 14: Beyond Basic Treatment for Breast Cancer

Bostwick III, J. "Breast Reconstruction After Mastectomy." *CA: A Cancer Journal for Clinicians.* 45(5):289–304, 1995.

Brody, G. S. "Breast Implants, Silicone: Safety and Efficacy." *eMedicine* (Online Journal at www.emedicine.com/plastic/topic500.htm). 3(1):1–25, 28 January 2002.

Bruning, N. *Breast Implants—Everything You Need to Know*, Third Edition. Alameda, CA: Hunter House, 2002.

Buchsel, P. D., and Kapustay, P. M. "Peripheral Stem Cell Transplantation." *Oncology Nursing: Patient Treatment and Support.* 2(2):1–14, 1995.

Carlson, G. W. "Breast Reconstruction: Surgical Options and Patient Selection." *Cancer.* 74(1, Supplement):436–439, 1994.

Haylock, P. J., and Curtiss, C. P. *Cancer Doesn't Have to Hurt: How to Conquer the Pain Caused by Cancer and Cancer Treatment.* Alameda, CA: Hunter House, 1997.

Institute of Medicine. *Safety of Silicone Breast Implants.* Washington, DC: Institute of Medicine National Academy Press, 2000.

Lewis, F. M., and Deal, L. W. "Balancing Our Lives: A Study of the Married Couple's Experience with Breast Cancer Recurrence." *Oncology Nursing Forum.* 22(6):943–953, 1995.

McGinn, K., and Moore, J. "Metastatic Breast Cancer: Understanding Current Management Options." *Oncology Nursing Forum.* 28 (3):507–512, 2001.

Chapter 15: Cancer of the Ovary

Canis, M., et al. "Risk of Spread of Ovarian Cancer after Laparoscopic Surgery." *Current Opinion in Obstetrics and Gynecology.* 31(1):9–14, 2001.

Lynch, H. T., and Casey, M. J. "Current Status of Prophylactic Surgery for Hereditary Breast and Gynecologic Cancers." *Current Opinion in Obstetrics and Gynecology.* 31(1):25–30, 2001.

Menon, U., and Jacobs, I. J. "Ovarian Cancer Screening in the General Population." *Current Opinion in Obstetrics and Gynecology.* 31(1):61–64, 2001.

Morgan, R. J., Copeland, L., Gershenson, D., Locker, G., McIntosh, D., Ozols, R., and Teng, N. "NCCN Ovarian Cancer Practice Guidelines." *Oncology.* 10 (11, Supplement):293–310, 1996.

PDQ: State of the Art Statement on Ovarian Cancer. National Cancer Institute: www.cancer.gov.

Piver, M. S. *Gilda's Disease: Sharing Personal Experiences and a Medical Perspective on Ovarian Cancer.* Amherst, NY: Prometheus Books, 1996.

Qazi, F., and McGuire, W. P. "The Treatment of Epithelial Ovarian Cancer." *CA: Cancer Journal for Clinicians.* 45:88–101, 1995.

Rubin, S. C., Benjamin, I., Behbakht, K., Takahashi, H., Morgan, M. A., et al. "Clinical and Pathological Features of Ovarian Cancer in Women with Germ-line Mutations of BRCA1." *New England Journal of Medicine.* 335(19):1413–1416, 1996.

Strauss, W., and Howe, N. *Generations: The History of America's Future, 1584 to 2069.* New York: William Morrow, 1992.

Teneriello, M. G., and Park, R. C. "Early Detection of Ovarian Cancer." *CA: A Cancer Journal for Clinicians.* 45:71–87, 1995.

U.S. Department of Health and Human Services, Public Health Service, National Institute of Health. *Ovarian Cancer: Screening, Treatment, and Follow-Up.* NIH Consensus Statement. 12(3): 5–7 April 1994.

Venn, A., Watson, L., Lumley, J., Giles, G., King, C., and Healy, D. "Breast and Ovarian Cancer Incidence After Infertility and In Vitro Fertilization." *Lancet.* 346:995–999, 1995.

Whysner, J., and Mohan, M. "Perineal Application of Talc and Cornstarch Powders: Evaluation of Ovarian Cancer Risk." *American Journal of Obstetrics and Gynecology.* 182(3):720–724, 2000.

Chapter 16: Cancer of the Uterus

American Cancer Society. *Cancer Facts and Figures—2002*. Atlanta, GA: 2002.

Bristow, R. E. "Endometrial Cancer." *Current Opinion in Oncology*. 11(5):388, 1999.

DeMello, A. B. "Uterine Artery Embolization." *AORN Journal*. 73(4):809–814, 2001.

DiSaia, P. J., and Creasman, W. T. *Clinical Gynecologic Oncology*, Third Edition. St. Louis, MO: C. V. Mosby, 1989.

Hubbard, J. L., and Holcombe, J. K. "Cancer of the Endometrium." *Seminars in Oncology Nursing*. 6(3):206–213, 1990.

PDQ: State of the Art Statement, Endometrial Cancer. National Cancer Institute, www.cancer.gov.

Sutton, G. P. "The Significance of Positive Peritoneal Cytology in Endometrial Cancer." *Oncology*. 4(6):21–26, 1990.

Chapter 17: Cancer of the Cervix and CIN

Andersen, B. L. "How Cancer Affects Sexual Functioning." *Oncology*. 4(6):81–93, 1990.

DiSaia, P. J., and Creasman, W. T. *Clinical Gynecologic Oncology*, Third Edition. St. Louis, MO: C. V. Mosby, 1989.

Dutton, C. J. "New Technology in Papanicolaou Smear Processing." *Clinical Obstetric and GYN*. 43(2):410–417, 2000.

Gross, A., and Ito, D. *Women Talk About Gynecological Surgery*. New York: HarperCollins, 1991.

Jenkins, B. "Patients' Reports of Sexual Changes After Treatment for Gynecologic Cancer." *Oncology Nursing Forum*. 15(3):349–354, 1988.

Janicek, M. F., and Averette, H. E. "Cervical Cancer: Prevention, Diagnosis and Therapeutics." *CA: A Cancer Journal for Clinicians*. 51(2):92–114, 2001.

Kaufman, R., Adam, E., and Vonka, V. "Human Papillomavirus Infection and Cervical Carcinoma." *Clinical Obstetric and GYN*. 43(2):363–380, 2000.

Nolte, S., and Hanjani, P. "Intraepithelial Neoplasia of the Lower Genital Tract." *Seminars in Oncology Nursing*. 6(3):181–189, 1990.

PDQ: State of the Art Statement: Cervical Cancer. National Cancer Institute, www.cancer.gov.

Pinto, A. P., and Crum, C. P. "Natural History of Cervical Dysplasia: Defining Progression and its Consequence." *Clinical Obstetric and GYN*. 43(2):352–362, 2000.

Sawaya, G. F., et al. "Current Approaches to Cervical-cancer Screening." *New England Journal of Medicine*. 344(21):1603–1607.

Smith, J. M. *Women and Doctors*. New York: Atlantic Monthly Press, 1992.

Yeo, A. S. S., et al. "Serum Micronutrients and Cervical Dysplasia in Southwestern American Indian Women." *Nutrition & Cancer*. 38(2):141–150, 2000.

Chapter 18: Cancer of the Vagina

Braun, M. L. *Still with Us: Research Needs of the DES-Exposed*. Presented to the National Institutes of Health Office of Research on Women's Health. Bethesda, MD: 12 June 1991.

Brooks, S. E., and Wakeley, K. E. "Current Trends in the Management of Carcinoma of the Cervix, Vulva, and Vagina." *Current Opinion in Oncology.* 11(5):383, 1999.

Chamorro, T. "Cancer of the Vulva and Vagina." *Seminars in Oncology Nursing.* 6(3):198–205, 1990.

"DES-Related Cancers Under Renewed Scrutiny." *Journal of the National Cancer Institute.* 84(8):565–566, 15 April 1992.

"DES Consensus Conference." *Journal of the National Cancer Institute.* 84(12):925–926, 17 June 1992.

DiSaia, P. J., and Creasman, W. T. *Clinical Gynecologic Oncology,* Third Edition. St. Louis, MO: C. V. Mosby, 1989.

Greenberg, E. R., Barnes, A. B., Resseguie, L., Barrett, J. A., et al. "Breast Cancer in Mothers Given Diethylstilbestrol in Pregnancy." *New England Journal of Medicine.* 311(22):1393–1398, 1984.

Melnick, S., Cole, P., Anderson, D., et al. "Rates and Risks of Diethylstilbestrol-Related Clear Cell Adenocarcinoma of the Vagina and Cervix: An Update. *New England Journal of Medicine.* 316(514): 1987.

Nolte, S., and Hanjani, P. "Intraepithelial Neoplasia of the Lower Genital Tract." *Seminars in Oncology Nursing.* 6(3):181–189, 1990.

PDQ: Vaginal Cancer: Information for Patients. National Cancer Institute, www.cancer.gov.

PDQ: State of the Art Statement: Vaginal Cancer: Information for Physicians. National Cancer Institute, www.cancer.gov.

Robboy, S. J., Noller, K. L., O'Brien, P., Kaufman, R. H., et al. "Increased Incidence of Cervical and Vaginal Dysplasia in 3,980 Diethylstilbestrol-Exposed Young Women." *Journal of the American Medical Association.* 252(21):2979–2983, 1984.

Smith, O. W., and Smith, G. V. S. "Diethylstilbestrol and Treatment of Complications of Pregnancy." *American Journal of Obstetrics and Gynecology.* 58:821–834, 1948.

Smith, J. *Women and Doctors.* New York: Atlantic Monthly Press, 1992.

Chapter 19: Cancer of the Vulva

Andersen, B. L., and Hacker, N. F. "Psychosexual Adjustment After Vulvar Surgery." *Obstetrics and Gynecology.* 62:459, 1983.

Brooks, S. E., and Wakeley, K. E. "Current Trends in the Management of Carcinoma of the Cervix, Vulva, and Vagina." *Current Opinion in Oncology.* 11(5):383, 1999.

Chamorro, T. "Cancer of the Vulva and Vagina." *Seminars in Oncology Nursing.* 6(3):198–205, 1990.

DiSaia, P. J. "Current Treatment of Small Vulvar Cancers. The Article Reviewed." *Oncology.* 4(8):26–28, 1990.

DiSaia, P. J., and Creasman, W. T. *Clinical Gynecologic Oncology.* St. Louis, MO: C. V. Mosby, 1989.

Grendys, E. C., and Fiorica, J. V. "Innovations in the Management of Vulvar Carcinoma." *Current Opinion in Obstetrics and Gynecology.* 12(1):15–20, 2000.

Hacker, N. F. "Current Treatment of Small Vulvar Cancers." *Oncology.* 4(8):21–25, 1990.

Homesley, H. D. "Current Treatment of Small Vulvar Cancers. The Article Reviewed." *Oncology*. 4(8):33, 1990.

Lamb, M. "Vulvar Cancer: Patient Information Booklet." *Oncology Nursing Forum*. 31(6):79–82, 1986.

Nolte, S., and Hanjani, P. "Intraepithelial Neoplasia of the Lower Genital Tract." *Seminars in Oncology Nursing*. 6(3):181–189, 1990.

PDQ: State of the Art Statement: Vulvar Cancer. National Cancer Institute, www.cancer.gov.

Phillips, G. L. "Current Management of Vulvar Melanoma." *Oncology*. 4(9):61–64, 1990.

Sandella, J. "Vulvar Self-Examination." *Oncology Nursing Forum*. 14(6):71–73, 1987.

Thiadens, S. R. J. *Lymphedema: An Information Booklet*. San Francisco, CA: National Lymphedema Network.

Chapter 21: Lung Cancer

Carney, D. N., and Hansen, H. H. "Non-small-cell Lung Cancer—Stalemate or Progress?" *New England Journal of Medicine*. 343(17):1261–2, 2000.

Fiore, M. C., Wetter, D. W., Bailey, W. C., et al. *Smoking Cessation Clinical Practice Guideline*. Rockville, MD: Agency for Health Care Policy and Research, Public Health Services, U.S. Dept. of Health and Human Services, 1996.

Keller, S. M., et al. "A Randomized Trial of Postoperative Adjuvant Therapy in Patients with Completely Resected Stage II or IIIA Non-small-cell Lung Cancer." *New England Journal of Medicine*. 343(17):1217–1222.

Patz, E. F., Goodman, P. C., and Bepler, G. "Screening for Lung Cancer." *New England Journal of Medicine*. 343(22):1627–1633.

PDQ. State of the Art Statement: Non-small cell lung cancer. National Cancer Institute, www.cancer.gov.

Petty, T. L., and Rollins, D. R. "A Critical look at Lung Cancer." *The Clinical Advisor*. February 2002.

Pieterman, R.M., et al. "Preoperative Staging of Non-small-cell Lung Cancer with Positron-emission Tomography." *The New England Journal of Medicine*. 343(4):254–261, 2000.

Chapter 23: Long-term and Late Effects

Carroll-Johnson, R. M., Gorman, L. M., and Bosh, N. J. (eds). *Psychosocial Nursing Care: Along the Cancer Continuum*. Pittsburgh, PA: Oncology Nursing Press, 1998.

Ganz, P. A. "Late Effects of Cancer and Its Treatment." *Seminars in Oncology Nursing*. 17(4):241–248, 2001.

Harpham, W. S. "Long-Term Survivorship: Late Effects." (In) Berger, A., et al (eds). *Principles and Practice of Supportive Oncology*. Philadelphia, PA: Lippincott-Raven Publishers, 1998, 889–907.

Leigh, S. A. "The Long-Term Cancer Survivor: A Challenge for Nurse Practitioners." *Nurse Practitioner Forum*. 9(3):192–196, 1998.

Mahon, S. M., Williams, M. T., and Spies, M. A. "Screening for Second Cancers and Osteoporosis in Long-Term Survivors." *Cancer Practice*. 8(6):282–290, 2000.

Mincey, B. A., Moraghan, T. J., and Perez, E. A. "Prevention and Treatment of Osteoporosis in Women with Breast Cancer." *Mayo Clinic Proceedings.* 75(8):821–829, 2000.

Nessim, S., and Ellis, J. *Cancervive: The Challenge of Life after Cancer.* Boston, MA: Houghton Mifflin Co., 2000.

Spingarn, N. D. *The New Cancer Survivors: Living with Grace, Fighting with Spirit.* Baltimore, MD: Johns Hopkins University Press, 1999.

Thaler-DeMers, D. "Sexuality, Fertility Issues, and Cancer." *Illness, Crisis & Loss.* 10(1):27–41, 2002.

Vachon, M. L. S. "The Meaning of Illness to a Long-Term Survivor." *Seminars in Oncology Nursing.* 17(4):279–283, 2001.

Chapter 24: Feelings after Treatment Ends

American Cancer Society. *Surviving Cancer: Proceedings of the Sixth National Conference on Cancer Nursing.* ACS Publication No. 4503.07. 1992.

Dow, K. H. "A Review of Late Effects of Cancer in Women." *Seminars in Oncology Nursing.* 11(2):128–136, 1995.

Welch-McCaffrey, D., Hoffman, B., Leigh, S., Loescher, L., and Meyskens, F. L. "Surviving Adult Cancers, Part 2: Psychosocial Implications." *Annals of Internal Medicine.* 111(6):517–524, 1989.

Chapter 25: After Treatment Ends: The Other Issues

Bachmann, G. A. "Nonhormonal Alternatives for the Management of Early Menopause in Young Women with Breast Cancer." *Journal of the National Cancer Institute/Monographs.* 16:161–167, 1994.

Barton, D., La Vasseur, B., Loprinzi, C., et al. "Venlafaxine for the Control of Hot Flashes: Results of a Longitudinal Continuation Study." *Oncology Nursing Forum.* 29(1):33–39, 2002.

Cohen, S. R., Payne, D. K., and Tunkel, R. S. "Lymphedema: Strategies for Management." *Cancer.* 92(4, supplement):980–987, 2001.

Dow, K. H. "A Review of Late Effects of Cancer in Women." *Seminars in Oncology Nursing.* 11(2):128–136, 1995.

Kalinowski, B. "Lymphedema." In S. Groenwald, M. Frogge, M. Goodman, and C. Yarbro (eds.) *Cancer Symptom Management.* Sudbury, MA: Jones and Bartlett, 1996, 433–463.

Kaplan, H. S. "The Neglected Issue: The Sexual Side Effects of Current Treatments for Breast Cancer." *Journal of Sex and Marital Therapy.* 18(1):3–19, 1992.

McKee, A. L., and Schover, L. R. "Sexuality Rehabilitation." *Cancer.* 92 (4, supplement):1008–1012, 2001.

Mellette, S. J. "The Cancer Patient at Work." *CA: A Cancer Journal for Clinicians.* 35(6):360–373, 1985.

Soffa, V. M. "Alternatives to Hormone Replacement for Menopause." *Alternative Therapies.* 2(2):34–39, 1996.

Young-McCaughan, S. "Sexual Functioning in Women with Breast Cancer After Treatment with Adjuvant Therapy." *Cancer Nursing.* 19(4):308–319, 1996.

Chapter 26: Cancer Is Still a Political Issue

Brady, J. *1 in 3: Women with Cancer Confront an Epidemic.* Pittsburgh, PA: Cleis Press, 1991.

Kasper, A. S., and Ferguson, S. J. *Breast Cancer: Society Shapes an Epidemic.* New York: St. Martin's Press, 2000.

Moss, R. W. *The Cancer Industry.* Brooklyn, NY: Equinox Press, 1996.

Pulcini, J. A., Neary, S. R., and Mahoney, D. F. "Health Care Financing." In Mason, D. J., Leavitt, J. K., and Chaffee, M. W. (eds.) *Policy and Politics in Nursing and Health Care,* Fourth Edition. Philadelphia, PA: Saunders, 2002, 241–297.

Stocker, M. (ed.). *Cancer as a Women's Issue.* Chicago, IL: Third Side Press, 1991.

White, L. C. *Merchants of Death: The American Tobacco Industry.* New York: Beech Tree Books, 1988.

RESOURCES

The following resources are some of the more helpful information sources available. Included are Internet sites, books and pamphlets, and information and support organizations. This is by no means a complete listing; any "browser" program will find other addresses. These were accessed in March 2002 and were accurate and available at that time:

COMPUTER RESOURCES (WEBSITES)

The **Internet** primarily provides information, although encouraging stories from cancer survivors and other resources are also available. The Internet requires a computer, modem, phone line, and Internet access software.

General

National Cancer Institute
www.cancer.gov (basic NCI website)
http://cis.nci.nih.gov (Cancer Information Service)
www3.cancer.gov/cancercenters/centerslist.html (list of cancer centers)
www/survivorship.cancer.gov (Office of Cancer Survivorship)

American Cancer Society
www.cancer.org (general and Cancer Survivors' Network)

OncoLink
http://oncolink.upenn.edu (many topics and links)

CancerBACUP (British cancer information resource)
www.bacup.org (many topics)

Association of Cancer Online Resources
www.acor.org

National Coalition for Cancer Survivorship
www.canceradvocacy.org (many topics; programs link to order *Cancer Survivor's Toolbox*)

Healthfinder
www.healthfinder.org (a general health website with good cancer information)

Drug cost assistance
www.cancersupportivecare.com/drug_assistance.html
www.accc-cancer.org/publications/hotlines.asp

Physician Data Query
www.cancer.gov

Finding an oncologist
www.asco.org ("find an oncologist" link)

Imaging studies
www.pinnacleimaging.com/procedures

Increased genetic risk
http://bcresources.med.unc.edu/genetic.htm
www.facingourrisk.org

Insurance coverage
www.accc-cancer.org/publications/patientbrochure.asp (online pamphlet: *Cancer Treatments Your Insurance Should Cover*)
www.hcfa.gov (information on Health Insurance Portability and Affordability Act, HIPAA)

Lymphedema
www.lymphnet.org

Medicines in clinical trials
www.phrma.org/searchcures/newmeds/webdb

Menopause
http://project-aware.org
www.power-surge.com

Pain
www.cancer-pain.org

Telling children
www.bacup.org/info/child/child-1.htm (online pamphlet)

Breast Cancer

National Alliance of Breast Cancer Organizations (NABCO)
www.nabco.org

National Breast Cancer Coalition
www.natlbcc.org (breast cancer activism)

Breast Cancer Org
www.breastcancer.org (up-to-date coverage on many topics)

Miscellaneous Sites
    Breast implants:
    www.fda.gov/cdrh/breastimplants
    STAR clinical trial:
    www.pinnacleimaging.com/breasthealth/star

Y-ME National Breast Cancer Organization
www.y-me.org/

Alternative/Complementary Therapies

Office of Cancer Complementary and Alternative Medicine
www.cancer.gov/occam

Dr. Andrew Weil/Santel Alternative Medicine Links
www.santel.lu/SANTEL/altmed.altmed.html

Dr. Bower's Complementary and Alternative Medicine Homepage
http://galen.med.virginia.edu/~pjb3s/Complementary HomePage.html

BOOKS AND PUBLICATIONS

This is a very limited list. Many free booklets are available from the Cancer Information Service of the National Cancer Institute (800-4-CANCER) and the American Cancer Society (800-ACS-2345) and are not listed here; some of them can also be read online on the organizations' websites. Some favorite books have gone out of print and we hope they will return to this list later.

General Cancer Information

Case, M., and Van Dernoot, P. *Helping Your Children Cope with Your Cancer: A Guide for Parents.* Long Island City, NY: Hatherleigh, 2002.

CURE: Cancer Updates, Research and Education. A magazine for patients and their caregivers. Individual subscription $20 (USA). Subscription information: CURE Editorial Office—phone: (214) 820-7126 or editor@curetoday.com. Or, website: www.curetoday.com.

Dollinger, M., Rosenbaum, E., and Cable, G. *Everyone's Guide to Cancer Therapy,* Fourth Edition. Kansas City, MO: Andrews and McMeel, 2002.

Facing Forward Series. *Life After Cancer Treatment.* U.S. Department of Health and Human Services, National Institutes of Health, National Cancer Institute. NCI Publication No. 02-2424, 2002.

Harpham, W. S. *After Cancer: A Guide to Your New Life.* New York: Harper Perennial, 1995.

Harpham, W. S. *Diagnosis Cancer: Your Guide Through the First Few Months,* Second Edition. New York: W. W. Norton, 1997.

Harpham, W. S. *When a Parent Has Cancer: A Guide to Caring for Your Children.* New York: HarperCollins Publishers, 1997.

Haylock, P. J., and Curtiss, C. P. *Cancer Doesn't Have to Hurt.* Alameda, CA: Hunter House, 1997.

Kushner, H. *When Bad Things Happen to Good People.* New York: Avon, 1997.

Lerner, M. *Choices in Healing.* Cambridge, MA: MIT, 1994.

Love, S., and Lindsey, K. *Dr. Susan Love's Hormone Book: Making Informed Choices about Menopause.* New York: Random House, 1997.

Morra, M., and Potts, E. *Choices: The New, Most Up-to-date Sourcebook for Cancer Information.* New York: Avon Books, 1994.

Surviving: A Cancer Patient Magazine. ($15/6 issues/year) c/o Stanford Health Care, Department of Radiation Oncology, Division of Radiation Therapy, Room A035, 300 Pasteur Drive, Stanford CA 94305.

Breast Health and Breast Cancer

American Cancer Society. *A Breast Cancer Journey: Your Personal Guidebook.* American Cancer Society, Atlanta, GA: 2001.

Bruning, N. *Breast Implants: Everything You Need to Know,* Third Edition. Alameda, CA: Hunter House, 2002.

Burt, J., and White, G. *Lymphedema: A Breast Cancer Patient's Guide to Prevention and Healing.* Alameda, CA: Hunter House, 1999.

Kahane, D. H. *No Less A Woman: Femininity, Sexuality & Breast Cancer,* Second Edition. Alameda, CA: Hunter House, 1995.

Kelly, P. T. *Assess Your True Risk of Breast Cancer.* New York: Owl Books, 2000.

Link, J. *The Breast Cancer Survival Manual: A Step-By-Step Guide for the Woman With Newly Diagnosed Cancer,* Second Edition. New York: Owl Books, 2000.

Love, S., and Lindsey, K. *Dr. Susan Love's Breast Book,* Third Edition. Cambridge, MA: Perseus, 2000.

Mayer, M., and Lamb, L. *Advanced Breast Cancer: A Guide to Living with Metastatic Disease,* Second Edition. Sebastopol, CA: Patient-Centered Guides, 1998

McGinn, K. A. *The Informed Woman's Guide to Breast Health*, Third Edition. Palo Alto, CA: Bull Publishing, 2001.

Stumm, D. *Recovering from Breast Surgery: Exercises to Strengthen Your Body and Relieve Pain.* Alameda, CA: Hunter House, 1995.

Tagliaferri, M., Cohen, I., and Tripathy, D. *Breast Cancer, Beyond Convention: The World's Foremost Authorities on Complementary and Alternative Medicine Offer Advice on Healing.* New York: Atria Books, 2002.

Weiss, M. C., and Weiss, E. *Living Beyond Breast Cancer: A Survivor's Guide for When Treatment Ends and the Rest of Your Life Begins.* New York: Times Books, 1998.

Cancer Therapies

Bruning, N. *Coping with Chemotherapy,* Revised Edition. New York: Avery Penguin Putnam, 2002.

Graham, ___, and Loner, ___. *Something's Got to Taste Good.* _____: Andrews & McMeel, 1981.

Handbook of Oncology Nutrition. Oncology Nutrition Dietetic Practice Group of the American Dietetic Association, 1999.

McKay, J., and Hirano, N., *The Chemotherapy & Radiation Therapy Survival Guide,* Second Edition. Oakland, CA: New Harbinger Publications, 1998.

Complementary and Alternative Therapies

Decker, G. M. (ed). *An Introduction to Complementary and Alternative Therapies.* Pittsburgh, PA: Oncology Nursing Press, 1999.

Gordon, J. S., and Curtin, S. *Comprehensive Cancer Care: Integrating Alternative, Complementary, and Conventional Therapies.* Cambridge, MA: Perseus Publishing, 2000.

Hammerschlag, C. A., and Silverman, H. D. *Healing Ceremonies: Creating Personal Rituals for Spiritual, Emotional, Physical and Mental Health.* New York: Berkley Publishing Group, 1997.

Khalsa, D.S., and Stauth, C. *Meditation as Medicine: Activate the Power of Your Natural Healing Force.* New York: Pocket Books, 2001.

Labriola, D. *Complementary Cancer Therapies: Combining Traditional and Alternative Approaches for the Best Possible Outcome.* Roseville, CA: Prima Health, 2000.

Moore, K., and Schmais, L. *Living Well with Cancer: A Nurse Tells You Everything You Need to Know About Managing the Side Effects of Your Treatment.* New York: G.P. Putnam's Sons, 2001.

Sagar, S. M. *Restored Harmony: An Evidence Based Approach for Integrating Traditional Chinese Medicine into Complementary Cancer Care.* Hamilton, Ontario: Dreaming DragonFly Communications, 2001.

Feelings and Relationships

Kushner, H. S. *When Bad Things Happen to Good People.* New York: Avon, 1997.

Surviving!: A Cancer Patient Newsletter. (6 times/year) c/o Stanford University Hospital, Department of Radiation Oncology, Division of Radiation Therapy, Room A035, 300 Pasteur Drive, Stanford, CA 94305.

Taking Time: Support Groups for People With Cancer and the People Who Care About Them (booklet). NIH Publication No. 88-2059. National Cancer Institute, 1996. (Available free from CIS)

Unconventional Cancer Therapies. Washington, D.C.: U.S. Government.

When Someone in Your Family Has Cancer. NIH Publication No.90-2685. National Cancer Institute, 1995. (For children; available free from CIS)

Survivorship and Practical Issues

Calder, K. J., and Pollitz, K. *What Cancer Survivors Need to Know About Health Insurance.* Silver Spring, MD, National Coalition for Cancer Survivorship, 1998.

Cancer Treatments Your Insurance Should Cover (pamphlet). Available as a download from the Association of Community Cancer Centers, www.accc-cancer.org.

Hoffman, B. (Ed.) *A Cancer Survivor's Almanac: Charting Your Journey.* National Coalition for Cancer Survivorship. Minneapolis, MN: Chronimed Publishing, 1996, 2003.

Klesges, R., and DeBon, M. *How Women Can Finally Stop Smoking.* Alameda, CA: Hunter House, 1994.

Mullan, B. D., and McGinn, K. A. *The Ostomy Book.* Palo Alto, CA: Bull Publishing, 1992.

Nessim, S., and Ellis, J. *Can Survive: The Challenge of Life after Cancer.* New York: Houghton Mifflin Co., 2000.

Ojeda, L. *Menopause Without Medicine*, Fourth Edition. Alameda, CA: Hunter House, 2000.

White, C. A. *Positive Options for Living with Your Ostomy.* Alameda, CA: Hunter House, 2002.

INFORMATION AND SUPPORT ORGANIZATIONS

American Cancer Society
1599 Clifton Rd. N.E.
Atlanta GA 30329   (800) ACS-2345
Website: www.cancer.org
Information and publications; local units also listed in phone book: Reach to
    Recovery; I Can Cope; Look Good, Feel Better, etc.

American Society of Plastic and Reconstructive Surgeons
(800) 635-0635
Names of local reconstructive surgeons, breast reconstruction brochures

Breast Cancer Action
55 New Montgomery, Ste 624   (877) 278-6722
San Francisco CA 94105   (415) 243-9301
Website: www.bcaction.org
San Francisco-based group; political activism, newsletter

Cancer Information Service (CIS)
(800) 4-CANCER (422-6237)
Website: www.cancer.gov
Service of National Cancer Institute: information over phone or mailed

Cancervive
(800) 4 TO CURE   (310) 203-9232
Survivorship information, some support groups

The Commonweal Cancer Help Program
PO Box 316
Bolinas CA 94924   (415) 868-0970
Website: www.commonweal.org
Bolinas, California,–based; family consulting, children's program, other projects

Conversations
(806) 355-2565
Ovarian cancer information clearinghouse, newsletter, support

DES Action
1615 Broadway #510
Oakland CA 94612   (510) 465-4011
Information and support for people with DES-related cancers

DES Cancer Network
514 10th St., NW, Ste. 400   (800) DES-NET4 (334-6384)
Washington DC 20004-1403   (202) 628-6330
Fax: (202) 628-6217
E-mail: desnetwrk@aol.com   Website: www.descancer.org

ENCOREplus
(800) 95-EPLUS

YWCA of USA, Office of Women's Health Initiatives
624 9th St. N.W., 3rd Fl.
Washington DC 20001-5303
Local groups, exercise programs, etc., for women with breast cancer
Food and Drug Administration (FDA)

FDA/CDRH, HFZ-210
5600 Fishers Ln.
Rockville MD 20857   (800) 532-4440
Current breast implant information

Gilda Radner Familial Ovarian Cancer Registry
(800) 682-7426

Susan B. Komen Breast Cancer Foundation
(800) IM AWARE (462-9273)
Website: www.komen.org
Breast cancer information; sponsors "Race for the Cure"

League of Women Voters
1730 M St. N.W.
Washington DC 20036   (202) 429-1965
Website: www.lwv.org
Annual resource guide, fact sheets, newsletter

National Alliance of Breast Cancer Organizations (NABCO)
9 E. 37th St., 10th Fl.
New York NY 10016   (888) 80-NABCO (806-2226)
Annual resource guide, fact sheets, newsletter

National Breast Cancer Coalition
1707 L St. N.W.
Washington DC 20036   (202) 296-7477
Political activism clearinghouse

National Coalition for Cancer Survivorship
1010 Wayne Ave., 5th Fl.
Silver Spring MD 20910 (301) 565-9670
Website: www.canceradvocacy.org
Newsletter, conferences, insurance and employment discrimination information
    and resources

National Lymphedema Network
Latham Sq. 1611 Telegraph Ave., Ste. 1111
Oakland CA 94612-2138
Hotline: (800) 541-3259 (510) 208-3200
Fax: (510) 208-3110
Website: www.lymphnet.org
Information clearinghouse, newsletter, annual conference

National Women's Health Network
514 10th St. N.W., Ste. 400
Washington DC 20004   (202) 347-1140

National Women's Health Resource Center
2425 L St. N.W., 3rd Fl.
Washington DC 20037   (202) 293-6045
Newsletter, literature searches, silicone-implant information

Oncology Nursing Society
125 Enterprise Dr.
Pittsburgh PA 15275-1214
(866) 257-4ONS (257-4667)
(412) 859-6100

Physician Data Query (PDQ)
Fax: (301) 402-5874
Website: www.cancer.gov

Society of Gynecologic Oncology
401 North Michigan Ave.
Chicago IL 60611   (800) 444-4441
Website: www.sgo.org
SGO website hosts Women's Cancer Network to inform women about gynecologic
    cancers

United Ostomy Association
(800) 826-9262
Information, support groups, newsletter, conferences

Wellness Community
2716 Ocean Park Blvd., Ste. 1040
Santa Monica CA 90405 (310) 314-2555
Local support groups and activities, all cancers

Western Union
(800) 325-6000
Public opinion message service

Y-ME Breast Cancer Hotline
212 W. Van Buren
Chicago IL 60607   (800) 221-2141
Support, education, some local chapters newsletter, some local chapters

INDEX

A

Achterberg, Jeanne, 156
acupressure, 127–128
acupuncture, 113, 128
adenocarcinomas, 61, 346, 373, 412
adenomatous polyposis coli (APC), 402
Adriamycin, 115
African American teens and smoking, 376
African Americans and cancer, 28–29, 203, 403, 471
age and cancer, 8, 27–28; breast cancer, 191; cervical cancer, 319; colorectal cancer, 403; ovarian cancer, 273, 276; uterine cancer, 302–303
AIDS, 10, 26, 123, 150, 151
alcohol, 16, 199, 403
alendronate sodium (Fosamax), 460
alkylating agents, 101–102
alopecia, 109–111
altretamine, 296
American Association for Cancer Research, 405
American Association of Sex Educators, Counselors and Therapists, 339
American Board of Genetic Counselors, 32
American Cancer Society (ACS), 21, 28, 46, 69, 82; and breast self-examination, 211, 212; *Cancer: Your Job, Insurance and the Law*, 462; and colorectal cancer screening, 406; and dietary recommendations, 132, 199, 208; and financial resources for cancer treatment, 119; *For the Woman Who Has Cancer and Her Partner*, 339; "I Can Cope", 82; "Look Good, Feel Better", 111, 184; National Task Force on Breast Cancer Control, 205; "Reach to Recovery", 80, 252, 253, 434; Tender Loving Care, 110; We Can Weekend, 149, 165
American Gastroenterological Association (AGA): 409–410
American Heart Association, 132
American Hospital Association, 85
American Journal of Obstetrics and Gynecology, 348
American Medical Directory, 70
American Music Therapy Association, 148
American Society of Clinical Oncology, 32, 69, 70
Americans with Disabilities Act, 462
amniography, 368
amphetamines, 27
anastrozole (Arimidex), 242
andro-estrogens, 17

anemia, 109
anger, 177–178, 439–441
angiogenesis, 12–13
anti-oncogene, 8–9, 192
antiangiogenesis, 163, 247
antibiotics, antitumor, 102
antidepressant medication, 177, 178, 459
antimetabolites, 101
antinausea medications, 112–113
antineoplastons, 157–158
antioxidants, 199, 375
anus, cancer of. *See* colorectal cancer
anxiety, 175–177
areola, 188, 259–260
arm mobility, regaining, 251–252
aromatase inhibitors, 242
aromatic amines, 21
arsenic, 21, 27
art therapy, 149
artery–vein system, 12
ascites, 276
Ashkenazi Jews and cancer, 193, 418
Asian women and cancer, 28, 203
aspergillus, 26
aspirin, 405
assertiveness, 183
Association of Genetic Nurses and Counselors (AGNC), 32
Association of Oncology Social Work, 73
axilla (armpit), 188
axillary surgery, 232–234

B

bacille Calmette-Guerin, 131
Bellergal, 459
Berkman, Sue, 479
Big Sky Cancer Recovery and Resource Center, 166–167
biological therapies, 14, 116–117, 296; for breast cancer, 246–247; for colorectal cancer, 418–419
biopsy, 51–60; breast, 195; complications from, 59; cone, 57; core, 53; feelings about, 59–60; fine needle aspiration (FNA), 52–53; Mammotome, 53; needle localization, 59; open, 57–59; punch, 55; stereotactic guided needle, 53–54
birth control pills. *See* contraceptives: oral
bladder cancer, 21

Block, Keith, 131–132
Bloomberg, Michael, 474
bone marrow, 107–109
brachytherapy, 97–98, 330
Brady, Judith, 482
Breast and Cervical Cancer Prevention and Treatment Act, 471
breast cancer, 186–208; biological therapies, 246–247; biopsy types, 51–60; and birth control pills, 196; and breastfeeding, 248–249; chemotherapy, 243–246; and childbearing, 195–196; detection, 209–219; diagnosis, 219–227; and diet, 198–199; and environmental factors, 200–201; family history, 30, 192–195; follow-up, 260–262; genetic factors, 30; hormonal therapy, 116, 241–243; and hormone replacement therapy, 196; inflammatory, 249–250; and lifestyle, 199–200; local treatments, 229–240; locally advanced, 249–250; and menstrual cycles, 195; metastasis, 263–265; and pregnancy, 247–248; prevention, 201–202; radiation therapy, 239–240; recovery, 251–260; recurrence, 262–265; risk factors, 191–201, 203–204; staging, 237; surgery, 229–240, 238–239; systemic treatment, 240–247; tests, 223; types, 222
Breast Cancer Prevention Trial (BCPT), 201
breast examination, professional, 219; self (BSE), 210–218, 262
breast implants, 200, 255–260; history of, 257–258
Breast Implants: Everything You Need to Know (Bruning), 260
breast prosthesis, 253–254
breast reconstruction, 254–255
breastfeeding, 191; and breast cancer, 248–249; and mammograms, 47; and ovarian cancer, 277
breasts: function of, 190–191; nonproliferative breast changes, 205; pain, 207–208; professional examination, 219; self-examination, 210–218; structure, 188–191
Bruning, Nancy, 260
Buchholz, William M., 436
Burt, Jeannie, 457
Burton, Lawrence, 161
Burzynski, Stanislaw, 157

C

Caisse, Rene, 144
calcifications, 43

calcium and colorectal cancer, 404–405
camptothecins, 297
Cancell, 159
cancer: alternative treatment, 120–170; causes, 15–36; classification of, 62–63; costs of treatment, 118–119; definition, 4; detection, 37–50; diagnosis, 51–65, 60–61; feelings about, 171–184, 432–446; grading, 37, 61, 63–64; growth, 11–14; hereditary factors, 30–31; infiltrating, 6; invasive, 6; local treatment, 86–98; long-term effects, 422–431; metastasis, 8; policy, 476–477; post-treatment issues, 447–465; prevention, 16; prognosis, 38, 64–65; research, 475–476; risk analysis, 31–36; staging, 37, 61–62; systemic treatment, 13–14, 99–119
Cancer and HIV Clinical Nutrition Pocket Guide (Wilkes), 396–397
cancer cells, 5-6; aneuploid, 63; diploid, 63; and radiation therapy, 93–94
Cancer Doesn't Have to Hurt (Haylock and Curtiss), 176, 265
Cancer Family Syndrome, 402
Cancer Information Service, 69, 79, 80, 82, 114, 194, 297
Cancer Survival Toolbox, The, 73, 119
Cancer Survivor's Almanac: Charting Your Journey, A (Ganz), 423
Cancer Treatments Your Insurance Should Cover, 119, 121
cancers. See listing for the specific type of cancer
Cantron, 159
capecitabine (Xeloda), 264, 417
capsular contracture, 256
carboplatin, 288, 296, 393
carcinogens, 8, 373–374
carcinoma in situ, 6, 221–227; cervical, 325–326; duct carcinoma in situ, 224–226, 232; Paget's disease of the nipple, 227, 249; vaginal, 342–344
carcinomas, 61; invasive, 6; non–small cell lung carcinoma (NSCLC), 383–384, 390–391; small cell lung carcinoma (SCLC), 383, 389–390
cardiac toxicity, 423
Casting for Recovery, 165
CAT scan. See computerized tomography
cell culture drug resistance testing, 101
cells, benign, 4; dysplasia, 6; granulosa, 274; growth, 5; hyperplasia, 5; Leydig, 274; malignant, 4; neoplasia, 5; Sertoli, 274; theca, 274;

trophoblastic, 161; tumor, 5. *See also* red blood cells; white blood cells
cellular treatments, 161
Centers for Disease Control, 196
cervical intraepithelial neoplasia (CIN), 40, 317–324; diagnosis, 321–323; risk factors, 319–320; treatment, 323–325
cervix, cancer of, 316–340; diagnosis, 27–28, 321–323; prevention, 320–321; recurrence, 332–333; risk factors, 27–28, 319–320; staging, 327–328; treatment, 328–339; types, 326
cervix, structure of, 317
chakra system, 128, 153
chaparral tea, 133, 144
chemoprevention, 16, 18–19
chemosensitivity assays, 101, 239
chemotherapy, 13, 99–115; adjuvant, 100, 243; for breast cancer, 243–246; for cervical cancer, 333; for colorectal cancer, 416–417; drug classifications, 101–102; and insurance coverage, 469–470; intra-arterial, 104; intraperitoneal, 104; for lung cancer, 393–394; neo-adjuvant therapy, 245; receiving, 103–105; routes, 104; side effects, 104–115, 245–246
Chernobyl, 22
childbearing, 452–454; and breast cancer, 247–248
children's reaction to cancer, 444
Chinese medicine, 127–128, 133
Chinese populations and cancer, 29
chorioadenoma destruens, 369
choriocarcinoma (GTN), 369–370
cisplatin, 287, 296, 393
Citizen's Guide to Radon, A, 22
Civilization, 123, 169
Clinical Gynecologic Oncology (DiSaia and Creasman), 335
clinical trials, 76, 117–118; in uterine cancer, 308–309
clonidine (Catapres), 459
coal tar, 27
Coenzyme Q_{10}, 158–159
cold cap, 110–111
colitis, chronic ulcerative, 402
College of American Pathologists, 205
colonoscopy, 409–410, 418
colorectal cancer, 400–419; diagnosis, 412–413; prevention, 404–405; recurrence, 418; risk factors, 400–404; screening for, 406–411;

staging, 412; symptoms, 411–412; treatment, 413–419
colostomy, 415
colostrum, 190
colposcopy, 321
comedo DCIS, 224
Commonweal, 165
Community Clinical Oncology Program (CCOP), 118
complementary and alternative therapies, 120–170; acupuncture, 127–128; dietary, 128–132; effectiveness, 167–169; herbal, 132–146; pharmacological agents, 157–164; physical, 149–154; psychological, 146–149; spirituality, 154–157
complexion changes, 111
computer-based technologies, 473–474
computerized thermal imaging (CTI), 50
computerized tomography (CAT), 48–49, 285, 286, 327
condyloma, 354
conization, 57, 322–323, 329
constipation, 114
contraceptives, barrier-type, 321; oral, 196, 277
control, regaining, 172–173, 182–183
Cooper's ligaments, 188
Coping, 173
coping strategies, 175–179. *See also* counseling, exercise, spirituality
core biopsy, 53
coronary artery disease, 423
Cosmetic, Toiletry and Fragrance Association Foundation, 111
costs of cancer care, 467–468
counseling, 77, 79, 174, 434
Couric, Katie, 418
Cousins, Norman, 148
Creasman, William T., 335
Crocinic Acid, 159
Crohn's disease, 402
cryosurgery, 324, 417
curette, 56
Curtiss, Carol, 176, 265
cyclophosphamide (Cytoxan), 110, 115, 244, 288, 393, 453; for breast cancer, 110, 244, 453; for lung cancer, 393; for ovarian cancer, 288; side effects, 115, 245
cysts, 53–54, 207
cytology, 39
cytotechnologist, 39–40

D

dehydration, 113
denial, 171–172
depression, 174, 178–179
DES. *See* diethylstilbestrol
DES Action, 82, 352, 434
DES Cancer Network, 349, 352
DES Registry, 349
dexrazoxane (Zinecard), 115, 245
Diamond, Susan, 173, 174
diarrhea, 114
dietary risk factors, 17, 21
Dietary Supplement Health and Education Act, 133
dietary therapy, 128–132
diethylstilbestrol (DES), 27, 198, 311; and vaginal cancer, 342, 348–353
digital rectal examination (DRE), 406–407
dilatation and curettage (D&C), 56, 302, 305
dimethyl sulfoxide (DMSO), 160
dioxin, 21–22
diphenhydramine (Benadryl), 459
Directory of Medical Specialists, 70
DiSaia, Philip, 335
DNA Ploidy, 63
docetaxel (Taxotere), 244, 393
Dr. Susan Love's Breast Book (Love), 205, 208
Dr. Susan Love's Hormone Book (Love), 310, 459
doctors, cancer specialties, 68; finding, 69; gynecologist, 268; oncologist, 13, 68; pathologist, 41; radiologist, 43, 300; relationship with patient, 72–74; and second opinions, 74–76; selecting, 69–71
doubling time, 11, 63
Down's syndrome, 31
doxorubicin (Adriamycin), 244, 393
drugs, unconventional, 157–164
duct carcinoma in situ, 224–226, 232
duct ectasia, 217
duct hyperplasia, 206
Duke's classification system, 62, 413
dysplasia, 6, 316, 317–324

E

Eastern medicine, 127–128
electrocautery, 324
electromagnetic fields, 24–25
embolization, 417
employment issues and cancer, 461–462
endocervical curettage (ECC), 322
endometrial cancer. *See* uterus, cancer of

endometrial hyperplasia, 301–302
endometriosis, 282
enemas, 131; barium, 286, 305, 409
Entelev, 159
Environmental Protection Agency (EPA), 22
environmental risk factors, 21–25
epoetin alfa, 109
Epogen, 109
erythropoietin, 109
essiac, 144
estradiol, 200
Estring, 338
estrogen, 190, 270
estrones, 17
ethnicity and cancer, 28–29
etoposide, 296, 394
Exceptional Cancer Patients (ECaP), 164
exemestane (Aromasin), 242
exercise, 17–18, 107, 149–151, 199, 403–404; and alternative cancer therapies, 149–151; and cancer risks, 17–18, 199; and chemotherapy, 107; and colorectal cancer, 403–404; post-breast surgery, 251–252; post-cancer recovery, 437

F

fallopian tubes, cancer of, 365–367; masses in, 282
familial adenomatous polyposis (FAP), 31
family reactions to cancer, 78–80, 442–444
fat cells, 188
fear, 175–177
fecal occult blood test, 407–408
Feinstein, Dianne, 475
Feinstein-Smith Cancer Bill, 475
fibroadenoma, 206
fibrocystic breast disease, 204–205
fibroid tumors, 299–301
FIGO. *See* International Federation of Gynecology and Obstetrics
filgrastim, 108, 246
financial aid, 118
fine needle aspiration (FNA), 52–53, 219
5-fluorouracil (5-FU), 244, 417
5-HT3 antagonists, 112
flow cytometry, 63
fluoxetine (Prozac), 459
folate and colorectal cancer, 405
Food and Drug Administration (FDA), 47, 123
France, 123
frozen section, 58

G

Ganz, Patricia, 423
gemcitabine, 394
Generations (Strauss and Howe), 268
genes, and biological therapy, 116–117,
    296–297; BRCA1, 9, 34, 192, 193–194, 278,
    365; BRCA2, 9, 34, 192, 193–194, 278, 365;
    BRCA3, 192; CHEK-2, 192; hMLH1, 34;
    p53, 9, 34
genetic counseling, 194
Genetic Nondiscrimination in Health Insurance
    and Employment Act, 33
genetic research, 472–473
genetic testing, 31–36
Germany, 123
Gerson Clinic, 163
Gerson diet, 129, 131
Gerson, Max, 129
gestational trophoblastic neoplasia (GTN), 367
Getting Well Again (Simonton), 123, 146
glandular therapy, 161
goal setting, 445–446
Goodman, Ellen, 474
Gotzsche, Peter, 44, 476–477
granisetron (Kytril), 112
granulocyte colony stimulating factor (G-CSF),
    108, 246
granulocyte-macrophage colony stimulating fac-
    tor (GM-CSF), 108
Great Britain, 123
Greek Cancer Cure, 164
grief, 178–179, 439–441
guaiac test, 407
guilt, 181
Gynecologic Oncology Group (GOG), 297, 370
gynecology, 268

H

hair loss, 109–111
Halsted radical mastectomy, 229–230
Handbook of Oncology Nutrition, 396
Hariton-Tzannis Alivizatos, 164
Harmony Hill, 166
Hay, Louise, 29-30, 156
Haylock, Pamela, 176, 265
Head First: The Biology of Hope (Cousins), 148
Heal Your Body (Hay), 29
Health and Healing (Whitaker), 158
health management organizations (HMOs), 15,
    69, 477—479
Healthy People 2010, 405

Heart and Estrogen/Progestin Replacement
    Study (HERS), 197
helicobacter pylori, 25–26
hematoma, 59
hemorrhagic cystitis, 245
Henig, Robin Marantz, 169
hepatic arterial perfusion, 417
HER-2/neu receptors, 64, 117
herbal therapy, 132–143
Herbst Registry, 352
hereditary risk factors, 30–31
His and Her Health, 339
Hispanic women and cancer, 28–29, 203, 320,
    403, 471
HIV, 25, 327, 396-397. *See also* AIDS
HMOs. *See* health management organizations
    (HMO)
homeopathy, 123
hormonal effects of radiation therapy, 428–429
hormonal therapy, 13–14, 115–116; for breast
    cancer, 241–243
hormone replacement therapy, 115, 191,
    197–198, 310–315; after menopause,
    457–458
hospitalist, 84
hospitalization, 83–85
Houston Chronicle, 472
How Women Can Finally Stop Smoking (Klesges
    and DeBon), 378, 379
Hoxsey, Harry, 144–145
Hoxsey therapy, 144–145
human papillomavirus (HPV), 35, 320–321; and
    cancer of the vulva, 354, 355; and vaginal
    cancer, 342
humor therapy, 148
hydatidiform mole, 367–369
hydrazine sulfate, 160
hydroxyprogesterone (Delalutin), 307
hypercalcemia, 264–265
hyperplasia, 5
hyperthermia, 263
hypnosis, 147
hysterectomy, 300, 306–307; for cervical cancer,
    329–330, 334–339; for CIN, 325; complica-
    tions from, 336–337; and sexuality issues,
    337–338; for uterine cancer, 306-307

I

ifosfamide, 296, 394
imaging techniques, 42–50; computerized ther-
    mal imaging (CTI), 50; computerized tomog-
    raphy (CAT), 48–49; digital mammography,

47–48; magnetic resonance imaging (MRI), 48–49; mammograms, 43–47; nuclear scans, 49–50; positron emission tomography (PET), 285; scintimammography, 50; T-scan imaging, 50; thermography, 50; ultrasound (sonography), 48; X-rays, 42–43
immune system, 10, 26
Immuno-Augmentative Therapy (IAT), 125, 161
implanted port, 105
implants. *See* breast implants
incentive spirometer, 92
infections, 25–26
inflammatory bowel disease, 402
information sources, 82–83
informed consent, 52
Informed Woman's Guide to Breast Health, The (McGinn), 208
initiators, 8
Institute of Medicine (IOM), 257, 471
insurance issues and cancer, 462–465, 471; Blue Cross/Blue Shield, 464; Consolidated Omnibus Budget Reconciliation Act of 1985 (COBRA), 463; Employee Retirement Income Security Act (ERISA), 464; health management organizations (HMOs), 463; Kassebaum-Kennedy Portability Bill, 463; Medicaid, 463, 468–471; Medicare, 463, 464, 468–471
integrative medicine, 120
Interdisciplinary Group for Cancer Care Evaluation, 261
interferon, 358
International Federation of Gynecology and Obstetrics (FIGO), 62, 273, 286
Internet sources of information, 83
intestines, diseases of, 282
intravenous pyelogram (IVP), 327
invasive mole, 369
Ireland, Jill, 439
irinotecan (Camptosar), 394, 417
Iscador, 145

J

Japanese: populations and cancer, 17, 22, 316
Jewish women and cancer, 193, 276, 319, 418
Jillian, Ann, 453
Jim's Juice, 159
Jones, Lovell, 472
Journal of the National Cancer Institute, 404
journal writing, 174

JS-101, 159
JS-114, 159

K

Kaiser Permanente, 31
Kassebaum-Kennedy Portability Bill, 119
Kaufman axillary treatment scale (KATS), 234
Kelley Clinic, 129
keloids, 90
Kessler, David, 257, 376
Khalsa, Dharma Singh, 147
ki, 128
Ki-67, 63
kidney cancer, 27
krebiozen, 164
Krieger, Dolores, 153, 156
Krippner, Stanley, 156
Kushner, Harold S., 175
Kytril, 112

L

laetrile, 161
Lancet, 44, 476
Landon, Michael, 129
laparotomy, 285, 345
laser vaporization, 325
latissimus dorsi flap (LATS), 259
legislation, 33
Lerner, Michael, 165
lesbians and cancer, 276
letrozole (Femara), 242
leucovorin, 417
leukemia, 23
Leukine, 108
leuprolide acetate, 296
levamisole (Ergamisol), 117, 417
lichen sclerosis, 356
"Life Beyond Cancer", 165
live cell therapy, 161
Livingston diet, 131
Livingston, Virginia, 131
Livingston-Wheeler Medical Clinic, 131
lobectomy, 392
lobular carcinoma in situ, 226–227
local invasion, 12
local treatments for cancer, 86–98
lomustine, 394
loop electrocautery excision procedure (LEEP), 322
lorazepam (Ativan), 113

Love, Medicine, and Miracles (Siegel), 30, 164, 180

Love, Susan, 41–42, 205, 310

Lukas Klinik, 145

lumpectomy, 229, 231–232

lung anatomy, 380–382

lung cancer, 373–399; detection, 384; diagnosis, 385; follow-up, 397–398; prevention, 375–380; and quality of life, 398–399; recurrence, 398; risk factors, 373–375; staging, 386–388; symptoms, 384–385; treatment, 388–397; types of, 382–384

lymph, 13, 455

lymph-node dissection, 232–233

lymph node sampling, 233

lymph nodes, 13, 61, 190

lymphangiogram, 344

lymphatic system, 12, 13

lymphedema, 232, 454–457

Lymphedema (Burt and White), 457

Lynch Syndrome, 402

M

MacDonald, Gayle, 153

macrobiotics, 130

macrophages, 108

magnet hospitals, 479

magnetic resonance imaging (MRI), 210, 285, 286, 327, 387

malignant transformation, 11

MammaCare Method, 214, 216

mammograms, 43–47, 210; diagnostic, 44; effectiveness, 44–46, 476; guidelines, 46–47; screening, 44

Mammography Quality Standards Act (MQSA), 47

Mammotome, 53

managed care. *See* health management organizations (HMOs)

marijuana (Marinol), 113

massage, 151–152

mastalgia (breast pain), 207–208

mastectomy, 229–232; and body image, 252–253; prophylactic, 35, 194–195

McQueen, Steve, 129

mediastinoscopy, 385

Medicaid/Medi-Cal, 70, 118, 468–471

Medicare, 70, 118, 468–471

medications and cancer risk, 10, 26–27

Medicine Hands: Massage Therapy for People with Cancer (MacDonald), 153

meditation, 147

Meditation as Medicine (Khalsa and Strauth), 147

medroxyprogesterone (Provera), 307, 312

mega-vitamin therapy, 130

megestrol acetate, 296

megestrol (Megace), 307

menopause: and breast cancer, 243–244; and breast function, 191; and hormone replacement therapy, 457–461; symptoms, 115; treatment of symptoms, 313–315, 458–461

menstruation, 115

mesothelioma, 373

metabolic therapy, 128–132

metastasis, 7, 61; distant, 12

methotrexate, 244

metoclopramide (Reglan), 113

Metzger, Deena, 441

microcalcifications, 43

micrometastasis, 233

microscopic nodal invasion, 62

microsurgical free flap procedures, 259

minorities and cancer, 471–472

mistletoe, 145

mitomycin, 393

mitosis, 63

modified radical mastectomy, 230–231

monoclonal antibodies, 116, 246–247, 296, 387

Montgomery's tubercles, 188

MRI. *See* magnetic resonance imaging

mucositis, 114

muscle flap reconstructive procedures, 258–260

mushrooms, medicinal, 133

music therapy, 148

myelocytic leukemia, 31

myomectomy, 300

N

nadir, 107

National Cancer Act, 475

National Cancer Institute (NCI), 45, 46, 475; and cancer policy, 476–477; Community Clinical Oncology Program (CCOP), 118; and complementary treatment, 126, 168; Comprehensive Cancer Centers, 75; Consensus Conference, 235; Cooperative Group Program, 370; and dietary recommendations, 132; Natural Products Branch, 144; Office of Cancer Survivorship, 422; Physician Data Query, 76, 82. *See also* Cancer Information Service

National Center for Complementary and Alternative Medicine, 126

National Coalition for Cancer Survivorship, 73, 119, 173, 434, 478, 481; *Facing Forward: A Guide for Cancer Survivors*, 462

National Cosmetology Association, 111

National Institute of Health, 126; Office of Research on Women's Health, 352

National Lymphedema Network, 457

National Research Council, 21

National Surgical Adjuvant Breast and Bowel Project, 202, 225

Native-American teens and smoking, 376

Native-American women and cancer, 320, 403, 471

nausea, 111–114

necrosis, 224

needle localization biopsy, 59

Nei Jing, 128

neoplasia, 5

nephrotoxicity, 428

Neupogen, 108, 246

neutropenia, 108

neutrophils, 108

New Age therapies. See complementary and alternative therapies

New England Journal of Medicine, 81, 319, 377, 418

New York Times, 45, 310

nipple, 188; Paget's disease of the nipple, 227, 249; reconstruction, 259–260

nipple discharge, 41, 217, 220

non–small cell lung carcinoma (NSCLC), 383–384, 390–391

nonsteroidal anti-inflammatory drugs, 405

nontunneled central catheter, 105

nurses, 32, 77, 415

nutrition, post-cancer, 437

O

obesity, 198

Office of Alternative Medicine (OAM), 126

Office of Technology Assessment (OTA), 125

Olsen, Ole, 44, 476–477

oncogenes, 9

oncologist, 13; gynecologic, 68; medical, 68; radiation, 68, 229; surgical, 68

Oncology Nursing Society, 31, 73; *Position on Quality Cancer Care*, 479–480

ondansetron (Zofran), 112

1 in 3: Women with Cancer Confront an Epidemic (Brady), 482

126-F, 159

oophorectomy, 35, 278, 279

open biopsy, 57–59

orthomolecular medicine, 130

osteoporosis, 309, 459–460

Ostomy Book, The (McGinn), 416

ovaries, cancer of, 272–298; biological therapies, 296; chemotherapy, 287–288, 292–293; detection, 279–281; diagnosis, 283–285; epithelial, 273; low malignant potential tumors, 289; natural history, 274–276; nonepithelial, 273–274, 275; prevention, 279; radiation therapy, 295; recurrence, 295–296; risk factors, 276–279; staging, 285–286, 288; symptoms, 281–282; treatment, 287–295

Oxaliplatin, 417

oxymedicine, 162–163

P

paclitaxel (Taxol), 244, 288–289, 296, 393

Paget's disease, of the nipple, 227, 249; of the vulva, 357

pain management, 90–91, 176

palliation, 86

pamidronate (Aredia), 265

Pancoast's syndrome, 395

panic attacks, 177

Pap smear, 27, 39–40, 54, 268–269, 304, 316; and diagnosis of cervical cancer, 321; and diagnosis of vaginal cancer, 342

parenchyma, 188

paroxetine (Paxil), 459

pathologic fractures, 394

pathologist, 40

Patient's Bill of Rights, 85

pau d'arco, 146

Pauling, Linus, 130

pelvic exenteration, 333–334, 345

Penguin Cold Cap Therapy System, 111

peripherally inserted central catheter (PICC), 105

peritoneal seeding, 275

permanent section, 58

personality and cancer, 29–30

PET. See positron emission tomography

pharmacological agents, 157–164

pharmaceutical industry, 467

phenacetin, 27

Philadelphia chromosome, 31
Philip Morris, 474
physical activity and cancer. *See also* exercise
physical therapists, 77
Plenosol, 145
pneumonectomy, 392
politics of women's cancers, 466–482
polyps, 401
Positive Options for Living with Your Ostomy
   (White), 416
positron emission tomography (PET), 285, 327,
   387
postmastectomy pain syndrome, 238
post-traumatic stress syndrome, 439
pregnancy, and breast cancer, 247–248; and
   breast function, 191; and mammography, 47;
   post-cancer, 452–454
prevention of cancer. *See* listing for the specific
   type of cancer
prochlorperazine (Compazine), 113
Procrit, 109
progesterone, 190, 270
promoters, 8
propanolol (Inderal), 459
prophylactic brain irradiation, 394
prophylactic surgery, 35
proto-oncogene, 8, 192
psoriasis, 27
psychological therapies, 146–149
psychoneuroimmunology (PNI), 147
psychotherapy, 77, 79, 174, 434
pulmonary fibrosis, 428
pulse rate, 151
punch biopsy, 55

Q

Qi gong (qigong), 150
quandrantectomy, 231

R

race and cancer, 28–29
radiation exposure, 22–23
radiation, radiofrequency, 23
radiation therapy, 12, 23, 93–98; for cervical
   cancer, 330–332, 333; for colorectal cancer,
   417–418; and insurance coverage, 470; for
   lung cancer, 394–397; side effects, 96–97,
   395–397; simulation, 95
radiologist, 43; interventional, 300

Radner, Gilda, 164, 272, 282, 439; Gilda
   Radner Familial Ovarian Cancer Registry,
   281, 296, 297
radon, 22
raloxifene (Evista), 194, 202, 242, 460–461
recombinant human interleukin-11, 109
Recovering from Breast Surgery (Stumm), 251
rectum, cancer of. See colorectal cancer
recurrence, fear of, 435–438
red blood cells, 107, 109
reflex sympathetic dystrophy, 393
reflexology, 127–128, 154
regional extension, 12
Rehabilitation Act of 1973, 462
Reiki, 128, 153
relationships, 442–445, 451–452
ReliefBand, 113, 128
religion, 154–157
Remen, Rachel Naomi, 156
remission of cancer, 100
reproductive system, 269–271
Resperin Corporation, 144
respiratory system, 380–382
retinoblastoma, 30
retinoids, 340
Richards, Peter, 228
risk analysis, 31–36
risk factors, 15–36. *See also* listing for the specific type of cancer
rituximab (Rituxan), 296
Roswell Park Cancer Institute, 31

S

S-phase fraction (SPF), 63
sarcomas, 61
sargramostim, 108
Scarff-Richardson-Bloom classification system,
   221
scars, 90
sclerosing adenosis, 206
scopes, bronchoscope, 55; colonoscope, 55; colposcope, 51, 54; culdoscope, 55; cystoscope,
   55; endoscope, 55; hysteroscope, 55; laparoscope, 51, 55, 285; proctosigmoidoscope, 55;
   sigmoidoscope, 51, 55
Scott, Diane W., 183, 443
screening tests, 38–39
second opinions, 74–76
secondhand smoke, 375
segmental resection, 231, 392

selective estrogen receptor modulator (SERM), 201, 241
selective serotonin uptake inhibitor (SSRI), 459
self-advocacy, 268–269
self-image, 181–184, 441–442, 448
Selye, Hans, 29
sentinal lymph node sampling (SLNS), 233–234
seroma, 59
serum (blood) tumor markers, 41–42
Sexual Health Network, 339
sexuality after cancer, 447–452
Sexuality and Cancer: For the Woman Who Has Cancer, and Her Partner, 450
shamanism, 155
shark cartilage, 163–164
Sharks Don't Get Cancer (Lane and Comac), 163
Sharks Still Don't Get Cancer (Lane and Comac), 163–164
Sheinkopf, Melinda, 173
Sheridan's Formula, 159
shiatsu, 127–128
Siegel, Bernie, 30, 164, 180
sigmoidoscopy, 408
Simonton, O. Carl, 156
skin cancers, 21, 23–24
small cell lung carcinoma (SCLC), 383, 389–390
Smith, Gordon, 475
Smith, John M., 335
smoking, 19–20, 404; and breast cancer, 199–200; cessation, 377–380; and lung cancer, 374–375; and teenagers, 375–377
Smoking Cessation Clinical Practice Guideline, 379, 380
specimen radiography, 59
Spiegel, David, 81
spinal cord compression, 395
spirituality, 154–157, 174
squamous cell hyperplasia, 356–357
Stauth, Cameron, 147
stem cell, research, 473; transplants, 265–266
stenosis, 323
stereotactic guided needle biopsy, 53–54
stomatitis, 114
stroma, 188, 274
strontium-89 chloride (Metastron), 265
Stumm, Diana, 251
suicide, 179
sun, exposure to, 23–24
sunburn, 23–24
sunscreen, 24
Sunstone Healing Center, 166

superior vena cava syndrome, 397
support groups, 80–82
surgery, 87–93; for breast cancer, 229–239; for cervical cancer, 328–330, 333–339; for colorectal cancer, 414–417; for lung cancer, 391–393; pain management, 90–91; recovery, 89–93; scars, 90; second-look, 290, 293–294, 297
Surviving, 436
Surviving Your HMO (Berkman), 479
survivorship, 429–431
systematic desensitization, 113
systemic treatment, 99–115

T

T'ai Chi, 149
Taking Time: Support for People with Cancer and the People Who Care About Them, 79
tamoxifen (Nolvadex), for breast cancer prevention, 194, 201–202; for breast cancer treatment, 241–242; for endometrial carcinoma 308; and heart disease, 460-461; and liver tumors, 27; for menopausal symptoms, 459; and osteoporosis, 460–461; for ovarian cancer, 296; and pregnancy, 453
technology and cancer, 472–473
teniposide, 394
therapeutic touch, 153
therapies, types of, 121–122
theratope cancer vaccine, 247
thoracotomy, 385
thrombocytopenia, 108–109
Time, 477
tissue expansion, 255–256
TNM classification, 62–63, 413
tobacco, 19–20, 474. *See also* smoking
tobacco industry, 474
Tomudex, 417
topotecan (Hycamtin), 296, 297, 393
touch therapy, 151–154
transverse rectus abdominus myocutaneous flap (TRAM), 258–259
trastuzumab (Herceptin), 117, 246–247, 264, 296
treatment goals, 86
treatment options, 13–14, 67
treatment team, 67
tumor board, 75
tumors, 5, 282; breast, 221, 223; fibroid, 299–301; and local treatment, 86–98; serum (blood) tumor markers, 41; staging, 61–62

tunneled central catheter, 105
tylectomy, 231

U

ultrasound (sonography), 210, 286
Unconventional Cancer Treatments (1990), 121
United Ostomy Association, 416
uranium, 22
urogram, 305
uterine artery embolization (UAE), 300
uterus, cancer of, 299–315; detection, 304; diagnosis, 56, 304; follow-up, 309; prevention, 304; recurrence, 307–308; risk factors, 302–304; staging, 306; treatment, 306–309; types of, 305–306

V

vagina, cancer of, 341–353; diagnosis, 344; follow-up, 346–347; prevention, 342; recurrence, 346; risk factors, 341–342; staging, 344; treatment, 345–347
vaginal fibrosis, 343
vaginal intraepithelial neoplasia (VAIN), 342–344
vaginal reconstruction, 346–347
vaginectomy, 345
Van Nuys Prognostic Index (VNPI), 225
venlafaxine (Effexor), 459
vesicants, 104
video-assisted thorascopic surgery (VATS), 385
Vietnamese women and cancer, 28–29, 316
vinblastine, 393
vinca alkaloids, 102
vinorelbine, 394
virtual colonoscopy, 418
viruses, 25, 327. *See also* human papillomavirus (HPV)
vitamin C, 130–131
vitamin E and colorectal cancer, 405
vomiting, 111–114
vulva, cancer of, 354–364; diagnosis, 359; follow-up, 362–363; and hygiene, 355; prevention, 355–356; recurrence, 362; risk factors, 354–355; staging, 360; symptoms, 358–359; treatment, 359–362
vulvar intraepithelial neoplasia (VIN), 357–358
vulvar self-exam (VSE), 356–358, 363
vulvectomy, 358, 360

W

walking, 151
Wall Street Journal, 349, 474
Weber, Treya Killam, 180
Weisenthal Cancer Group, 101
Wellness Community, The, 82, 164, 265
When Bad Things Happen to Good People (Kushner), 175
When Someone in Your Family Has Cancer, 80
Whitaker, Julian, 158
white blood cells, 107, 108, 114
White, Gwen, 457
White House Commission on Complementary and Alternative Medicine Policy, 120–121
wigs, 110
Wilkes, Gail, 397
Wilms' tumor, 30
Woman's Decision: Breast Care, Treatment, and Reconstruction, A (Berger and Bostwick), 260
Women and Doctors (Smith), 335
Women's Health Initiative, 26, 197, 198, 310, 457
Wound, Ostomy, and Continence Nurse (WOCN), 415

X

X rays, 22–23. *See also* imaging techniques
xenoestrogens, 200

Y

Y-ME Breast Cancer Support Program, 82, 260, 434, 481
yoga, 150

Z

Zofran, 112
zoledronic acid (Zometa), 265